Emerging Topics in Statistics and Biostatistics

Emerging Topics in Statistics and Biostatistics

Ding-Geng Chen • Carlos A. Coelho
Editors

Biostatistics Modeling and Public Health Applications

Study Design and Analysis Methodology in Health Sciences, Volume 1

Springer

Editors
Ding-Geng Chen
College of Health Solutions
Arizona State University
Phoenix, AZ, USA

Carlos A. Coelho
Department of Mathematics
NOVA University of Lisbon
Caparica, Portugal

ISSN 2524-7735 ISSN 2524-7743 (electronic)
Emerging Topics in Statistics and Biostatistics
ISBN 978-3-031-69692-3 ISBN 978-3-031-69690-9 (eBook)
https://doi.org/10.1007/978-3-031-69690-9

This Springer imprint is published by the registered company Springer Nature Switzerland AG
The registered company address is: Gewerbestrasse 11, 6330 Cham, Switzerland

Preface

This book aims to discuss a wide range of emerging topics in biostatistical modeling with applications to public health. It serves as a comprehensive resource for students, researchers, and professionals seeking to deepen their understanding of biostatistical methods and their practical applications in public health. The contributing authors are a distinguished group of scholars and researchers from leading academic institutions and research institutes around the world. Their collective expertise covers various aspects of biostatistical modeling and public health data analysis, offering readers diverse insights and advanced knowledge.

By bringing together these scholars and researchers, the book provides a thorough exploration of contemporary issues and innovative approaches in biostatistical modeling. Topics covered include advanced biostatistical techniques, the integration of biostatistics with other scientific disciplines, and the application of these methods to real-world public health problems. The interdisciplinary nature of the contributions aims to stimulate further collaborations between the fields of mathematics, statistics, and public health, fostering a multidisciplinary approach to addressing complex health challenges.

Furthermore, the book emphasizes the importance of biostatistics in improving public health outcomes, showcasing case studies and examples that illustrate the practical impact of statistical modeling on health policy, disease prevention, and health promotion. By highlighting these applications, the book not only enhances the reader's theoretical understanding but also provides practical tools and methodologies that can be applied in various public health settings.

Overall, we intend to have this book to be an invaluable resource for anyone involved in biostatistics and public health, offering a platform for the exchange of ideas and the development of new research collaborations. It aims to inspire future research and innovation in the field, ultimately contributing to the advancement of public health through improved statistical practices.

The chapters of the book are organized into three parts with Part I (five chapters) presenting some emerging topics in biostatistical modeling, Part II (two chapters) delving into the emerging development in imaging data analysis, and Part III (five chapters) presenting the public health applications. Each chapter is self-contained with references at the end for easy access.

Part I (Biostatistical Modeling) includes five chapters. In Chap. 1, Rabab Elnaiem, Thomas Mathew, and Xiaoyu Dong discuss a most important development on bioequivalence. They state that for the assessment of average bioequivalence, the two one-sided t-test (TOST) is widely used. The test is known to be very conservative for large values of the variance, suggesting that the TOST is likely to have type I error probabilities close to the nominal level if the test is implemented using a significance level larger than the nominal level. In this chapter, a bootstrap calibration is proposed to estimate the required significance level. Numerical results show that a bootstrap-calibrated TOST provides better type I error probabilities, and hence increased power. The test may be an attractive alternative to the scaled average bioequivalence test, especially since the latter cannot be implemented using data from a 2×2 crossover design, whereas such data are adequate for carrying out the bootstrap calibrated TOST. The bootstrap-calibrated TOST is easy to understand and implement, unlike some of the theoretical improvements of the TOST available in the literature. The bootstrap-calibrated TOST can be adopted for the assessment of multivariate average bioequivalence. Finally, the bootstrap calibration methodology is applied for obtaining an accurate test procedure for the assessment of scaled average bioequivalence for highly variable drugs with data generated using a four-period crossover design.

In Chap. 2, Isabel Natario reviews the Bayesian framework on hypothesis testing. She states that in a Bayesian framework, statistical inference relies on posterior distributions of unknown quantities and parameters of the models used for fitting data. From these, point estimators, credible intervals, and posterior probabilistic statements can be produced. However, unlike the frequentist approach, null hypothesis testing does not hold the same importance neither is a consensus matter between Bayesian statisticians, that regard the frequentist significance tests with reservation, admitting that they might serve a more complementary role to parameter estimation. Bayesian statistics, quite critics of p-values, suggests an investigation of the alternative hypotheses using the Bayes factor, only dependent on the observed data, for evaluating evidence in favor of the null hypothesis and being quite intuitive, forming a bridge to those interested in testing. Hypothesis tests have become completely essential in applied studies in areas such as biology, health, and psychology, even though their generalized use is sometimes a problem, and the change in paradigm often stumbles in this particular difference between approaches. This work reviews the most common Bayesian approach for hypothesis testing, the Bayes factor, more robust and less demanding on assumptions and sample sizes than the frequentist approach, reflecting on its disadvantages, including sensitivity to prior distributions and computational difficulties, and misuses related to wrong interpretations. Two examples are detailed with R implementation.

In Chap. 3, Mahboubeh Akbari, Najmeh Nakhaei Rad, Ding-Geng Chen, and Vahid Fakoor present an overview of the length-biased sampling which has been widely used in various fields, including economics, industrial reliability, applications in etiology, and studies related to epidemiology, genetics, and cancer screening. The assessment of the relationship between risk factors and survival time in the presence of biased data, particularly length-biased right-censored (LBRC) data, has long been a statistical challenge. Since the structure of observed length-biased data differs from that of the target population, using traditional methods to estimate covariate effects based on the observed length-biased data is inappropriate. This chapter focuses on discussing existing methods for estimating regression coefficients under commonly used semiparametric models, specifically the Cox proportional hazard (Cox) and accelerated failure time (AFT) models, when dealing with LBRC data. To compare the efficacy of available methods, a simulation study is conducted. In summary, the results indicate that all the estimating methods proposed to accommodate LBRC data exhibit better performance than the traditional approach for estimating coefficients of Cox model, which ignores bias in sampling. Furthermore, the composite partial likelihood method outperforms all other methods in terms of bias and standard error. For the AFT model, the inverse weighted estimating equation approach is more efficient in the presence of LBRC data compared to other existing methods. Additionally, to illustrate the practical performance of these methods, a real dataset is analyzed.

In Chap. 4, Yue Cui and Solomon Harrar present nonparametric models for incomplete multivariate data in quality of life outcomes. They state that in studies of efficacies of intervention modalities, outcomes measured in ordinal scales such as Quality of Life (QOL) outcomes are routinely used as primary endpoints. The standard data analysis strategy computes composite overall and domain scores, and conducts a mixed-model analysis for evaluating efficacy or monitoring medical conditions as if these scores were in continuous metric scale. However, assumptions of parametric models like continuity and homoscedasticity can be severely violated in these cases. Furthermore, it is more challenging when there are missing values on some of the variables. In this chapter, they proposed a purely nonparametric approach in the sense that meaningful and, yet, nonparametric effect size measures are developed. They proposed an estimator for the effect size and developed its asymptotic properties. The Asthma Randomized Trial of Indoor Wood Smoke data were used to illustrate applications of the proposed methods.

In Chap. 5, Tshiamo Kgoale, Albert Whata, Justine Nasejje, Najmeh Nakhaei Ra, and Tshilidzi Mulaudzi discuss the causal inference in the survival analysis framework to evaluate the survival probabilities under the influence of time-dependent covariates. Incorporating potential outcomes and propensity scores in survival analysis, they examined treatment effects at both a population level and an individual level, leading to a more nuanced comprehension of treatment outcomes. The accuracy of the treatment effect estimators within the framework is assessed, focusing on the DeepSurv, DeepHit, and the multi-task learning deep neural network (MTL-DNN) models. Notably, the DeepHit model applied to both real and simulated datasets outperformed with an average concordance statistic (C-statistic) of 0.9997. This surpasses the C-statistic of DeepSurv and MTL-DNN, which are 0.8928 and 0.9996, respectively. These results showed that the deep learning models have exceptional discrimination and agreement between observed and predicted survival probabilities. In addition, the bias values for DeepSurv (0.0174), DeepHit

(0.0114), and MTL-DNN (0.0108) are notably small and comparable, indicating that these models provide accurate and unbiased estimates of treatment effects. Consequently, this research underscores the superior predictive accuracy of these deep learning models, suggesting their potential to enhance decision-making and deepen our understanding of treatment outcomes in survival analysis.

Part II (Imaging Data Analysis) includes two chapters. In Chap. 6, Xuze Zhang, Yuichi Goto, Benjamin Kedem, and Shuo Chen discuss the detection and testing of the significance of quadratic interactions in brain functional connectivity with applications to blood oxygen level-dependent signals or time series from schizophrenia patients and from healthy controls. The underlying tool is the measure of lagged coherence which extends the pervasive and widely used measure of coherence between time series pairs from different brain regions.

In Chap. 7, Habte Tadesse Likassa and Ding-Geng Chen present the recent concerns in biomedical image processing which revolve around robustly detecting outliers and noise. To address these concerns, they proposed a robust principal component analysis (RPCA) with affine transformation (AT) and rank prior information (RPI). This method leverages convex optimization to enhance the quality of retinal images while mitigating the impact of outliers and occlusions. Simulation results demonstrated the superiority of our proposed methods over state-of-the-art works, which is particularly evident in three different retinal images sourced from public databases.

Part III (Public Health Applications) includes five chapters. In Chap. 8, Denekew Bitew Belay, Ding-Geng Chen, and Sintayehu Agegnehu Matintu present a Susceptible-Exposed-Infected-Recovered-Death (SEIRD) mathematical modeling and its four extensions with two scenarios for modeling the malaria transmission with monthly malaria cases along with death rates obtained from WHO reports as an initial value. They applied these models with and without intervention scenarios to study the malaria disease transmission dynamics. With this mathematical malaria transmission modeling, they showed that the disease continues to be the leading cause of morbidity and mortality in the region unless strict intervention and control mechanisms are taken with increased efforts. In addition, they found that the basic reproduction number (R_0) is greater than one, which showed that malaria will continue to be a public health problem and requires a tangible improvement in the eradication of the epidemic.

In Chap. 9, Mohammad Arashi and Samuel Manda discuss the difficulties from the process of selecting variables for generalized longitudinal predictive modeling due to potential connections among observations and issues related to the true distribution of the response variable. In this chapter, they employ an efficient selection mechanism within the flexible generalized semiparametric longitudinal model, where they consider the possibility of nonlinear connections between predictors and the response variable. They focus on modeling CD4 levels in the Human Immunodeficiency Virus (HIV) and address the current limitations in selecting variables for regression modeling. Their analysis revealed noteworthy interaction effects that must be considered when conducting CD4 regression modeling.

In Chap. 10, Haile Mekonnen Fenta, Ding-Geng Chen, and Temesgen Zewotir brought our attention to the important point in analyzing the spatial data in accounting the spatial autocorrelation through the weight matrix. In the Bayesian context, the intrinsic conditional autocorrelation prior distribution has been used to model spatial autocorrelation. The authors used the most recent Demographic and Health Surveys (DHS) data from 33 sub-Saharan African (sSA) countries. The Bayesian generalized geo-additive mixed effects model was fitted to incorporate the linear, nonlinear, and spatial effects of childhood mortality. The spatial components were smoothed by the two-dimensional spline and the continuous variables were modeled by penalized splines. The model inference was made based on Integrated Nested Laplace Approximation (INLA), and the parameter sensitivity for priors was validated. A total of 352,322 under-five children were included in the study. The overall prevalence of under-five mortality in sSA was 6.04% with countries Chad (9.79%), Nigeria (9.68%), and Sierra Leon (8.99%) recording the highest prevalence. The likelihood of dying was prominently high among children decreasing in urban residence (AOR = 0.94; 95% CI = 0.90–0.99). Similarly, a significant association with risk of U5M was found which includes child-level covariates (sex, birth order, place of delivery, and dietary diversity) and household-level covariates (mother education, wealth index, autonomy of mothers, source of water, sanitation facilities, and cooking fuels).

In Chap. 11, Tsirizani Kaombe and Gracious Hamuza discuss the survey design effect. If regression methods are used for prediction of under-five mortality, not much is known about the effect of ignoring the sample design in the estimates. This chapter is concerned with estimating and comparing the bias a researcher commits when using unweighted and weighted logistic regression methods to predict under-five mortality rate in Malawi through the national survey. They used data from 2004, 2010, and 2015–2016 Malawi demographic and health surveys, as well as UNICEF annual mortality monitoring data. The survey weights were considered at two stages: during model fitting and when computing overall predicted mortality rate. The results showed that there was higher accuracy in estimation when the weights were applied during calculation of overall predicted probability of child death given a fitted logit model, than during model fitting. They recommend incorporating survey cluster-weights when computing the overall predicted probability of event, without regard of the weights during model fitting, for binary data models whose goal is the prediction of event probability.

In Chap. 12, Sheyla Rodrigues Cassy and Samuel Manda present multivariate spatial analysis. It is noted that most spatial analyses of health survey data have employed univariate spatial modeling for specific diseases even if the studies diseases are epidemiologically interrelated. Joint spatial modeling of several interrelated outcomes has both epidemiological and statistical benefits including identifying specific and shared spatial risk patterns and improvement in the statistical power by borrowing strength from neighboring areas. Also, despite recent methodological research in spatial analyses of complex health survey data, a majority of the analyses do not account for the survey designs. This chapter brings these two issues in an integrated approach with an application to estimate the geographic distribution of childhood-related diseases in sub-Saharan Africa based on health survey data.

The successful publication of this book would have been impossible without the invaluable support and contributions of many people. We would like to express our heartfelt gratitude to them. Firstly, and most importantly, we extend our sincere appreciation to all the chapter authors listed in the "List of Contributors" for their high-quality contributions to this book. Secondly, and most sincerely, we like to thank the reviewers for their professional service and contribution to this book. Thirdly, we sincerely thank Anne Rubio for her professional assistance to communicate with contributing authors on all aspects of reviewing and production. Furthermore, we owe a special debt of gratitude to Faith Su, the Editor for Statistics Books at Springer, for her exceptional guidance and support throughout the entire publication process. Their expertise and dedication were instrumental in bringing this book to fruition.

This book was initiated as a professional product, when Professor Ding-Geng Chen was invited by "The Centro de Matemática e Aplicações" of Nova University of Lisbon (NOVA Math) for his academic visit during the period from April 30, 2023, to May 12, 2023. With this publication, Professor Chen would like to thank all the researchers and staff members of NOVA Math for their hospitality and professional collaborations.

To strive for continuous improvement, we are open to receiving suggestions from our readers for further enhancements. Please feel free to contact the editors. Your input is always invaluable and we look forward to receiving your comments on this book.

Phoenix, AZ, USA — Ding-Geng Chen
Caparica, Portugal — Carlos A. Coelho

List of Reviewers

Masoumeh Akbari
Department of Statistics, University of Mazandaran, Babolsar, Iran
Email: m.akbari@umz.ac.ir.

Lubna Amro
Department of Statistics, TU Dortmund University, Dortmund, Germany.
Email: lubna.amro@tu-dortmund.de

Patrícia Bermudez
Centre of Statistics and its Applications (CEAUL), Faculty of Sciences of the University of Lisbon. Lisbon, Portugal
Email: pcbermudez@fc.ul.pt

Zelalem G. Dessie
Department of Statistics, Bahir Dar University, Bahir Dar, Ethiopia
School of Mathematics, Statistics and Computer Science, College of Agriculture Engineering and Science, University of KwaZulu-Natal, Durban, South Africa
Email: zelalem_getahune@yahoo.com

Hassan Doosti
School of Mathematical and Physical Sciences, Macquarie University, Faculty of Science and Engineering, Macquarie University
Email: hassan.doosti@mq.edu.au

Konstantinos Fokianos
Department of Mathematics & Statistics, University of Cyprus
Nicosia 1678, CYPRUS
Email: fokianos@ucy.ac.cy

K. Krishnamoorthy
Mathematics Department
University of Louisiana at Lafayette
Lafayette, LA 70504, USA
E-mail: krishna@louisiana.edu

Fairouz Makhlouf
Division of Biometrics VIII, US FDA
10903 New Hampshire Ave
Silver Spring, MD 20993, USA
E-mail: fairouz.makhlouf@fda.hhs.gov

Malick Mbodj
Office of Biostatistics, US FDA
10903 New Hampshire Ave
Silver Spring, MD 20993, USA
E-mail: Malick.Mbodj@fda.hhs.gov

Justine B. Nasejje
University of the Witwatersrand Johannesburg: Johannesburg, Gauteng, South Africa.
Email address: justine.nasejje@wits.ac.za

Luigi Salmaso
Department of Management and Engineering, University of Padova, Vicenza, Italy
Email: luigi.salmaso@unipd.it

Awoke Seyoum
Department of Statistics, Bahir Dar University, Bahir Dar, Ethiopia
Email address: bisrategebrail@yahoo.com

Yegnanew A. Shiferaw
Department of Statistics, University of Johannesburg, South Africa
Email address: yegnanews@uj.ac.za

Giovani Silva
Centre of Statistics and its Applications (CEAUL), Instituto Superior Técnico. University of Lisbon. Lisbon, Portugal.
Email: giovani.silva@tecnico.ulisboa.pt

Paula Simões
Center for Mathematics and Applications (NOVA Math), NOVA University of Lisbon. Lisbon, Portugal;

Centro de Investigação, Desenvolvimento e Inovação da Academia Militar (CINAMIL), Instituto Universitário Militar. Lisbon, Portugal
Email: pc.simoes@campus.fct.unl.pt

Georg Zimmerman
Team Biostatistics and Big Medical Data, Lab for Intelligent Data Analytics Salzburg, Paracelsus Medical University, Salzburg, Austria
Research and Innovation Management, Paracelsus Medical University, Salzburg, Austria.
Email: georg.zimmermann@pmu.ac.at

Contents

Editors and Contributors

About the Editors

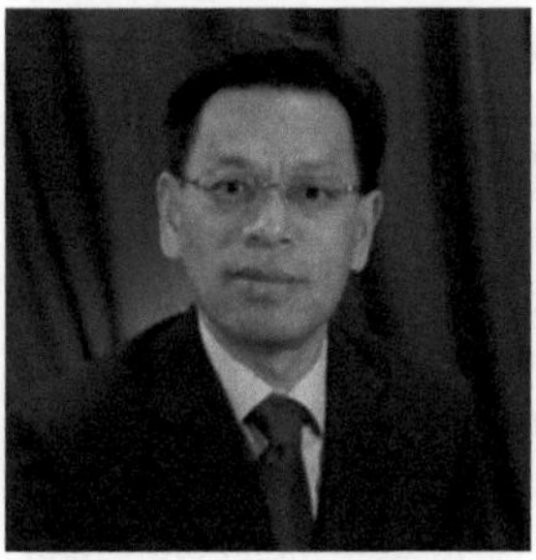

Ding-Geng Chen is a Fellow of the American Statistical Association and is currently the Executive Director and Professor of Biostatistics in the College of Health Solutions at Arizona State University. He is also an Extraordinary Professor and the SARChI Research Chair in Biostatistics at the University of Pretoria and an Honorary Professor at the University of KwaZulu-Natal, South Africa. Dr. Chen was a Professor of biostatistics at the University of North Carolina at Chapel Hill, a Professor of Biostatistics at the University of Rochester Medical School, and the Karl E. Peace Endowed Eminent Scholar Chair in Biostatistics at Georgia Southern University. He is a senior biostatistics consultant for biopharmaceuticals and government agencies with extensive expertise in biostatistics, clinical trials, and public health statistics and data sciences. Dr. Chen has more than 200 referred professional publications and co-authored/co-edited 40 books on clinical trial methodology, meta-analysis, data science, causal inference, and public health research.

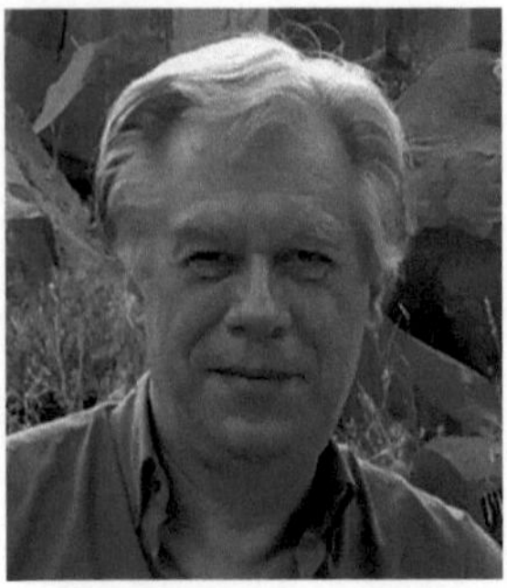

Carlos A. Coelho is a Full Professor of Statistics in the Mathematics Department of NOVA School of Science and Technology at NOVA University of Lisbon. He holds a Ph.D. in Biostatistics from the University of Michigan, Ann Arbor, MI, where he was a Fulbrighter. His main area of research is Multivariate Analysis, namely the development of likelihood ratio tests for elaborate covariance structures and for MANOVA models, also with elaborate covariance structures, together with the study of the exact distribution and the development of near-exact distributions for the associated test statistics. Related to this area, other areas of interest are Mathematical Statistics and Distribution Theory, as well as Estimation, Univariate and Multivariate Linear, and Generalized Linear and Mixed Models. More recently, he also got interested in tests for high dimensionality and the application of Multivariate Analysis techniques to Statistical Disclosure Control problems. Carlos A. Coelho has served as Associate Editor on the Editorial Boards of *Discussiones Mathematicae—Probability and Statistics*, *REVSTAT-Statistical Journal*, the *Journal of Interdisciplinary Mathematics*, and the *Journal of Applied Statistics*, and currently serves on the Editorial Boards of the *Journal of Statistical Theory and Practice* and the *American Journal of Mathematical and Management Sciences*. He is also Associate Editor of the Springer Book series Emerging Topics in Statistics and Biostatistics and a member of the International Council of the "Business World" Library of the Tsenov Academy of Economics (Svishtov, Bulgaria). Currently, Carlos A. Coelho also serves as President of Fulbrighters Portugal, the Portuguese Fulbright Alumni Association.

Contributors

Mahboubeh Akbari Department of Statistics, University of Pretoria, Pretoria, South Africa

Mohammad Arashi Department of Statistics, Faculty of Mathematical Sciences, Ferdowsi University of Mashhad, Mashhad, Iran
Department of Statistics, Faculty of Natural and Agricultural Sciences, University of Pretoria, Pretoria, South Africa

Denekew Bitew Belay Department of Statistics, Bahir Dar University, Bahir Dar, Ethiopia
Department of Statistics, University of Pretoria, Pretoria, South Africa

Sheyla Rodrigues Cassy DMI, Faculdade de Ciências, Universidade Eduardo Mondlane, Maputo, Mozambique

Ding-Geng Chen Department of Statistics, University of Pretoria, Pretoria, South Africa
College of Health Solution, Arizona State University, Phoenix, AZ, USA

Shuo Chen Maryland Psychiatric Research Center, School of Medicine, University of Maryland, College Park, MD, USA

Yue Cui Department of Mathematics, Missouri State University, Springfield, MO, USA

Xiaoyu Dong Data Sciences Institute, Takeda, Cambridge, MA, USA

Rabab Elnaiem University of Maryland Baltimore County, Baltimore, MD, USA

Vahid Fakoor Department of Statistics, School of Mathematical Sciences, Ferdowsi University of Mashhad, Mashhad, Iran

Haile Mekonnen Fenta Department of Statistics, University of Pretoria, Pretoria, South Africa
Department of Statistics, Bahir Dar University, Bahir Dar, Ethiopia

Yuichi Goto Faculty of Mathematics, Kyushu University, Japan

Gracious A. Hamuza National Statistics Office, Zomba, Malawi

Solomon W. Harrar Dr. Bing Zhang Department of Statistics, University of Kentucky, Lexington, KY, USA

Tsirizani M. Kaombe Department of Mathematical Sciences, School of Natural and Applied Sciences, University of Malawi, Zomba, Malawi

Benjamin Kedem Department of Mathematics and Institute for Systems Research, University of Maryland, College Park, MD, USA

Tshiamo Kgoale Department of Mathematical Sciences, Sol Plaatje University, Kimberley, South Africa

Habte Tadesse Likassa College of Health Solutions, Arizona State University, Phoenix, AZ, USA

Samuel Manda Department of Statistics, Faculty of Natural and Agricultural Sciences, University of Pretoria, Pretoria, South Africa

Thomas Mathew University of Maryland Baltimore County, Baltimore, MD, USA

Sintayehu Agegnehu Matintu Department of Mathematics, Injibara University, Injibara, Ethiopia

Tshilidzi Mulaudzi University of Venda, Limpopo, South Africa

Justine B. Nasejje School of Statistics and Actuarial Science, University of Witwatersrand, Johannesburg, South Africa

Isabel Natário Department of Mathematics of NOVA School of Sciences and Technology & NOVA MATH, Caparica, Portugal

Najmeh Nakhaei Rad Department of Statistics, University of Pretoria, Pretoria, South Africa

Albert Whata Department of Statistics, University of Pretoria, Pretoria, South Africa

Temesgen T. Zewotir School of Mathematics, Statistics and Computer Science, College of Agriculture Engineering and Science, University of KwaZulu-Natal, Durban, South Africa

Xuze Zhang Department of Mathematics and Institute for Systems Research, University of Maryland, College Park, USA

Part I
Biostatistical Modeling

Chapter 1
Bootstrap Calibrated Tests for Average Bioequivalence and Scaled Average Bioequivalence

Rabab Elnaiem, Thomas Mathew, and Xiaoyu Dong

1.1 Introduction

The assessment of the bioequivalence between a brand name drug (or reference drug) and a generic copy (or test drug) is a topic that has received considerable attention in the literature. Crossover designs are used to generate the data, and the variables on which data are obtained are the area under the blood concentration-time curve (denoted by AUC), the maximum blood concentration (denoted by $C_{\max}$) of the active drug ingredient, or the time to reach the maximum concentration (denoted by $T_{\max}$). Usually the log-transformed data are modeled and analyzed. Univariate bioequivalence assessment consists of the modeling and analysis of the data on any single variable, and multivariate bioequivalence assessment consists of the joint modeling and analysis of the data on all the three variables, or any two of them. For bioequivalence assessment, a widely used criterion is that of average bioequivalence. A canonical form for testing univariate average bioequivalence consists of two independent random variables D and S^2 having the distributions

$$D \sim N(\mu, c^2\sigma^2), \text{ and } v\frac{S^2}{\sigma^2} \sim \chi^2_v, \tag{1.1}$$

where c^2 is a known constant, and χ^2_v denotes the central chisquare distribution with df $= v$. The value of the constant c^2 and the df v both depend on the crossover

R. Elnaiem · T. Mathew (✉)
University of Maryland Baltimore County, Baltimore, MD, USA
e-mail: relnaiem1@umbc.edu; mathew@umbc.edu

X. Dong
Data Sciences Institute, Takeda, Cambridge, MA, USA
e-mail: cassie.dong@takeda.com

D.-G. Chen, C. A. Coelho (eds.), *Biostatistics Modeling and Public Health Applications*, Emerging Topics in Statistics and Biostatistics,
https://doi.org/10.1007/978-3-031-69690-9_1

design used to generate the data, the sample sizes, and the model used to analyze the data; a brief derivation of (1.1) appears in Sect. 1.2.1 for a 2×2 crossover design, and in Section 3 for a four-period crossover design. Here μ is actually the difference between the population mean responses based on the brand name drug and its generic copy. As already noted, the population means and the canonical form (1.1) are usually based on log-transformed responses (ln(AUC), for example). Here we shall not give detailed background information; reference may be made to the books Patterson and Jones (2017), Chow and Liu (2009), and Hauschke et al. (2007).

In terms of the canonical form (1.1), the average bioequivalence hypothesis can be stated as

$$H_0 : |\mu| \geq \delta \ \text{ vs } \ H_1 : |\mu| < \delta, \tag{1.2}$$

where the usual choice is $\delta = \ln(1.25)$. The rejection of H_0 leads to the conclusion of average bioequivalence. The widely used two one-sided t-test (TOST) consists of concluding average bioequivalence if

$$\frac{D+\delta}{cS} > t_v(\alpha) \quad \text{and} \quad \frac{D-\delta}{cS} < -t_v(\alpha),$$

where $t_v(\alpha)$ is the upper α percentile of the t-distribution with df $= v$, α being the significance level. The test can also be expressed using a single test statistic; we conclude average bioequivalence if

$$\frac{|D|-\delta}{cS} < -t_v(\alpha). \tag{1.3}$$

Clearly, the TOST is easy to understand and implement; however, the test is known to be conservative as the variance σ^2 in (1.1) becomes large. In fact it can be theoretically shown that the type I error probability of the TOST approaches zero as σ becomes large, and it approaches the nominal level α as σ approaches zero. This suggests that if the TOST is carried out using a significance level larger than the nominal level α, the resulting test is likely to have a type I error probability close to α. However, the significance level to be used will depend on σ, and hence we will use a bootstrap calibration to estimate the required significance level from the data. The methodology is explained in the next section. Our numerical results show that the resulting test does maintain the type I error probability satisfactorily. Application of the proposed procedure for multivariate bioequivalence testing is also indicated.

When the responses for the reference drug exhibit a large variability, a *reference-scaled* criterion or a *mixed-scaled* criterion is often recommended; see Tothfalusi and Endrenyi (2012), Tothfalusi and Endrenyi (2017), Davit (2012), Tothfalusi and Endrenyi (2009), and Deng and Zhou (2020). We refer to these articles and also Chapter 7 in Patterson and Jones (2017) for earlier references and further background information. A drug with an intra-subject coefficient of variation greater than 30% is considered highly variable. A difficulty in using the TOST for such drugs is that the conservatism of the TOST makes it difficult to conclude bioequivalence even if bioequivalence holds. For such drugs, instead of μ, one option is to consider the US FDA (2022) recommended *mixed-scaled* criterion $\mu/[\max(0.25, \sigma_{WR})]$, where σ^2_{WR} is the within-subject variance corresponding to the reference drug. We note that the scale factor used in the criterion becomes equal to σ_{WR} when it is too large, i.e., when it is more than 0.25. A practical recommendation for implementing the mixed-scaled criterion is to choose between the quantities 0.25 and σ_{WR} in the denominator of the criterion based on the magnitude of $\hat{\sigma}_{WR}$, where $\hat{\sigma}^2_{WR}$ is an unbiased estimator of σ^2_{WR}. The US FDA Food and Drug Administration (2022) document recommends a threshold of 0.294 for $\hat{\sigma}_{WR}$ in order to choose between 0.25 and σ_{WR} in the reference-scaled criterion. We shall thus consider the hypotheses

$$
\begin{aligned}
H_0 : \frac{|\mu|}{\sigma_{WR}} \geq \delta_s \text{ vs } H_1 : \frac{|\mu|}{\sigma_{WR}} < \delta_s, \text{ if } \hat{\sigma}_{WR} \geq 0.294 \\
H_0 : \frac{|\mu|}{0.25} \geq \delta_s \text{ vs } H_1 : \frac{|\mu|}{0.25} < \delta_s, \text{ if } \hat{\sigma}_{WR} < 0.294,
\end{aligned}
\tag{1.4}
$$

where δ_s is a specified threshold. In contrast to the *mixed-scaled* criterion given above, a *reference-scaled* criterion scales $|\mu|$ with σ_{WR} only. We refer to Patterson and Jones (2012) for some comments on the scaled average bioequivalence criterion. In Sect. 1.3, we shall discuss a test for this hypothesis using the idea of a *modified large sample* (MLS) procedure, coupled with a bootstrap calibration. Numerical results will be reported to show that the resulting test satisfactorily maintains the type I error probability. Here it should be noted that even though our focus is on the two bioequivalence criteria specified in (1.2) and (1.4), other criteria have been considered in the literature; see the book Chow and Liu (2009) and the articles Tsong and Shen (2007), Dong and Tsong (2014a), and Dong and Tsong (2014b) (the last two articles discuss criteria based on tolerance intervals).

It appears that when faced with a large variability, one can consider two options for bioequivalence assessment: (i) use a calibrated TOST that takes care of the conservatism of the TOST resulting from the large variability or (ii) use a scaled criterion that suitably expands the bioequivalence limits. Here we would like to point out that with a standard two-period crossover design, it is not possible to estimate σ^2_{WR} due to the lack of replication, a fact that is well known in the literature. Thus, in order to test the hypotheses in (1.4), it is necessary to use a crossover design having more than two periods; we will be considering a four-period crossover design in Sect. 1.3. In other words, option (ii) is not possible under a two-period design. The need to have appropriate procedures to analyze bioequivalence data from a 2×2 crossover design, when the data exhibit high variability, has been noted in the literature; see Kang and Vahl (2017), Maurer et al. (2018), and Molins et al. (2021). In particular Kang and Vahl (2017) have cited several applications, including applications in veterinary medicine, where crossover designs having more than two periods present practical difficulties. We shall not repeat their arguments here; please see Section 1 in Kang and Vahl (2017). The above articles also make a strong case for having procedures that provide accurate type I error probabilities. In their work Kang and Vahl (2017) have addressed the type I error issue by developing an alternative test procedure using the concept of fiducial quantities. However, it was necessary to assume the absence of a subject-by-formulation interaction in order to develop the test. The later papers in Maurer et al. (2018) and Molins et al. (2021) have explored the use of a two-stage adaptive design under a 2×2 crossover design, when the data are likely to exhibit high variability. This appears to be an attractive option if one decides to do an interim analysis and, if necessary, proceed to a second stage by enrolling more subjects. These articles and other relevant literature cited by the authors demonstrate the need to address the issues of high variability and undesirable type I error probabilities when bioequivalence data are generated using a 2×2 crossover design. Our bootstrap calibrated TOST appears to be a satisfactory option that addresses the above issues. Furthermore, like the TOST, the bootstrap calibrated TOST is also a procedure that is easy to understand and implement.

1.2 Bootstrap Calibration of the TOST

We want to first note that several successful attempts have been made to modify the TOST so as to fix its conservatism; these include Munk (1993), Munk (1999), Munk (2000), Brown et al. (1997), Berger and Hsu (1996), Munk et al. (2000), and Cao and Mathew (2008). Even though some important theoretical developments are reported in several of these papers, the modified tests often appear to be rather complicated to understand and implement; in any case, they lack the simplicity of the TOST. In fact some discussants of the article Berger and Hsu (1996) have noted that from a practical perspective, some of the improved tests are too complicated. Here we want to attempt yet another modification of the TOST based on the bootstrap. Our motivation is twofold: First of all, the bootstrap modification we propose is simple to understand and easy to implement; we feel that the modified test is a "TOST-like test" that is almost as simple as the TOST. Second, the methodology can be applied to other problems pertinent to bioequivalence assessment; in particular, we shall demonstrate its applicability for testing scaled average bioequivalence.

We shall first explain the bootstrap calibrated TOST for univariate bioequivalence testing and then briefly discuss the multivariate case. For a general discussion of bootstrap calibration, we refer to Chapter 18 in Efron and Tibshirani (1993).

1.2.1 The Univariate Case

Recall that the purpose is to estimate a significance level larger than the nominal level α so that when the TOST is carried out using such an estimated significance level, the type I error probability will be closer to the nominal level α, compared to the TOST. Algorithm 1.1 explains the bootstrap calibration, i.e., the methodology for estimating the significance level using the bootstrap. Here the bootstrapping is done parametrically. The algorithm is presented referring to the canonical form (1.1), the hypotheses in (1.2), and the rejection rule given in (1.3).

Algorithm 1.1 The bootstrap calibrated TOST

1. Generate M parametric bootstrap samples (D_{i*}, S_{i*}^2) according to

$$D_{i*} \sim N(\delta, c^2 S^2) \text{ and } \upsilon \frac{S_{i*}^2}{S^2} \sim \chi_\upsilon^2,$$

   $i = 1, 2, ..., M$.
2. Compute M values of the test statistics: $\frac{|D_{i*}|-\delta}{cS_{i*}}$, $i = 1, 2, ..., M$.
3. Numerically select $\hat{\alpha}$ so that the proportion

$$\frac{|D_{i*}| - \delta)}{cS_{i*}} < -t_\upsilon(\hat{\alpha})$$

   is close to α. Note that $\hat{\alpha}$ is data dependent.
4. Now carry out the TOST using the significance level $\hat{\alpha}$. The corresponding rejection rule is

$$\frac{|D| - \ln(1.25)}{cS} < -t_\upsilon(\hat{\alpha}).$$

Type I Error and Power

We shall now report estimated type I error probabilities and power of the TOST and the bootstrap calibrated TOST, estimated using 20,000 simulated samples when the data are obtained on n subjects using a 2×2 crossover design. Let us denote by y_{jT} and y_{jR}, respectively, the responses to T and R for the jth subject, $j = 1, 2, ..., n$. These could be the log-transformed AUC, for example. We assume the models

$$y_{jT} = \mu_T + \eta_{jT} + e_{jT}$$
$$y_{jR} = \mu_R + \eta_{jR} + e_{jR},$$

where $(\eta_{jT}, \eta_{jR})'$ is a bivariate random effect corresponding to the jth subject, and e_{jT} and e_{jR} represent within-subject random errors. We assume

$$(\eta_{jT}, \eta_{jR})' \sim N(0, \Sigma_B),\ e_{jT} \sim N(0, \sigma_{WT}^2) \text{ and } e_{jR} \sim N(0, \sigma_{WR}^2),$$

and all the random variables are independent, $j = 1, 2, ..., n$. Let

$$D_j = y_{jT} - y_{jR},\ D = \frac{1}{n}\sum_{j=1}^{n} D_j,\ S^2 = \frac{1}{n-1}\sum_{j=1}^{n}(D_j - D)^2.$$

Then D and S^2 are independent, and

$$D \sim N\left(\mu_T - \mu_R, \frac{\sigma^2}{n}\right),\ (n-1)\frac{S^2}{\sigma^2} \sim \chi^2_{n-1}, \tag{1.5}$$

where σ^2 is a function of the variances σ^2_{WT}, σ^2_{WR}, and the elements of the matrix Σ_B. Thus we now have the canonical form (1.1) with $\mu = \mu_T - \mu_R$, $c^2 = \frac{1}{n}$, and $v = n - 1$.

Figures 1.1 and 1.2 give plots of the estimated type I error probabilities of the TOST and the calibrated TOST, when a 5% nominal level is used. In Fig. 1.1, the type I error probabilities are plotted against the df = $n-1$, and in Fig. 1.2, the plot is against the standard deviation σ. The type I error probabilities have been estimated using 20,000 simulated samples, and for the bootstrap calibration, 10,000 parametric bootstrap samples were used (i.e., we chose M = 10,000 in Algorithm 1.1). In order to arrive at $\hat{\alpha}$, we considered a grid of values in the interval [0.05, 0.5] with a step size of 0.005. The setup used for the simulation is the canonical form (1.5) corresponding to a 2×2 crossover design. The plots in Figs. 1.1 and 1.2 help us to assess the effect of the bootstrap calibration when the sample size n increases and when the standard deviation σ increases. It should be clear that the TOST and its calibrated version exhibit similar performance in terms of type I error probabilities for small values of σ. However, we notice marked differences between the two tests for larger values of σ, especially for a larger sample size. The plots clearly show that in terms of type I error probability, the bootstrap calibration of the TOST is a significant improvement over the TOST, especially for large values of σ and for large sample sizes. It should be noted that the bootstrap calibrated TOST is also conservative for large values of σ and small sample sizes.

Figures 1.3 and 1.4 give the plots of the power curves of the TOST and the calibrated TOST in the same setups that were used in order to estimate the type I error probability. The powers were evaluated at the alternative values $\mu = 0$ and $\mu = 0.2$. It is clear that the power is a decreasing function of σ and an increasing function of the sample size n, as can be anticipated. Furthermore, the difference between the powers of the two tests becomes more pronounced when σ gets large; once again, this is to be expected due to the extreme conservatism of the TOST for large values of σ. We also note that for large values of σ, the difference between the powers increases with the sample size. As an overall conclusion, we can state that for large sample sizes and for large values of σ, there is a significant advantage in using the calibrated TOST.

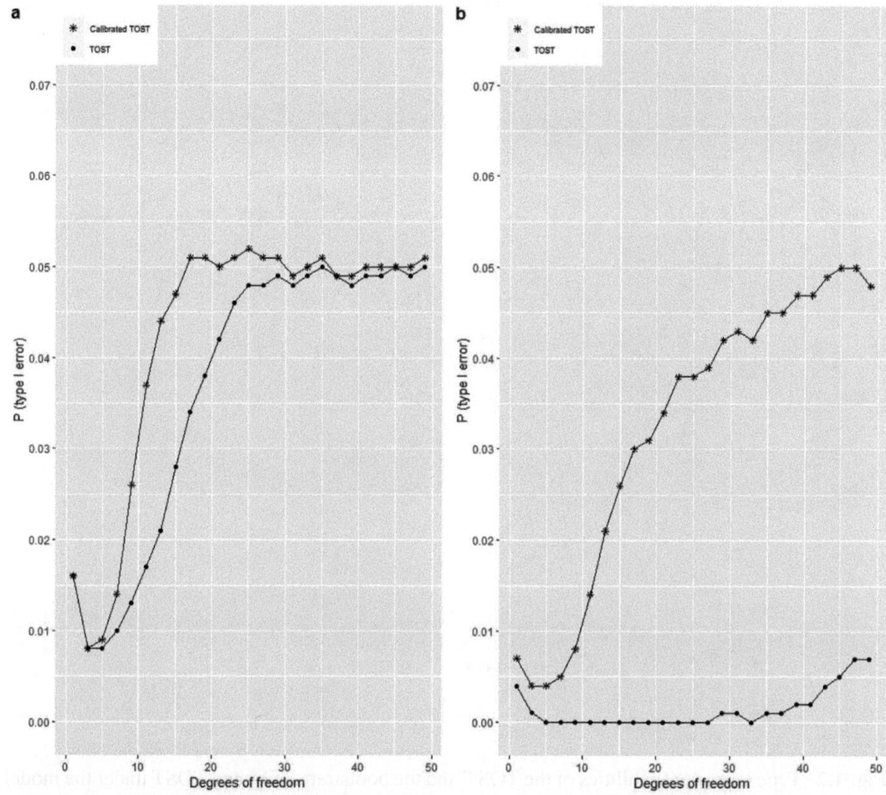

Fig. 1.1 Type I error probabilities of the TOST and the bootstrap calibrated TOST under the model (1.5), plotted against the degrees of freedom $n - 1$, corresponding to a 5% significance level for $\sigma = 0.5$ (left panel) and $\sigma = 1$ (right panel)

An Example

We shall briefly present an example to illustrate the bootstrap calibrated TOST. The example is taken from Chow and Liu (2009). Here the data are based on a four-sequence, four-period crossover study to compare a test formulation with a reference formulation of the drug Verapamil used to control angina and to treat high blood pressure. A total of 23 healthy volunteers were used in the study. Data on the AUC are given in Table 12.3.3 of Chow and Liu (2009). Based on the log-transformed AUC data, we have the point estimates $D = -0.0196$ and $S^2 = 0.059$. Furthermore, $c^2 = 0.04375$, and we make the standard choice $\delta = \log(1.25)$. The model used, along with the derivations necessary to arrive at the above quantities, is given in Sect. 1.3. For the TOST, the test statistic has the value -4.0054. Since $t_{19}(0.05) = 1.7291$, we reject the null hypothesis and conclude average bioequivalence using the TOST. Note that there is no need to apply a bootstrap calibration here; if we do, the conclusion will be the same.

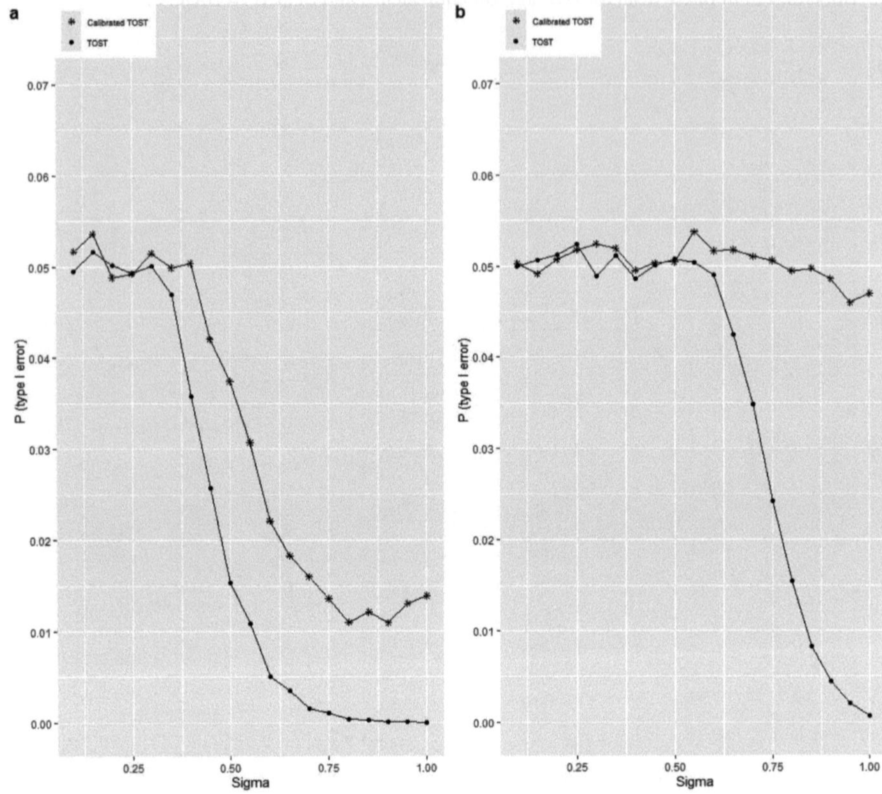

Fig. 1.2 Type I error probabilities of the TOST and the bootstrap calibrated TOST under the model (1.5), plotted against the standard deviation σ, corresponding to a 5% significance level for $n = 12$ (left panel) and $n = 36$ (right panel)

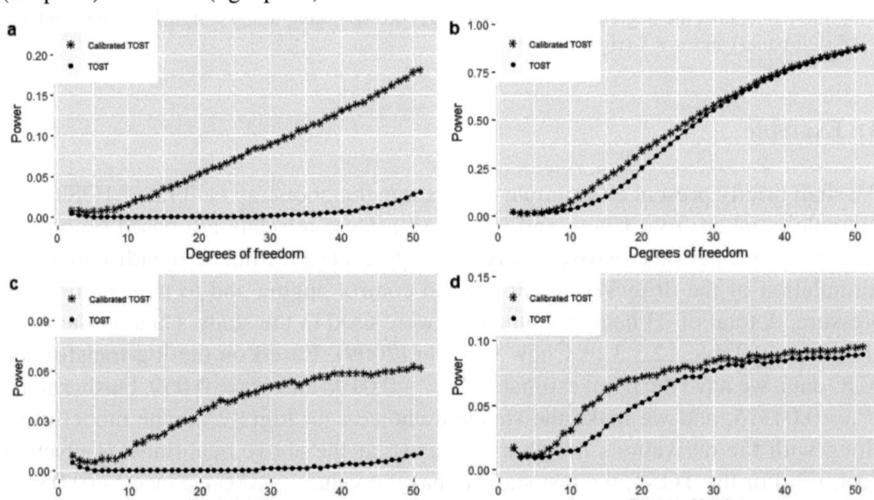

Fig. 1.3 Powers of the TOST and the bootstrap calibrated TOST, plotted against the degrees of freedom $n-1$, for the two alternatives $\mu = 0$ and 0.2, and for $\sigma = 0.5$ and 1, for a 5% significance level; (**a**) $\mu = 0$, $\sigma = 1$, (**b**) $\mu = 0$, $\sigma = 0.5$, (**c**) $\mu = 0.2$, $\sigma = 1$, and (**d**) $\mu = 0.2$, $\sigma = 0.5$

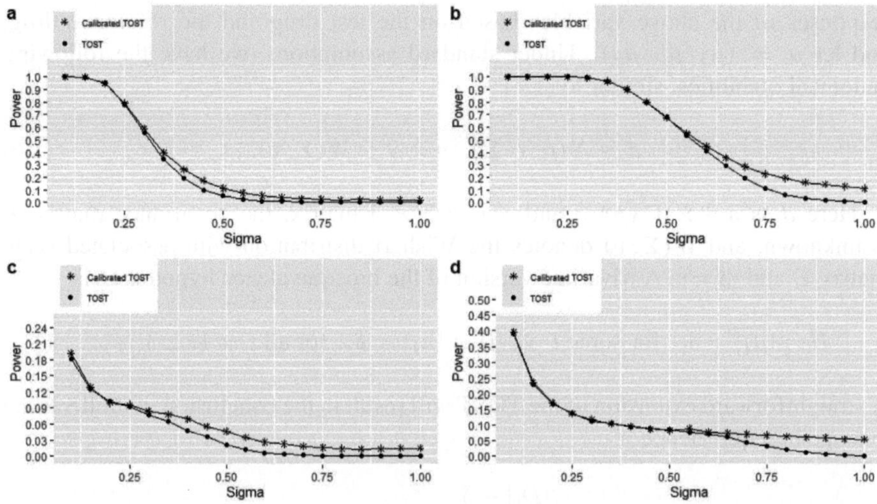

Fig. 1.4 Powers of the TOST and the bootstrap calibrated TOST, plotted against the standard deviation σ, for two alternatives $\mu = 0$ and 0.2, and for $n = 12$ and 36, for a 5% significance level; **(a)** $\mu = 0$, $n = 12$, **(b)** $\mu = 0$, $n = 36$, **(c)** $\mu = 0.2$, $n = 12$, and **(d)** $\mu = 0.2$, $n = 36$

In order to see the effect of bootstrap calibration, we considered the same design, and the same summary statistics, except that we assume a few larger values for S^2. The assumed values of S^2 and the results of the analysis are presented in the following table. We have provided the values of the test statistic corresponding to each assumed sample variance, and the estimated significance level $\hat{\alpha}$ to be used, where the latter was obtained by applying bootstrap calibration. In all the cases presented below, the TOST resulted in a conclusion against bioequivalence (i.e., the null hypothesis was not rejected). However, the calibrated TOST resulted in the rejection of the null hypothesis, thereby concluding average bioequivalence.

S^2	0.32	0.37	0.41	0.45	0.49
Test statistics	−1.7199	−1.5995	−1.5194	−1.4503	−1.3899
$\hat{\alpha}$	0.065	0.075	0.080	0.090	0.100

We note that the estimated significance level $\hat{\alpha}$ increases with S^2, as expected.

1.2.2 The Multivariate Case

In multivariate bioequivalence testing, we test the equivalence hypothesis on two or three variables: the three variables being $\ln AUC$, $\ln C_{\max}$, and $\ln T_{\max}$. Let μ_1, μ_2, and μ_3, respectively, denote the differences between the population mean responses of the above variables based on the test drug and the reference drug, and let $\mu = (\mu_1, \mu_2, \mu_3)'$. Under standard assumptions, we have the following canonical quantities, similar to (1.1):

$$d \sim N(\mu, c^2\Sigma), \; v \times S \sim W(\Sigma, v). \tag{1.6}$$

Here d is a 3×1 vector and S is a 3×3 matrix, the covariance matrix Σ is unknown, and $W(\Sigma, v)$ denotes the Wishart distribution with associated scale matrix Σ and df = v. A trivariate version of the bioequivalence hypotheses is

$$H_0 : |\mu_i| \geq \delta, \;\text{ for some } i \;\text{ vs }\; H_1 : |\mu_i| < \delta, \;\text{ for all } i = 1, 2, 3. \tag{1.7}$$

A straightforward extension of the TOST will result in the conclusion of multivariate average bioequivalence if

$$\frac{|D_i| - \delta}{c\sqrt{S_{ii}}} < -t_v(\alpha), \tag{1.8}$$

where S_{ii} is the ith diagonal element of S, i = 1, 2, 3. Note that we are actually carrying out the TOST three times, for the three variables. Thus the bootstrap calibration has to be carried out three times as well. The bootstrap calibrated test will conclude multivariate average bioequivalence if

$$\frac{|D_i| - \delta}{c\sqrt{S_{ii}}} < -t_v(\hat{\alpha}_i), \tag{1.9}$$

i = 1, 2, 3. It is important to note that the bootstrap calibration is carried out separately for each component, resulting in possibly different significance levels $\hat{\alpha}_i$ for the different components, i = 1, 2, 3. Obviously, the test can be adopted to the bivariate case as well, for example, using the data on ln AUC and ln $C_{\max}$ only.

The multivariate bioequivalence problem is investigated in Wang et al. (1999). The authors have applied the univariate size α test due to Brown et al. (1997) for each component hypothesis, and their numerical results show the improved power of the resulting test, compared to the test given in (1.8). For the bootstrap calibrated TOST defined by (1.9), numerical results on the power are given in Table 1.1 for $\mu = 0$ in the bivariate case and in the trivariate case for the sample size 24, assuming that the diagonal elements of Σ are all equal. In the table, ρ denotes the correlation in the bivariate case and a common correlation in the trivariate case. The numerical results in Table 1.1 show that the bootstrap calibrated multivariate TOST gives significantly improved power compared to the same test without calibration. Only positive values of the correlation were considered in the simulation, and we note that the powers of the TOST and the calibrated TOST increase with the correlation.

Table 1.1 The empirical powers of the TOST and the calibrated TOST (denoted by TOST*) in the bivariate and trivariate cases for sample size 24 and $\alpha = 0.05$; σ_{ii} denotes the diagonal elements of Σ in (1.6) and ρ denotes the correlations in Σ, assumed to be common in the trivariate case

	Bivariate case					
	$\sigma_{11} = \sigma_{22} = 0.2$		$\sigma_{11} = \sigma_{22} = 0.4$		$\sigma_{11} = \sigma_{22} = 0.6$	
ρ	TOST	TOST*	TOST	TOST*	TOST	TOST*
0.0	0.9995	0.9996	0.4633	0.4944	0.0183	0.0605
0.1	0.9995	0.9995	0.4644	0.4946	0.0186	0.0614
0.2	0.9995	0.9995	0.4681	0.4989	0.0193	0.0629
0.3	0.9995	0.9995	0.4743	0.5045	0.0205	0.0648
0.4	0.9995	0.9995	0.4834	0.5128	0.0222	0.0669
0.5	0.9994	0.9995	0.4951	0.5257	0.0250	0.0713
0.6	0.9994	0.9995	0.5110	0.5406	0.0291	0.0779
0.7	0.9994	0.9995	0.5310	0.5593	0.0354	0.0867
0.8	0.9994	0.9995	0.5569	0.5845	0.0452	0.1010
0.9	0.9995	0.9996	0.5933	0.6191	0.0622	0.1278
	Trivariate case					
	$\sigma_{11} = \sigma_{22} = \sigma_{33} = 0.2$		$\sigma_{11} = \sigma_{22} = \sigma_{33} = 0.4$		$\sigma_{11} = \sigma_{22} = \sigma_{33} = 0.6$	
ρ	TOST	TOST*	TOST	TOST*	TOST	TOST*
0.0	0.9991	0.9992	0.3165	0.3483	0.0029	0.0150
0.1	0.9991	0.9992	0.3186	0.3504	0.0030	0.0150
0.2	0.9991	0.9992	0.3255	0.3578	0.0032	0.0155
0.3	0.9992	0.9993	0.3379	0.3699	0.0039	0.0172
0.4	0.9992	0.9993	0.3544	0.3864	0.0049	0.0184
0.5	0.9992	0.9993	0.3753	0.4060	0.0066	0.0223
0.6	0.9992	0.9993	0.4028	0.4346	0.0086	0.0264
0.7	0.9992	0.9994	0.4380	0.4690	0.0126	0.0337
0.8	0.9994	0.9994	0.4819	0.5119	0.0201	0.0466
0.9	0.9994	0.9994	0.5419	0.5696	0.0371	0.0767

1.3 Highly Variable Drugs and Scaled Average Bioequivalence

Highly variable drugs and the corresponding hypotheses based on a mixed-scaled criterion were briefly discussed in the introduction, and the relevant hypotheses were stated in (1.4). The hypotheses can equivalently be stated as

$$H_0 : \frac{\mu^2}{\sigma_{WR}^2} \geq K \text{ vs } H_1 : \frac{\mu^2}{\sigma_{WR}^2} < K, \text{ if } \hat{\sigma}_{WR}^2 \geq (0.294)^2$$

$$H_0 : \frac{\mu^2}{0.25^2} \geq K \text{ vs } H_1 : \frac{\mu^2}{0.25^2} < K, \text{ if } \hat{\sigma}_{WR}^2 < (0.294)^2, \quad (1.10)$$

where σ^2_{WR} denotes the variance of the response ($\ln(AUC)$, for example) to the reference drug, $\hat{\sigma}^2_{WR}$ denotes its unbiased estimator, and K is a specified threshold. One choice for the threshold is $K = \left(\frac{\ln(1.25)}{0.25}\right)^2$; see the US FDA Food and Drug Administration (2022) document (pp. 19–20).

In order to test the hypotheses in (1.10), it is necessary to obtain the unbiased estimator $\hat{\sigma}^2_{WR}$ for σ^2_{WR}; a 2×2 crossover design is inadequate for this purpose. Here we shall consider a four-period crossover design, so that each subject receives two administrations of each of the two formulations T and R. Suppose there are s sequences in the design, with n_i subjects in the ith sequence, $i = 1, 2, ..., s$. Consequently, we now have an $s \times 4$ crossover design. We shall use the notation Y_{ijkl} to denote the lth observation corresponding to the formulation k given to the jth subject in the ith sequence, $l = 1, 2$; $k = T, R$; $j = 1, 2, ..., n_i$ and $i = 1, 2, ..., s$. We shall assume the following model for Y_{ijkl}; the model is considered in Chinchilli and Esinhart (1996) and is also given in the US FDA Food and Drug Administration (2001) document (Appendix G).

$$Y_{ijkl} = \mu_k + \gamma_{ikl} + \eta_{ijk} + \epsilon_{ijkl}, \quad k = R, T, \tag{1.11}$$

where μ_k is the average effect due to the kth formulation, γ_{ikl} is a fixed effect corresponding to the lth application of treatment k in the ith sequence, and $\eta_{ij} = (\eta_{ijT}, \eta_{ijR})'$ is a bivariate random effect that is normally distributed with zero mean and covariance matrix Σ_B:

$$\Sigma_B = \begin{pmatrix} \sigma^2_{BT} & \rho\sigma_{BT}\sigma_{BR} \\ \rho\sigma_{BT}\sigma_{BR} & \sigma^2_{BR} \end{pmatrix}. \tag{1.12}$$

Furthermore, the ϵ_{ijkl}s are normally distributed with mean zero and variance σ^2_{Wk}. The η_{ij}s and the ϵ_{ijkl}s are all assumed to be independent. The fixed effect γ_{ikl}s are assumed to satisfy the following estimability condition:

$$\sum_{i=1}^{s}\sum_{l=1}^{2} \gamma_{ikl} = 0, \; k = T, R.$$

Canonical quantities and their distributions under the model (1.11) are given by (see Appendix B)

$$D \sim N\left(\mu = \mu_T - \mu_R, c^2\sigma^2\right), \; A = \begin{pmatrix} A_{11} & A_{12} \\ A_{21} & A_{22} \end{pmatrix} \sim W(\Sigma, v),$$

$$\frac{vS^2}{\sigma^2} \sim \chi^2_v, \; \frac{SS_{WR}}{\sigma^2_{WR}} \sim \chi^2_v, \tag{1.13}$$

where D and S^2 are independent, and so are D, A, and SS_{WR}. In (1.13), $W(\Sigma, v)$ denotes the Wishart distribution with degrees of freedom v, and associated covariance matrix Σ. Expressions for the parameter matrix Σ, the variance σ^2, and the constants c^2 and v are given in Appendix B.

In order to test the hypotheses in (1.10), we shall proceed as follows. Let $\hat{\sigma}^2_{WR} = \frac{SS_{WR}}{v}$, so that $\hat{\sigma}^2_{WR}$ is an unbiased estimator of σ^2_{WR}; see (1.13). Following the guidance in FDA Food and Drug Administration (2022)(pp. 19-20), we first check if $\hat{\sigma}^2_{WR} \geq (0.294)^2$. If so, we test the hypotheses in (1.10) using σ^2_{WR} as the scaling factor. If not, we test the hypotheses in (1.10) using $(0.25)^2$ as the scaling factor. Thus the testing problem can be written as

$$H_0 : \mu^2 - K\sigma^2_{WR} \geq 0, \text{ vs } H_1 : \mu^2 - K\sigma^2_{WR} < 0, \text{ if } \hat{\sigma}^2_{WR} \geq (0.294)^2$$

$$H_0 : \mu^2 - K \times (0.25)^2 \geq 0, \text{ vs } H_1 : \mu^2 - K \times (0.25)^2 < 0, \text{ if } \hat{\sigma}^2_{WR} < (0.294)^2. \quad (1.14)$$

In each case, we conclude bioequivalence if the corresponding null hypothesis is rejected. The test procedure consists of first computing a $100(1-\alpha)\%$ upper confidence limit for $\mu^2 - K\sigma^2_{WR}$ or for $\mu^2 - K(0.25)^2$; we note that computing an upper confidence limit for the latter quantity amounts to computing the same for μ^2. The corresponding null hypothesis is rejected at significance level α when the upper confidence limit is less than zero. The required upper confidence limits will be computed using a *modified large sample* (MLS) procedure. The MLS approach is meant to provide approximate confidence limits (one-sided or two-sided) for a linear combination of parameters, when confidence limits are available for the individual parameters. The approach was proposed in Graybill and Wang (1980). A detailed discussion and numerous applications are available in the book Burdick and Graybill (1992); see also Section 1.3 in Krishnamoorthy and Mathew (2009). An outline of the MLS approach is given in Appendix A. In the context of evaluating bioequivalence for highly variable drugs, the MLS idea is used in Tothfalusi et al. (2001); see also Section 7.3 in Patterson and Jones (2017). While computing the upper confidence limit, a bootstrap calibration will be applied in order to have accurate performance in terms of type I error probabilities. We shall now provide details of what we have just outlined.

Recall that under the model (1.11) for the $s \times 4$ crossover design under consideration, unbiased estimates of μ and σ^2_{WR} are given by $\hat{\mu} = D$ and $\hat{\sigma}^2_{WR} = SS_{WR}/v$, respectively, where the relevant statistics have been defined earlier. A $100(1-\alpha)\%$ upper confidence limit for μ^2, say $\hat{\mu}^2_U$, and a $100(1-\alpha)\%$ lower confidence limit for σ^2_{WR}, say $\hat{\sigma}^2_{WR,L}$, respectively, are given by

$$\hat{\mu}^2_U = \left(|D| + t_{(1-\alpha)} \times cS\right)^2, \; \hat{\sigma}^2_{WR,L} = \frac{SS_{WR}}{\chi^2_v(1-\alpha)}, \quad (1.15)$$

where S^2 is defined in (1.19) and $\chi_v^2(1-\alpha)$ denotes the $100(1-\alpha)$th percentile of the chisquare distribution with df $= v$. The upper confidence limit $\hat{\mu}_U^2$ given above is taken from Hsu et al. (1994). Applying the MLS methodology (outlined Appendix A), a $100(1-\alpha)\%$ upper confidence limit for $\mu^2 - K\sigma_{WR}^2$ is the quantity UB_1 given below in (1.16). We shall define the upper confidence bounds UB_1, UB_2 and UB as follows:

$$UB_1 = \left\{D^2 - K\hat{\sigma}_{WR}^2\right\} + \sqrt{\left\{\hat{\mu}_U^2 - D^2\right\}^2 + K^2\left\{\hat{\sigma}_{WR,L}^2 - \hat{\sigma}_{WR}^2\right\}^2}$$

$$UB_2 = \hat{\mu}_U^2 - K(0.25)^2$$

$$UB = \begin{cases} UB_1 \text{ if } \hat{\sigma}_{WR}^2 \geq (0.294)^2 \\ UB_2 \text{ if } \hat{\sigma}_{WR}^2 < (0.294)^2. \end{cases} \tag{1.16}$$

We reject H_0 in (1.10) and conclude scaled average bioequivalence if $UB < 0$.

Our numerical results show that the test proposed above, based on the MLS approach, is reasonably accurate in terms of maintaining the type I error probability; however, it can sometimes be conservative. This conservatism is perhaps due to two reasons. First of all, note that we need to test the first or second set of hypothesis in (1.14) depending on whether or not $\hat{\sigma}_{WR}^2 \geq (0.294)^2$; the upper confidence bound UB in (1.16) has been defined accordingly. Second, the MLS upper confidence bound UB_1 in (1.16) is only an approximate upper confidence bound. We shall thus apply a bootstrap calibration in order to improve the type I error probability performance. Similar to the case of the calibrated TOST, the calibration is done in order to determine the estimated confidence level to be used in order to compute the required upper confidence limit. Algorithm 1.2 in Appendix C explains the methodology for obtaining the bootstrap calibrated MLS upper confidence bound.

Table 1.2 gives the type I error probabilities of the test based on the MLS upper bound and the calibrated MLS upper bound. These have been estimated using 5000 simulated samples with $M = 1000$ bootstrap samples for the bootstrap calibration. In order to arrive at the required confidence level, say $1-\hat{\alpha}$, we considered a grid of α-values in the interval [0.04, 0.3] with a step size of 0.005. The values of σ_{BT}, σ_{WT}, σ_{BR}, and σ_{WR} used in the simulation are specified in the table. In addition, referring to the matrix Σ_B, we used a correlation of 0.80 while generating the data. We note that the MLS-based test maintains the type I error probability fairly accurately in most scenarios. In a few instances where the test is conservative, the bootstrap calibration provides an improvement.

Table 1.2 The empirical type I error rates of the MLS test and its bootstrap calibrated version (MLS*) for scaled average bioequivalence; $\alpha = 0.05$

σ_{BT}	σ_{WT}	σ_{BR}	σ_{WR}	Sample size	MLS	MLS*
0.1	0.15	0.2	0.25	12	0.0507	0.0502
				24	0.0485	0.0504
				32	0.0507	0.0503
0.15	0.2	0.25	0.3	12	0.0498	0.0512
				24	0.0482	0.0500
				32	0.0505	0.0501
0.2	0.25	0.3	0.35	12	0.0498	0.0502
				24	0.0482	0.0500
				32	0.0505	0.0512
0.25	0.3	0.35	0.4	12	0.0488	0.0514
				24	0.0478	0.0499
				32	0.0481	0.0501
0.3	0.35	0.4	0.45	12	0.0481	0.0511
				24	0.0481	0.0501
				32	0.0489	0.0511
0.4	0.35	0.3	0.25	12	0.0398	0.0512
				24	0.0463	0.0489
				32	0.0490	0.0513
0.45	0.4	0.35	0.3	12	0.0419	0.0513
				24	0.0466	0.0491
				32	0.0497	0.0502
0.5	0.45	0.4	0.35	12	0.0423	0.0512
				24	0.0467	0.0495
				32	0.0499	0.0507
0.55	0.5	0.45	0.4	12	0.0440	0.0513
				24	0.0464	0.049
				32	0.0496	0.0512
0.6	0.55	0.5	0.45	12	0.0446	0.0513
				24	0.0463	0.0486
				32	0.0498	0.0502

1.3.1 Example (Continued)

Let us reconsider the example in Sect. 1.2.1 where we have a four-sequence, four-period crossover study; the corresponding data on the AUC are given in Table 12.3.3 of Chow and Liu (2009). In addition to the summary statistics reported earlier, we also have the estimates $\hat{\sigma}^2_{WT} = 0.1271$, $\hat{\sigma}^2_{BT} = 0.20785$, $\hat{\sigma}^2_{WR} = 0.07450$, $\hat{\sigma}^2_{BR} = 0.27908$. For testing the hypotheses in (1.10), we first note that $\hat{\sigma}_{WR} = 0.2729 < 0.294$. Thus the hypotheses simplify to

$$H_0 : \mu^2 - K(0.25)^2 \geq 0 \text{ vs } H_1 : \mu^2 - K(0.25)^2 < 0,$$

where $K = \left(\frac{\ln(1.25)}{0.25}\right)^2 = 0.79669$. In order to test the above hypotheses, we shall use the upper confidence bound UB_1 for $\mu^2 - K(0.25)^2$, given in (1.16). Applying the MLS procedure, the 95% upper confidence bound is computed as $UB_1 = -0.01715$. Since $UB_1 < 0$, we conclude scaled average bioequivalence. The bootstrap calibration also led to the same conclusion of scaled average bioequivalence.

Let us now refer back to the example as discussed in Sect. 1.2.1, where we recall that when the variance $S^2 = 0.32$, the TOST and its calibrated version resulted in different conclusions: The TOST resulted in a conclusion against bioequivalence, whereas the calibrated version was in favor of bioequivalence. This is not surprising in view of the conservatism of the TOST for large values of the variance. Choosing $\hat{\sigma}^2_{BR} = 0.54008$ (which will result in $S^2 = 0.32$) and keeping all the other estimates the same as before, the 95% MLS upper confidence bound is computed as $UB_1 = -0.00148$. Since $UB_1 < 0$, we conclude scaled average bioequivalence. Thus for a large value of the variance S^2, the bootstrap calibrated TOST for testing the usual average bioequivalence and the test for scaled average bioequivalence both led to a conclusion in favor of bioequivalence, contrary to the conclusion from the TOST. A somewhat similar conclusion regarding the adequacy of a 2×2 crossover design is also noted in Section 3 in Kang and Vahl (2017). We have commented on this further in the brief discussion that follows.

1.4 Discussion

In the assessment of bioequivalence, the TOST is widely recommended and extensively used; its simplicity is a major attraction. However, due to its conservatism, there is the possibility of drawing a conclusion against bioequivalence, when bioequivalence does hold. Theoretical and numerical results have shown that the conservatism of the TOST occurs when the variability is large. Motivated by this observation, several successful attempts have been made in order to address the conservatism of the TOST; some of the relevant literature was cited earlier. However, the resulting tests lack the simplicity of the TOST, and the tests do not seem to have made an impact on the practice of bioequivalence testing; see some of the discussions following the article Berger and Hsu (1996). In this chapter, we have pursued a simple idea to fix the conservatism of the TOST: Since the TOST is conservative when the variance gets large, use a significance level that is larger than the nominal level and is also variance dependent. Since the variance is unknown, employ the bootstrap in order to estimate the variance-dependent significance level, and then carry out the TOST using the significance level so estimated. The resulting test is just as simple as the TOST, except that the estimated significance level has to be numerically obtained. As expected, the estimated significance level can be larger than the nominal level; this is noted in the example in Sect. 1.2.1. The example also presents situations where the TOST will lead to a conclusion against average bioequivalence, whereas the bootstrap calibrated TOST results in a conclusion in favor of average bioequivalence.

Faced with an increased variability, an option recommended and widely investigated in the literature is the use of a scaled average bioequivalence criterion, which amounts to widening the bioequivalence limits by making it variance dependent. In this chapter, we have addressed this scenario also, and a test is recommended using the idea of a modified large sample procedure, coupled with a bootstrap calibration. Without the bootstrap calibration, we noticed that the test can sometimes result in conservative type I error probabilities. Scaled average bioequivalence based on mixed-scaled criteria is discussed in Deng and Zhou (2020), and the authors have suggested some step-wise procedures to address the issue of type I error inflation. Bootstrap calibration appears to be a simple and unified approach to accomplish this.

Based on the present work, it appears to us that two options are available while trying to assess bioequivalence in the presence of a large variability. The first option is to use the usual average bioequivalence criterion and the bootstrap calibrated TOST. The second option is to use a scaled average bioequivalence criterion. Both options may lead to the same conclusion, and this is noted in the context of the example presented in Sect. 1.3. When the sample variance was somewhat large, both options led to the same conclusion, in favor of bioequivalence, even though the TOST led to a conclusion against bioequivalence. However, the calibrated TOST has an advantage: It can be carried out using data from a 2×2 crossover design. This is not possible with the scaled average bioequivalence test, since the scaling factor cannot be estimated using data from a 2×2 crossover design (the example we have considered is a four-period crossover design). In other words, the bootstrap calibrated TOST appears to be an attractive option to assess bioequivalence using the usual average bioequivalence criterion; it is simple to understand and implement, and it addresses the conservatism of the TOST. It should also be noted that practical considerations may make it difficult to use a crossover design having more than two periods even if high variability is anticipated. This is noted in the introduction, citing Kang and Vahl (2017), Maurer et al. (2018), and Molins et al. (2021), elaborating on the importance of the 2×2 crossover design in veterinary medicine Kang and Vahl (2017), note that "Crossover designs with a relatively long duration could not be conducted on growing animals or those who suffer physiological stress under prolonged confinement and repeated dosing" (see Section 1 in their paper). These authors have developed a test for the reference-scaled average bioequivalence criterion under the assumption that the subject-by-formulation interaction is zero. However, this assumption cannot be verified under a 2×2 crossover design; our bootstrap calibrated TOST does not require this assumption.

R codes for implementing the bootstrap calibrated tests proposed in this chapter are available in Appendix D.

Acknowledgments We are grateful to a reviewer for the detailed comments which clarified some of the ideas and improved the presentation of the material.

Data Availability Statement
All data used in this chapter are available in the published literature.

Appendix A: The Modified Large Sample (MLS) Procedure

In order to present the MLS idea, consider k unknown variance parameters σ_i^2 ($i = 1, 2, ..., k$) and independent random variables $S_1^2, ..., S_k^2$ such that $m_i S_i^2/\sigma_i^2 \sim \chi^2_{m_i}$, $i = 1, ..., k$. Clearly, $\hat{\sigma}_i^2 = S_i^2$ is an unbiased estimator of σ_i^2. Furthermore, exact $100(1-\alpha)\%$ upper and lower confidence limits for σ_i^2 are given by $\frac{m_i\widehat{\sigma}_i^2}{\chi^2_{m_i;\alpha}}$ and $\frac{m_i\widehat{\sigma}_i^2}{\chi^2_{m_i;1-\alpha}}$, respectively. Here $\chi^2_{m;\gamma}$ denotes the 100γth percentile of a central chisquare distribution with df = m. These upper and lower confidence bounds can also be expressed, respectively, as $\widehat{\sigma}_i^2 + \sqrt{\widehat{\sigma}_i^4\left(\frac{m_i}{\chi^2_{m_i;\alpha}} - 1\right)^2}$ and $\widehat{\sigma}_i^2 + \sqrt{\widehat{\sigma}_i^4\left(1 - \frac{m_i}{\chi^2_{m_i;1-\alpha}}\right)^2}$. Now suppose we want an approximate upper confidence limit for the linear combination $\sum_{i=1}^k c_i\sigma_i^2$, where each c_i could be positive or negative. A $100(1-\alpha)\%$ MLS upper confidence bound for $\sum_{i=1}^k c_i\sigma_i^2$ is given by

$$\sum_{i=1}^k c_i\widehat{\sigma}_i^2 + \sqrt{\sum_{i=1}^k c_i^2\widehat{\sigma}_i^4\left(\frac{m_i}{u_i} - 1\right)^2}, \tag{1.17}$$

where

$$u_i = \begin{cases} \chi^2_{m_i;\alpha}, & c_i > 0, \\ \chi^2_{m_i;1-\alpha}, & c_i < 0. \end{cases}$$

Similarly, a $100(1-\alpha)\%$ MLS lower confidence bound for $\sum_{i=1}^k c_i\sigma_i^2$ is obtained as

$$\sum_{i=1}^k c_i\widehat{\sigma}_i^2 + \sqrt{\sum_{i=1}^k c_i^2\widehat{\sigma}_i^4\left(\frac{m_i}{l_i} - 1\right)^2}, \tag{1.18}$$

where

$$l_i = \begin{cases} \chi^2_{m_i;1-\alpha}, & c_i > 0, \\ \chi^2_{m_i;\alpha}, & c_i < 0. \end{cases}$$

For a $100(1-\alpha)\%$ two-sided MLS confidence interval, the limits are obtained as the $\left(1-\frac{\alpha}{2}\right)$ MLS lower confidence bound and the $\left(1-\frac{\alpha}{2}\right)$ MLS upper confidence bound.

Appendix B: Derivation of the Canonical Quantities in (1.13)

The derivation is given in McNally et al. (2003). For $k = T, R$, define

$$\bar{Y}_{ijk} = \frac{1}{2}\left(Y_{ijk1} + Y_{ijk2}\right),\ D_{ij} = \bar{Y}_{ijT} - \bar{Y}_{ijR},\ \bar{D}_i = \frac{1}{n_i}\sum_j D_{ij}, D = \frac{1}{s}\sum_i \bar{D}_i$$

$$E_{ijR} = \frac{1}{\sqrt{2}}\left(Y_{ijR1} - Y_{ijR2}\right),\ \bar{E}_{iR} = \frac{1}{n_i}\sum_j E_{ijR},$$

$$SS_{WR} = \sum_i\sum_j (E_{ijR} - \bar{E}_{iR})^2$$

$$SS_I = \sum_i\sum_j (D_{ij} - \bar{D}_i)^2,\ \bar{Y}_{i\star k} = \frac{1}{n_i}\sum_j \bar{Y}_{ij}$$

$$A = \sum_{i=1}^{s}\sum_{j=1}^{n_i}\begin{pmatrix}\bar{Y}_{ijT} - \bar{Y}_{i\star T}\\ \bar{Y}_{ijR} - \bar{Y}_{i\star R}\end{pmatrix}\begin{pmatrix}\bar{Y}_{ijT} - \bar{Y}_{i\star T}\\ \bar{Y}_{ijR} - \bar{Y}_{i\star R}\end{pmatrix}' = \begin{pmatrix}A_{11} & A_{12}\\ A_{21} & A_{22}\end{pmatrix},$$

$$\Sigma = \Sigma_B + \frac{1}{2}\text{diag}\left(\sigma_{WT}^2, \sigma_{WR}^2\right) = \begin{pmatrix}\sigma_{11} & \sigma_{12}\\ \sigma_{21} & \sigma_{22}\end{pmatrix},$$

$$c^2 = \frac{1}{s^2}\sum_{i=1}^{s}\frac{1}{n_i},\ v = \sum_{i=1}^{s} n_i - s$$

$$S^2 = \frac{1}{v}\left(A_{11} + A_{22} - 2A_{12}\right),\ \sigma^2 = \sigma_{11} + \sigma_{22} - 2\sigma_{12}, \tag{1.19}$$

where Σ_B is given in (1.12).

Appendix C: Algorithm for the Bootstrap Calibrated MLS Procedure

The confidence level to be estimated using bootstrap calibration will be denoted by $1-\gamma$.

Algorithm 1.2 The bootstrap calibrated MLS upper confidence bound

1. From the given data, compute the quantities D, A, and SS_{WR}. Let

$$\hat{\Sigma} = \frac{A}{v} = \begin{pmatrix} \hat{\sigma}_{11} & \hat{\sigma}_{12} \\ \hat{\sigma}_{21} & \hat{\sigma}_{22} \end{pmatrix}.$$

2. For q = 1, 2, ..., M, generate M parametric bootstrap samples

$$D_q^* \sim N\left(D, c^2 S^2\right), \; A_q^* \sim W(\hat{\Sigma}, v), \; \frac{SS_{WR,q}^*}{\hat{\sigma}_{WR}^2} \sim \chi_v^2, \; . \tag{1.20}$$

3. For q = 1, 2, ..., M, let

$$A_q^* = \begin{pmatrix} A_{11,q}^* & A_{12,q}^* \\ A_{21,q}^* & A_{22,q}^* \end{pmatrix}, \; S_q^{2*} = (A_{11,q}^* + A_{22,q}^* - 2A_{12,q}^*)/v,$$

$$\hat{\sigma}_{WR,q}^{2*} = \frac{SS_{WR,q}^*}{v},$$

and compute the $100(1-\gamma)\%$ confidence bounds (where $1-\gamma$ will be determined by bootstrap calibration)

$$\hat{\mu}_{U,q}^{2*} = \left(|D_q^*| + t_{(1-\gamma)} \times cS_q^*\right)^2, \; \hat{\sigma}_{WR,L,q}^{2*} = \frac{SS_{WR,q}^*}{\chi_v^2(1-\gamma)}. \tag{1.21}$$

4. For each q = 1, 2, ..., M, compute the $100(1-\gamma)\%$ upper confidence bounds $UB_{1,q}^*$ and $UB_{2,q}^*$ given by

$$UB_{1,q}^* = \left\{D_q^{*^2} - K\hat{\sigma}_{WR,q}^{2*}\right\} + \sqrt{\left\{\hat{\mu}_{U,q}^{2*} - D_q^{*^2}\right\}^2 + K^2\left\{\hat{\sigma}_{WR,L,q}^{2*} - \hat{\sigma}_{WR,q}^{2*}\right\}^2}$$

$$UB_{2,q}^* = \hat{\mu}_{U,q}^{2*} - K(0.25)^2$$

$$UB_q^* = \begin{cases} UB_{1,q}^* \text{ if } \hat{\sigma}_{WR,q}^{2*} \geq (0.294)^2 \\ UB_{2,q}^* \text{ if } \hat{\sigma}_{WR,q}^{2*} < (0.294)^2. \end{cases} \tag{1.22}$$

We note that $UB_{1,q}^*$, $UB_{2,q}^*$ and UB_q^* in (1.22) are similar to the corresponding upper bounds given in (1.16).

5. Compute the M $100(1-\gamma)\%$ upper confidence limits $UB_{1,q}^*$, q = 1, 2, ..., M, in (1.22) for a grid of values of γ, and check the proportion of times $UB_{1,q}^* < 0$.

Choose a value of γ that makes this proportion close to α. Denote the resulting value of γ by $\hat{\alpha}$.

6. Compute the upper confidence bound UB given in (1.16) corresponding to the confidence level $100(1 - \hat{\alpha})\%$. The upper confidence bound so obtained is the bootstrap calibrated MLS upper confidence bound. Conclude scaled average bioequivalence if the bootstrap calibrated MLS upper confidence bound is less than zero.

Appendix D: Program Code

Program Code

```
#-------------------Calibrated TOST-----------------------
# Notation:
# Bootstrap_TOST is a function that returns the estimated alphahat
# n= sample size , s=number of sequences, for example in a 4x4 design,
  s=4
# D is the estimate of the difference of averages, M is the number of
  simulations
# alpha is a grid of alpha values, S_square  is the estimate of the
  variance.
Bootstrap_TOST <- function(alpha,D,n,s,S_square,M,c){
  v <- n-s ; d1  <-  numeric (length(alpha)); Sigma_stra
  <- rchisq(M, v)*  (S_square/v)
  Dstar <-  rnorm(M,0.2231,sqrt(S_square)*c)
  for(j in 1:length(alpha)){
    counter1 <- 0 ; TT1 <- numeric(M)
    for (i in 1:M) {
      TT1[i] <- (abs(Dstar[i]) - 0.2231)/(c*sqrt(Sigma_stra[i]))
      if (TT1[i] < - qt(1-alpha[j],v))
        counter1 <- counter1 +  1
    }
    d1[j] <- abs(counter1/M-0.05)
  }
  T_TOST_Calibrated <- (abs(D) - 0.2231)/(c*sqrt(S_square))
  AlphaHat1 <- alpha[which.min(d1)]
  if ( T_TOST_Calibrated < -  qt(1-0.05,v)) {
    Des1= "TOST Reject H0"} else {
      Des1= "TOST Fail to reject H0 "
    }
  if (T_TOST_Calibrated < -  qt(1-AlphaHat1,v)) {
    Des2 = "TOST^* Reject H0 "} else {
      Des2= "TOST^* Fail to reject H0 "
    }
  return (list(Test_stat= T_TOST_Calibrated, Des1 = Des1, Des2= Des2))
}
#------ To reproduce the result of the example, run the following lines:
--------
n1=6 ; n2=n1 ; n3=n1 ; n4=5 ; D_AUC=-0.0196 ; alpha_0 =
```

(continued)

```
seq(0.05,0.5,0.005)
n = n1+n2+n3+n4 ; s=4 ; c <- sqrt( (1/s^2)*( (1/n1) + (1/n2) +(1/n3) +
(1/n4)  ))
set.seed(1234)
out <- Bootstrap_TOST(n=n, D=D_AUC, S_square=0.059, M=10^3,
alpha=alpha_0, s=s, c=c)
out
set.seed(1234)
out <- Bootstrap_TOST(n=n, D=D_AUC, S_square=0.32, M=10^3, alpha=alpha_0,
s=s, c=c)
out
set.seed(1234)
out <- Bootstrap_TOST(n=n, D=D_AUC, S_square=0.37, M=10^3, alpha=alpha_0,
s=s, c=c)
out
set.seed(1234)
out <- Bootstrap_TOST(n=n, D=D_AUC, S_square=0.41, M=10^3, alpha=alpha_0,
s=s, c=c)
out
set.seed(1234)
out <- Bootstrap_TOST(n=n, D=D_AUC, S_square=0.45, M=10^3, alpha=alpha_0,
s=s, c=c)
out
set.seed(1234)
out <- Bootstrap_TOST(n=n, D=D_AUC, S_square=0.49, M=10^3, alpha=alpha_0,
s=s, c=c)
out
#-------------------MLS Procedure----------------------
# MLS is the function that returns the upper bound.
# Calibrated_MLS is the function that returns the calibrated upper bound.
# Calibration is the function that returns the estimated alphahat
# Notation:
# n=sample size, M=number of simulations, s=number of sequences, D = the
  estimate of
# the difference of averages, sigmaBT=standard deviation of the between
  subject
# variability for the test, sigmaBR=standard deviation of the between
  subject
# variability for the reference, sigmaWT=standard deviation of the within
  subject
# variability for the test , sigmaWR=standard deviation of the within
  subject
# variability for the reference, alpha is a grid of alpha values
# ---- The MLS function ----
MLS <- function(n,sigmaBR,sigmaBT,K,sigmaWT,sigmaWR,rho,alpha,s,D){
  v <- n-s;  cSquare <- 1/n
  sigma11 <- sigmaBT^2 + (0.5 * sigmaWT^2)
  sigma22 <- sigmaBR^2 + (0.5 * sigmaWR^2)
  sigma12 <- rho * sigmaBT * sigmaBR
  sigmaR <- sigmaWR + sigmaWT
  sigma <- sigma11 + sigma22 - (2 * sigma12)
  Ssquare <- sigma11 + sigma22 - (2 * sigma12)
  sigmaWRL <- sqrt(sigmaWR^2 / qchisq(1-alpha,v))
  SigmaHat <- matrix(c(sigma11,sigma12,sigma12,sigma22),nrow=2,ncol=2,
  byrow = TRUE)
  muSquare <- ( abs(D) + qt(1-alpha, n-1) * sqrt( Ssquare*cSquare) )^2
```

(continued)

```
    UB1StarOne <- D^2 - K * ( sigmaWR^2)
    UB1StarTwo <- (muSquare - D^2)^2 + K^2* ((sigmaWRL^2 - sigmaWR^2)^2 )
    UB1Star <- UB1StarOne + sqrt( UB1StarTwo )
    UB2Star <-  muSquare - K * 0.25^2
    if(sigmaWR^2 >= 0.294^2)
    { UBStar <- UB1Star }
    else
    {UBStar <- UB2Star}
    return(list(Upper=UBStar))
  }
  #-------------------The calibration function----------------------
  Calibration <- function(N,n,sigma11,sigma12,sigma22,K,sigmaWR,alpha,s,
  DStarHat){
    v <- n-s;  cSquare <- 1/n
    sigma <- sigma11 + sigma22 - (2 * sigma12)
    SigmaHat <- matrix(c(sigma11,sigma12,sigma12,sigma22),nrow=2,ncol=2,
    byrow = TRUE)
    AStar <- rWishart(N,v,SigmaHat)
    SSwRStar <- (rchisq(N,v)*sigmaWR^2)
    if (sigmaWR^2 >= 0.294^2)
    { D <- sqrt( K * sigmaWR^2) }
    else { D <- sqrt(K * 0.25^2)}
    DStar <- rnorm(N,DStarHat,sqrt(sigma*cSquare))
    distance <- numeric(length (alpha))
    for (i in 1:length(alpha)){
      SSquare <- numeric(N)
      sigma22HatStar <- numeric(N)
      sigmaWRSquareHatStar <- numeric(N)
      muSquareHatStar <- numeric(N)
      sigma22HatStarL <- numeric(N)
      SStartSquare <- numeric(N)
      sigmaWRHatStarL <- numeric(N)
      UB1Star <- numeric(N)
      UB2Star <- numeric(N)
      UBStar <- numeric(N)
      UB1StarOne <- numeric(N)
      UB1StarTwo <- numeric(N)
      for(w in 1:N){
        SStartSquare[w] <- (AStar[1,1,w] + AStar[2,2,w] -
        ( 2 * AStar[1,2,w])) / v
        sigma22HatStar[w] <- AStar[2,2,w] / v
        sigmaWRSquareHatStar[w] <-  SSwRStar[w] / v
        muSquareHatStar[w] <- ( abs(DStar[w]) + qt(1-alpha[i], n-1) *
        sqrt(SStartSquare[w] *cSquare) )^2
        sigma22HatStarL[w] <- AStar[2,2,w] / qchisq(1-alpha[i],v)
        sigmaWRHatStarL[w] <- SSwRStar[w] / qchisq(1-alpha[i],v)
        UB1StarOne[w] <- DStar[w]^2 - K * (sigmaWRSquareHatStar[w])
        UB1StarTwo[w] <- (muSquareHatStar[w] - DStar[w]^2)^2 + K^2*
        ( (sigmaWRHatStarL[w] - sigmaWRSquareHatStar[w])^2 )
        UB1Star[w] <- UB1StarOne[w] + sqrt( UB1StarTwo[w] )
        UB2Star[w] <-  muSquareHatStar[w] - K * 0.25^2
        if(SSwRStar[w] >= 0.294^2)
        { UBStar[w] <- UB1Star[w] }
        else
        {UBStar[w] <- UB2Star[w]}
      }
```

(continued)

```
    distance[i] <- abs(mean(UBStar < 0) - 0.05)
  }
  return(alpha[which.min(distance)])
}
#-------------------The calibrated MLS function-----------------------
Calibrated_MLS <- function(N,n,sigmaBR,sigmaBT,K,sigmaWT,sigmaWR,rho,
alpha,s){
  v <- n-s; cSquare <- 1/n
  sigma11 <- sigmaBT^2 + (0.5 * sigmaWT^2)
  sigma22 <- sigmaBR^2 + (0.5 * sigmaWR^2)
  sigma12 <- rho * sigmaBT * sigmaBR
  sigmaR <- sigmaWR + sigmaWT
  sigma <- sigma11 + sigma22 - (2 * sigma12)
  Ssquare <- sigma11 + sigma22 - (2 * sigma12)
  SigmaHat <- matrix(c(sigma11,sigma12,sigma12,sigma22),nrow=2,ncol=2,
  byrow = TRUE)
  alphahat <- Calibration(N=N,n=n,sigma11=sigma11,sigma12=sigma12,
  sigma22=sigma22,K=K,
                         sigmaWR=sigmaWR,alpha=alpha,s=s,DStarHat=D)
  sigmaWRL <- sqrt(sigmaWR^2 / qchisq(1-alphahat,v))
  muSquare <- ( abs(D) + qt(1-alphahat, n-1) * sqrt( Ssquare*cSquare) )^2
  UB1StarOne <- D^2 - K * (sigmaWR^2)
  UB1StarTwo <- (muSquare - D^2)^2 + K^2* ((sigmaWRL^2 - sigmaWR^2)^2 )
  UB1Star <- UB1StarOne + sqrt( UB1StarTwo )
  UB2Star <-  muSquare - K * 0.25^2
  if(sigmaWR^2 >= 0.294^2)
  { UBStar <- UB1Star }
  else
  {UBStar <- UB2Star}
  return(list(Upper=UBStar,alphahat=alphahat))
}
n1=6 ; n2=6 ; n3=6 ; n4=5 ; M=10^3 ;s=4 ; D =- 0.0196 ; K= 0.79669
rho=0.8 ; alpha=0.05 ; S_square=0.059 ; n = n1+n2+n3+n4
sigmaWT=sqrt(0.1271) ; sigmaBT = sqrt(0.20785)
sigmaWR=sqrt(0.07450) ; sigmaBR = sqrt(0.27908)
out <- MLS(n,sigmaBR,sigmaBT,K,sigmaWT,sigmaWR,rho,alpha,s,D)
if (out$Upper < 0){
  print( "MLS procedure reject H0")} else  {
    print("MLS procedure fail to reject H0")
  }
out
sigmaBR = sqrt(0.54008)
out <- MLS(n,sigmaBR,sigmaBT,K,sigmaWT,sigmaWR,rho,alpha,s,D)
if (out$Upper < 0){
  print( "MLS procedure reject H0")} else  {
    print("MLS procedure fail to reject H0")
  }
out
```

Appendix E: Index

Highly variable drugs, modified large sample (MLS) procedure, multivariate bioequivalence, two one-sided t-test (TOST).

References

Berger, R. L., & Hsu, J. C. (1996). Bioequivalence trials, intersection-union tests and equivalence confidence sets. *Statistical Science, 11*, 283–319.

Brown, L. D., Huang, J. T., & Munk, A. (1997). An unbiased test for the bioequivalence problem. *The Annal of Statistics, 25*, 2345–2367.

Burdick, R. K., & Graybill, F. A. (1992). *Confidence intervals on variance components*. Dekker.

Cao, L., & Mathew, T. (2008). A simple numerical approach towards improving the two one-sided test for average bioequivalence. *Biometrical Journal, 50*, 205–211.

Chow, S.-C, & Liu, J.-P. (2009). *Design and analysis of bioavailability and bioequivalence studies* (3ird ed.). Chapman and Hall/CRC.

Chinchilli, V. M., & Esinhart, J. D. (1996). Design and analysis of intra-subject variability in cross-over experiments. *Statistics in Medicine, 15*, 1619–1634.

Davit, B. M., et al. (2012). Implementation of a reference-scaled average bioequivalence approach for highly variable generic drug products by the US Food and Drug Administration. *The AAPS Journal, 14*, 915–924.

Deng, Y., & Zhou, X.-H. (2020). Methods to control the empirical type I error rate in average bioequivalence tests for highly variable drugs. *Statistical Methods in Medical Research, 29*, 1650–1667.

Dong, X., & Tsong, Y. (2014a). Equivalence assessment for interchangeability based on two-sided tests. *Journal of Biopharmaceutical Statistics, 24*, 1312–1331.

Dong, X., Tsong, Y., & Shen, M. (2014b). Equivalence tests for interchangeability based on two one-sided probabilities. *Journal of Biopharmaceutical Statistics, 24*, 1332–48.

Efron, B., & Tibshirani, R. J. (1993). *An introduction to the bootstrap*. Chapman & Hall.

Graybill, A. F., & Wang, C. M. (1980). Confidence intervals on nonnegative linear combinations of variances. *Journal of the American Statistical Association, 75*, 869–873.

Hauschke, D., Steinijans, V., & Pigeot, I. (2007). *Bioequivalence studies in drug development: Methods and applications*. Wiley.

Hsu, J. C., Hwang, J. T., Liu, H., & Ruberg, S. J. (1994). Confidence intervals associated with tests for bioequivalence. *Biometrika, 91*, 103–114.

Kang, Q., & Vahl, C. I. (2017). Testing for bioequivalence of highly variable drugs from TR-RT crossover designs with heterogeneous residual variances. *Pharmaceutical Statistics, 16*, 361–377.

Krishnamoorthy, K., & Mathew, T. (2009). *Statistical tolerance regions: Theory, applications, and computation*. Wiley.

Maurer, W., Jones, B., & Chen, Y. (2018). Controlling the type I error rate in two-stage sequential adaptive designs when testing for average bioequivalence. *Statistics in Medicine, 37*, 1587–1607.

McNally, R. J., Iyer, H., & Mathew, T. (2003). Tests for individual and population bioequivalence based on generalized p-values. *Statistics in Medicine, 22*, 31–53.

Molins, E., Labes, D., Schütz, H., Cobo, E., & Ocaña, J. (2021). An iterative method to protect the type I error rate in bioequivalence studies under two-stage adaptive 2×2 crossover designs. *Biometrical Journal, 63*, 122–133.

Munk, A. (1993). An improvement on commonly used tests in bioequivalence Assessment. *Biometrics, 49*, 1225–1230.

Munk, A. (1999). A note on unbiased testing for the equivalence problem - another Christmas tree. *Statistics and Probability Letters, 41*, 401–406.

Munk, A. (2000). An unbiased test for the average equivalence problem - the small sample case. *Journal of Statistical Planning and Inference, 87*, 69–86.

Munk, A., Brown, L. D., & Hwang, J. T. G. (2000). The bioequivalence problem - finding a compromise between theory and practice. *Biometrical Journal, 42*, 531–552.

Patterson, S. D., & Jones, B. (2012). Viewpoint: observations on scaled average bioequivalence. *Pharmaceutical Statistics, 11*, 1–7.

Patterson, S. D., & Jones, B. (2017). *Bioequivalence and statistics in clinical pharmacology* (2nd ed.). Chapman and Hall/CRC.

Tothfalusi, L., & Endrenyi, L. (2012). Sample sizes for designing bioequivalence studies for highly variable drugs. *Journal of Pharmaceutical Sciences, 15*, 73–84.

Tothfalusi, L., & Endrenyi, L. (2017). Algorithms for evaluating reference scaled average bioequivalence: Power, bias, and consumer risk. *Statistics in Medicine, 36*, 4378–4390.

Tothfalusi, L., Endrenyi, L., & Arieta, A. G. (2009). Evaluation of bioequivalence for highly variable drugs with scaled average bioequivalence. *Clinical Pharmacokinetics, 48*, 725–743.

Tothfalusi, L., Endrenyi, L., Midha, K., Rawson, M., & Hubbard, J. (2001). Evaluation of the bioequivalence of highly-variable drugs and drug products. *Pharmaceutical Research, 18*, 728–733.

Tsong, Y., & Shen, M. (2007). An alternative approach to assess exchangeability of a test treatment and the standard treatment with normally distributed response. *Journal of Biopharmaceutical Statistics, 17*, 329–338.

U.S. Food and Drug Administration (2001). Center for Drug Evaluation and Research. Guidance for Industry: Statistical Approaches to Establishing Bioequivalence. Available at: http://www.fda.gov/downloads/Drugs/Guidances/ucm070244.pdf

U.S. Food and Drug Administration (2022). Center for Drug Evaluation and Research. Guidance for Industry: Statistical Approaches to Establishing Bioequivalence. Available at: https://www.fda.gov/media/163638/download

Wang, W., Hwang, J. T. G., & Dasgupta, A. (1999). Statistical tests for multivariate bioequivalence. *Biometrika, 86*, 395–402.

Chapter 2
Hypothesis Testing Within Bayesian Inference

Isabel Natário

2.1 Introduction

Hypothesis tests are quite entangled with the practice of statistics, especially in the applied areas that depend on statistics to take conclusions on their studies. Despite this, in fact, statistical tests differ a lot between frequentist and Bayesian approaches and, even within the Bayesians, this is an area of a great controversy and few agreements (Robert, 2022). The generalized use of hypothesis tests, having become completely essential in applied works, is then sometimes a problem, and the change in paradigm often stumbles in the particular differences between approaches.

Several research studies argue about the advantage of the Bayesian hypothesis tests over the frequentist ones, the latter considering in their construction data that have not been observed (Tendeiro & Kiers, 2019) and the frequent (bad) use of the p-value measure (Wasserstein & Lazar, 2016). The Bayesian hypothesis tests consist of the choice of the hypothesis that better fits data and not of the choice of the true hypothesis. This fit is usually based both on marginal likelihoods and also on posterior probabilities that the parameters lie in certain intervals, as these distributions are naturally conditioned on each of the different hypotheses. The problem with the approach based on marginal likelihoods is that they tend to be influenced by the prior model, which the likelihood may take time to compensate (Robert, 2022).

The previous problem has led to the development of Bayes factor (Jeffreys, 1935; Kass & Raftery, 1995), a Bayesian tool for hypothesis testing that compares marginal likelihoods between the different hypotheses instead of posterior prob-

I. Natário (✉)
Department of Mathematics of NOVA School of Sciences and Technology & NOVA MATH, Caparica, Portugal
e-mail: icn@fct.unl.pt

D.-G. Chen, C. A. Coelho (eds.), *Biostatistics Modeling and Public Health Applications*, Emerging Topics in Statistics and Biostatistics,
https://doi.org/10.1007/978-3-031-69690-9_2

abilities, dependent on the prior model. However, there is not an agreement on which the best approach is, being the Bayes factor criticized for missing a direct connection with the posterior and of not being able to offer an easy interpretation of the support's strength to a certain hypothesis by means of its magnitude. Some authors suggest the use of both approaches (Berger, 2008, 2011).

It is today undeniable that there has been a considerable increase of hypothesis testing within Bayesian applications, using the Bayes factor (Tendeiro & Kiers, 2019). Bayes factor allows to quantify evidence in favour of the null hypothesis, and it can be updated in face of more data and does not require hypotheses to match nested models, among others (Kass & Raftery, 1995). However, there are some times theoretical and practical difficulties in its calculation, due to improper priors, vague priors (with a tendency to favour the null hypothesis) and the assessment of the marginal likelihoods that might be difficult to compute (Li et al., 2014).

In this work the Bayes factor is described and its practical implementation in two specific situations considered (Sect. 2.2): t-tests for mean equality in normal populations and Spearman correlation tests. Through these examples we expect to illustrate the strengths and weaknesses of Bayes factors for hypothesis testing, from which stands out providing evidence in favour of the null hypothesis just based on data (Wei et al., 2022) and the difficulty in having a unified framework for testing procedures and computations. Results are presented in Sect. 2.3 and discussed in Sect. 2.4.

2.2 Bayes Factor

According to the influential work of Kass and Raftery in 1995 (Kass & Raftery, 1995), the Bayesian approach to statistical tests was introduced by Jeffreys in 1935, committed to compare prediction between models corresponding to different hypothesis. The Bayesian methodology provides evidences in favour of the null hypothesis based on data, prior information and model's uncertainties through the use of the Bayes factor.

Kass and Raftery's excellent work laid the first grounds on the use of the Bayes factor for testing, both conceptually and computationally. Assuming that data x appeared under one of the two hypothesis H_0 and H_1, according to a probability distribution $P(x|H_0)$ or $P(x|H_1)$, and assuming prior probabilities for each hypothesis, $P(H_0)$ and $P(H_1) = 1 - P(H_1)$, the posterior probabilities, updating the prior information with the data, are obtained as

$$P(H_0|x) = \frac{P(x|H_0)P(H_0)}{P(x)} \quad \text{and} \quad P(H_1|x) = \frac{P(x|H_1)P(H_1)}{P(x)}.$$

These can be converted into odds:

$$\frac{P(H_0|x)}{P(H_1|x)} = \frac{P(x|H_0)}{P(x|H_1)}\frac{P(H_0)}{P(H_1)} \quad \Leftrightarrow \quad \frac{P(H_0|x)}{P(H_1|x)} = B_{01}\frac{P(H_0)}{P(H_1)}.$$

The quantity B_{01} is the Bayes factor in favour of hypothesis H_0, transforming prior odds into posterior odds by product. It is also the ratio between the posterior odds of H_0 and its prior odds:

$$B_{01} = \frac{\frac{P(H_0|x)}{P(H_1|x)}}{\frac{P(H_0)}{P(H_1)}}.$$

Notice the symmetry of the Bayes factor that might be considered in favour of the hypothesis H_1:

$$B_{10} = \frac{\frac{P(H_1|x)}{P(H_0|x)}}{\frac{P(H_1)}{P(H_0)}}.$$

If both hypotheses have the same prior probability, the Bayes factor is just the posterior odds in favour of H_0.

Note that the Bayes factor is the ratio of probabilities of data conditional on hypotheses and not probabilities of the hypotheses being correct (Tendeiro & Kiers, 2019). So, conclusions have to be on whether data are more or less plausible of being observed under each hypothesis.

Kass and Raftery suggest a classification of very strong evidence against H_0 if $B_{10} > 150$, strong evidence against H_0 if $20 < B_{10} < 150$, positive evidence against H_0 if $3 < B_{10} < 20$ and not worth more than a bare mention evidence against H_0 if $1 < B_{10} < 3$.

2.3 Bayes Factor in Examples

This section describes two quite different examples that allow us to perceive the complexity of the methodological and practical approach behind a Bayesian hypothesis test based on the Bayes factor.

2.3.1 Bayesian t-Test for Comparing the Means of Two Normal Populations

Rouder et al. (2009) developed a Bayes factor alternative to a t-test, favouring one hypothesis over the other, only based on data. In the present work, this is used to compare the means of two paired normal populations, testing

$$H_0 : \mu = 0 \ \ vs \ \ H_1 : \mu \neq 0,$$

where μ is the difference mean. Following the authors, consider $y_1, \ldots, y_n$ to be the observed differences Y between the paired populations, assumed to follow a normal distribution parameterized by the standardized effect size $\delta = \frac{\mu}{\sigma}$, where σ^2 is the corresponding variance

$$Y \sim \text{Normal}(\sigma\delta, \sigma^2).$$

The null hypothesis is then

$$H_0 : \delta = 0 \ \ vs \ \ H_1 : \delta \neq 0.$$

This parameterization allows an intrinsic scale about the ranges that may help to set the prior, although if the prior is too variable, the marginal likelihood in the Bayes factor will be lowered, which tends to favour the null hypothesis (Rouder et al., 2009). A large discussion on this provided by the authors suggests the use of a standard Cauchy prior distribution for δ. The authors further add that it is possible to tune the scale of the prior on the effect size, incorporating the goals of specific experimental contexts, using a scale factor r:

$$\delta \sim r \times \text{Standard-Cauchy}.$$

We take r to be $\sqrt{2}$ (medium scale), 1 (standard Cauchy, wide scale) and $\frac{\sqrt{2}}{2}$ (ultrawide scale) in the example presented here, Morey et al. (2011). For comparison purposes, it is further considered a Normal(0,0.001) prior distribution for δ. A noninformative Jeffreys prior is placed on the variance of the normal population

$$\left(\sigma^2\right)^{-1} \sim \text{Gamma}(0.0001, 0.0001).$$

Within this setting, Gibbs sampler is used, through JAGS software (Plummer, 2003), to obtain the posterior distribution of δ and obtaining the Bayes factors. See the Appendix for code.

This test was performed to simulated data, comparing paired populations with the same mean and different standard deviations (Case 1), with different means and same standard deviations (Case 2) and with different means and different standard deviations (Case 3). Normal distributions were considered for the populations, with means taken to be more far apart or closer, and standard deviations considered as small or moderate, see Table 2.1. Additionally, data were also generated from a gamma distribution, to be compared with normal simulated data, standing for 'imperfect data', having the same mean and standard deviation, Fig. 2.1.

Three sized samples were considered, corresponding to $n = 20$, $n = 50$ or $n = 100$. The Bayes factors B_{10} (comparing H_1 to H_0) for the tests corresponding to the situations described in the first row of Table 2.1 are depicted in Table 2.2, for

Table 2.1 Population distributions used for simulating data

Compares (Dist 1)	Case 1 (Dist 2)	Case 2 (Dist 2)	Case 3 (Dist 2)
Normal(10, 2^2)	Normal(10, 4^2)	Normal(16, 3.2^2)	Normal(16, 6.4^2)
Normal(10, 2^2)	Normal(10, 8^2)	Normal(12, 2.4^2)	Normal(12, 9.6^2)
Normal(10, 2^2)	Gamma(6.25,1.6)[a]	Gamma(25,0.64)[b]	Gamma(6.25,2.56)[c]

[a]($\mu = 10, \sigma = 4$); [b]($\mu = 16, \sigma = 3.2$); [c]($\mu = 16, \sigma = 6.4$)

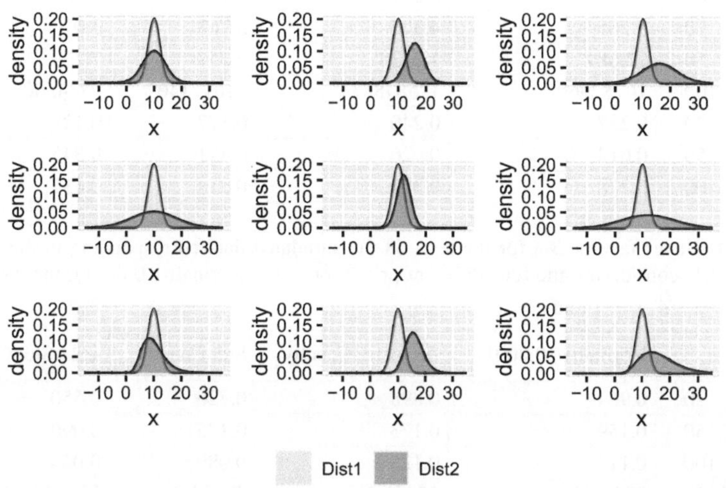

Fig. 2.1 Distributions used to simulate data. Dist 1 identifies the Normal(10, 2^2) distribution chosen as the first population and Dist 2 the distribution for the second population according to Table 2.1

Table 2.2 Bayes factors B_{10} for the tests on the simulated data corresponding to the first line of Table 2.1, considering the four different priors for δ, the Normal(0, 0.0001), the $r\times$Standard Cauchy, $r = \frac{\sqrt{2}}{2}$, $r = 1$ and $r = \sqrt{2}$

Case	n	Normal(0, 0.0001)	$\frac{\sqrt{2}}{2}\times$Std. Cauchy	Std. Cauchy	$\sqrt{2}\times$Std. Cauchy
1	20	0.253	0.266	0.197	0.143
1	50	0.207	0.223	0.162	0.117
1	100	0.263	0.286	0.207	0.149
2	20	25635.7	18132.9	21332.3	22881.3
2	50	6.064e+10	3.853e+10	4.483e+10	4.708e+10
2	100	1.808e+27	1.260e+27	1.535e+27	1.706e+27
3	20	23.880	17.744	16.664	14.359
3	50	1312634	859406.8	883374.5	814217.9
3	100	5.206e+9	3.610e+9	3.517e+09	3.082e+9

each of the four different priors considered for δ, Normal(0, 0.0001), $\frac{\sqrt{2}}{2}\times$ Standard Cauchy, Standard Cauchy and $\sqrt{2}\times$ Standard Cauchy. From here we can see that,

Table 2.3 Bayes factors B_{10} for the tests on the simulated data corresponding to the second line of Table 2.1, considering the four different priors for δ, the Normal(0, 0.0001), the $r\times$Standard Cauchy, $r = \frac{\sqrt{2}}{2}$, $r = 1$ and $r = \sqrt{2}$

Case	n	Normal(0, 0.0001)	$\frac{\sqrt{2}}{2}\times$Std. Cauchy	Std. Cauchy	$\sqrt{2}\times$Std. Cauchy
1	20	0.240	0.254	0.187	0.136
1	50	0.238	0.255	0.186	0.134
1	100	0.229	0.249	0.180	0.129
2	20	5.265	4.302	3.763	3.070
2	50	12.689	11.438	9.357	7.224
2	100	16782960	12584883	11617146	9734560
3	20	0.227	0.240	0.177	0.128
3	50	0.612	0.626	0.471	0.345
3	100	0.278	0.301	0.218	0.157

Table 2.4 Bayes factors B_{10} for the tests on the simulated data corresponding to the third line of Table 2.1, considering the four different priors for δ, the Normal(0, 0.0001), the $r\times$Standard Cauchy, $r = \frac{\sqrt{2}}{2}$, $r = 1$ and $r = \sqrt{2}$

Case	n	Normal(0, 0.0001)	$\frac{\sqrt{2}}{2}\times$Std. Cauchy	Std. Cauchy	$\sqrt{2}\times$Std. Cauchy
1	20	0.964	0.898	0.720	0.550
1	50	0.159	0.173	0.125	0.090
1	100	0.113	0.125	0.089	0.064
2	20	35451.0	25421.2	30152.7	32624.1
2	50	7.006e+11	4.621e+11	5.487e+11	5.911e+11
2	100	5.775e+22	3.618e+22	4.243e+22	4.490e+22
3	20	147.282	101.012	102.195	93.787
3	50	20716.5	14742.1	14152.9	12290.4
3	100	3.595e+10	2.437e+10	2.415e+10	2.147e+10

independently of the sample size, the hypothesis favoured is always the one that was expected (H_0 for Case 1 and H_1 for Cases 2 and 3).

The Bayes factors B_{10} for the tests corresponding to the situations described in the second row of Table 2.1 are depicted in Table 2.3, for each of the four different priors for δ. From here we can see that for Case 1 the null hypothesis H_0 is always favoured as expected, independently of the sample size. For case 2, the alternative hypothesis H_1 is favoured, more expressively for larger sample sizes and for smaller scales r. For Case 3, independently of the sample size, the hypothesis favoured is always the null hypothesis H_0, unlike the expected.

The Bayes factors B_{10} for the tests corresponding to the situations described in the last row of Table 2.1 are depicted in Table 2.4, for each of the four different priors for δ. Also here, independently of the sample size, the hypothesis favoured is always the expected one (H_0 for Case 1 and H_1 for Cases 2 and 3). To sum up, nearer mean values of populations or increasing variability of one of the populations hinders the good performance of the Bayes factor. In this example, the MCMC simulations of the needed posterior distributions could be obtained through the JAGS software, fed afterward in the R package `bridgesampling`, (Gronau et al., 2020), to obtain marginal likelihoods, which enabled the calculations of the Bayes factor.

2.3.2 Bayesian Spearman's Rank Test

Following van Doorn et al. (2020), a rank-based hypothesis testing for the Spearman's coefficient of correlation ρ_S, relying on the Bayes factor to favour one hypothesis over the other (Spearman's correlation test), is used here to evaluate correlation on simulated data. The authors base their approach on latent normal models, allowing transforming ordinal into parametric problems. Let $x = (x_1, \ldots, x_n)$ and $y = (y_1, \ldots, Y_n)$ be data measurements on the same items, and let $r^x = (r_1^x, \ldots, r_n^x)$ and $r^y = (r_1^y, \ldots, r_n^y)$ denote their corresponding ranks values. Spearman's correlation ρ is given by

$$\rho_S = \frac{\mathrm{Cov}(r^x, r^y)}{\sigma_{r^x}\sigma_{r^x}}.$$

Associated with the ranks r^x and r^y are considered unobserved latent normal scores z^x and z^y, respectively, dependent on parameter ρ_S. The observed ranks are related to these scores in such a way that the ordinal information is preserved, through the data model

$$f(r^x, r^y | z^x, z^y).$$

The prior model is given by

$$\pi(z^x, z^y | \rho_S) \times \pi(\rho_S),$$

representing $\pi(z^x, z^y | \rho_S)$ the latent prior structure, taken to be a centred bivariate normal density with unit variances and correlation ρ_S. The prior distribution for ρ_S is taken to be a uniform distribution.

Using the MCMC sampler developed by the authors van Doorn et al. (2020), it is possible to obtain the scores and Spearman's correlation posterior distribution, from which the Bayes factor for the test

$$H_0 : \rho_S = 0 \;\; vs \;\; H_1 : \rho_S \neq 0$$

is obtained (also programmed by the authors), see the Appendix for code.

This test is here applied to data sets of sizes $n = 10$, $n = 25$ and $n = 50$, simulated from:

1. Case 1 (negative correlation on normal models, $\rho = -0.6$): a bivariate normal distribution with mean vector and covariance matrix given, respectively, by

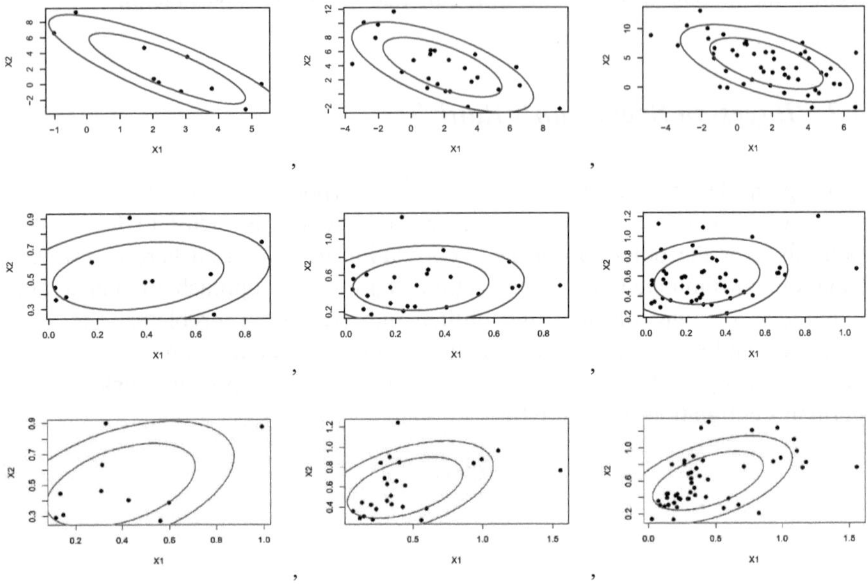

Fig. 2.2 Simulated data for Spearman's correlation test. Line 1 corresponds to Case 1 (negative correlation on normal models, $\rho = -0.6$), Line 2 corresponds to Case 2 (independence on gamma models, $\rho = 0$) and Line 3 corresponds to Case 3 (positive correlation on gamma copula model, $\rho = 0.6$). Within each line, from left to right the sample size varies from $n = 10$, $n = 25$ and $n = 50$

$$\mu = \begin{bmatrix} 2 \\ 4 \end{bmatrix} \qquad \Sigma = \begin{bmatrix} 9 & -10.8 \\ -10.8 & 16 \end{bmatrix}.$$

2. Case 2 (independence on gamma models, $\rho = 0$): Independent Gamma(2,4) and Gamma(4,7) distributions are considered and data paired.
3. Case 3 (positive correlation on gamma copula model, $\rho = 0.6$): a bivariate gamma copula model with shape vector $(2, 4)^T$, rate vector $(5, 7)^T$ and correlation $\rho = 0.6$.

The simulated data can be seen in Fig. 2.2.

In Table 2.5 the results of Bayesian Spearman's correlation test are presented. The Bayes factor B_{10}, comparing H_1 to H_0, and the estimate of the correlation coefficient (posterior mean, $\hat{\rho}_S$) are depicted for each one of the simulated data set described before.

These results show that the test did well for the bivariate normal distribution, independent of the sample size, as well as for the independent gamma distributed data. However, for the Gamma copula data, for the smallest sample size ($n = 10$), the test did not work out, and the correlation was not correctly estimated. This situation improved with the increase of the sample size, although the correlation

Table 2.5 Estimated correlation coefficient and Bayes factors B_{10} for the tests on the simulated data depicted in Fig. 2.2, corresponding to different sample sizes of three different cases: Case 1 (negative correlation on normal models, $\rho = -0.6$), Case 2 (independence on gamma models, $\rho = 0$) and Case 3 (positive correlation on gamma copula model, $\rho = 0.6$)

Case	n	B_{01}	$\hat{\rho}_S$
1	10	12.737	−0.695
1	25	98.746	−0.561
1	50	5233.531	−0.569
2	10	0.433	0.183
2	25	0.270	0.110
2	50	0.486	0.199
3	10	0.448	0.178
3	25	4.048	0.411
3	50	185.898	0.501

estimate is not perfect. This test, even for the not so large sample sizes, takes some minutes to run.

2.4 Discussion

The classical approach for hypothesis testing has been recently quite criticized, much because conclusions rely on non-observed data and of the sampling methods used. Bayes factor is the Bayesian approach to hypothesis testing, which provides evidence in favour of the null hypothesis, based on data, existing prior information and accounting for uncertainty in the choice of models (Kass & Raftery, 1995). It is possible to use Bayes factor for any statistical test we might think of. However it is not without pain. Computationally, it might be much harder and time consuming to implement. It might also be affected by small sample sizes, especially if model chosen is not adequate to data. Prior distributions must be chosen, and it is not an automatic procedure. More, if the priors are too vague, the null hypothesis might be favoured by the Bayes factor (Lindley paradox). Bayes factors might be difficult to interpret if they are not too large or too small and also because they are not posterior model probabilities (Tendeiro & Kiers, 2019). Even within the Bayesians it is not a consensus that it is a good idea to test, although the applied areas are very much into test, as a way to have objective results. The main issue is that the Bayes factor cannot be used as a simple tool, needing adaptation and programming in different situations, a big disadvantage to no proficiency users. This is very clear in the two examples presented in this chapter. And this is a challenge to be solved, generalize the use of the Bayes factor for the most common statistical situations, and include these in a common testing framework.

Acknowledgments This work is funded by national funds through the FCT—Fundação para a Ciência e a Tecnologia, I.P., under the scope of the projects: UIDB/00297/2020 (https://doi.org/10.54499/UIDB/00297/2020) and UIDP/00297/2020 (https://doi.org/10.54499/UIDP/00297/2020) (Center for Mathematics and Applications).

Appendix

Code for Bayesian t-test example (the same distribution). (Adapted from Wei et al., 2022).

```
library(bridgesampling)
library(R2jags)

#T-test

RES<-NULL

for (n in c(20,50,100)){  #For different n

  #Simulate data

  set.seed(123)

  #Same distribution, same mean, different sd
  y1<- rnorm(n,10,2)
  y2<- rnorm(n,10,8)

  #Same distribution, different mean, same sd
  y3<- rnorm(n,12,2.4)

  #Same distribution, different mean, different sd
  y4<- rnorm(n,12,9.6)


  # compute difference scores
  d<-matrix(NA,ncol=3,nrow=length(y1))
  d[,1] <- y1 - y2
  d[,2] <- y1 - y3
  d[,3] <- y1 - y4
  n <- dim(d)[1]

  #-----------------------------------------------------------------------
  # JAGS models
  #-----------------------------------------------------------------------

  code_H1 <-
  ''model {
  delta ~ dnorm(0,0.001)            # prior
  inv_sigma2 ~ dgamma(0.0001, 0.0001) # prior
  sigma <- 1 / sqrt(inv_sigma2)       # convert precision to sigma
  for (i in 1:n) {
     d[i] ~ dnorm(sigma * delta, inv_sigma2) # likelihood
  }
  }''

  code_H1.star <-
```

```
  ''model {
delta ~ dt(0, 1 / r ^ 2, 1)          # prior (mu=0, scale=r^2, df=1)
inv_sigma2 ~ dgamma(0.0001, 0.0001) # prior
sigma <- 1 / sqrt(inv_sigma2)        # convert precision to sigma
for (i in 1:n) {
   d[i] ~ dnorm(sigma * delta, inv_sigma2) # likelihood
}
}''

code_H0 <-
  ''model {
inv_sigma2 ~ dgamma(0.0001, 0.0001) # prior
for (i in 1:n) {
   d[i] ~ dnorm(0, inv_sigma2)       # likelihood
}
}''
#-----------------------------------------------------------------------
# fit models
#-----------------------------------------------------------------------

set.seed(1)

for (case in 1:3){
  jags_H1 <- jags(data = list(d = d[,case], n = n),
              parameters.to.save = c(''delta'', ''inv_sigma2''),
              model.file = textConnection(code_H1), n.chains = 3,
              n.iter = 16000, n.burnin = 1000, n.thin = 1)

  #For the rscale argument, several named values are recognized:
  ''medium'', ''wide'',
  #and ''ultrawide''. These correspond to r scale values of sqrt(2)/2, 1
  and sqrt(1)
  #respectively.

  jags_H1.star<-list(NULL)

  jags_H1.star[[1]] <- jags(data = list(d = d[,case], n = n,
                r = 1 /  sqrt(2)),
                parameters.to.save = c(''delta'',
                ''inv_sigma2''),
                model.file = textConnection(code_H1.star),
                n.chains = 3,
                n.iter = 16000, n.burnin = 1000, n.thin = 1)

  jags_H1.star[[2]] <- jags(data = list(d = d[,case], n = n, r = 1 ),
                         parameters.to.save = c(''delta'',
                         ''inv_sigma2''),
                         model.file = textConnection(code_H1.star),
                         n.chains = 3,
                         n.iter = 16000, n.burnin = 1000, n.thin = 1)

  jags_H1.star[[3]] <- jags(data = list(d = d[,case], n = n, r = sqrt(2)),
                         parameters.to.save = c(''delta'',
                         ''inv_sigma2''),
                         model.file = textConnection(code_H1.star),
                         n.chains = 3,
                         n.iter = 16000, n.burnin = 1000, n.thin = 1)

  jags_H0 <- jags(data = list(d = d[,case], n = n),
                parameters.to.save = ''inv_sigma2'',
```

```
model.file = textConnection(code_H0), n.chains = 3,
             n.iter = 16000, n.burnin = 1000, n.thin = 1)

#---------------------------------------------------------------------------
# specify unnormalized log posterior functions
#---------------------------------------------------------------------------

log_posterior_H1 <- function(pars, data) {

  delta <- pars[''delta'']           # extract parameter
  inv_sigma2 <- pars[''inv_sigma2''] # extract parameter
  sigma <- 1 / sqrt(inv_sigma2)    # convert precision to sigma

  out <-
    dnorm(delta, 0.001, log = TRUE) +         # prior
    dgamma(inv_sigma2, 0.0001, 0.0001, log = TRUE) +     # prior
    sum(dnorm(data$d, sigma * delta, sigma, log = TRUE)) # likelihood

  return(out)

}

log_posterior_H1.star <- function(pars, data) {

  delta <- pars[''delta'']           # extract parameter
  inv_sigma2 <- pars[''inv_sigma2''] # extract parameter
  sigma <- 1 / sqrt(inv_sigma2)    # convert precision to sigma

  out <-
    dcauchy(delta, scale = data$r, log = TRUE) +         # prior
    dgamma(inv_sigma2, 0.0001, 0.0001, log = TRUE) +     # prior
    sum(dnorm(data$d, sigma * delta, sigma, log = TRUE)) # likelihood

  return(out)

}

log_posterior_H0 <- function(pars, data) {

  inv_sigma2 <- pars[''inv_sigma2''] # extract parameter
  sigma <- 1 / sqrt(inv_sigma2)    # convert precision to sigma

  out <-
    dgamma(inv_sigma2, 0.0001, 0.0001, log = TRUE) + # prior
    sum(dnorm(data$d, 0, sigma, log = TRUE))         # likelihood

  return(out)

}

#---------------------------------------------------------------------------
# specify lower and upper bounds for the parameters
#---------------------------------------------------------------------------

lb_H1 <- rep(-Inf, 2)
ub_H1 <- rep(Inf, 2)
names(lb_H1) <- names(ub_H1) <- c(''delta'', ''inv_sigma2'')
lb_H1[[''inv_sigma2'']] <- 0

lb_H0 <- 0
ub_H0 <- Inf
```

```
      names(lb_H0) <- names(ub_H0) <- "inv_sigma2"

      #-----------------------------------------------------------------------
      # compute log marginal likelihoods
      #-----------------------------------------------------------------------

      set.seed(12345)

      bridge_H1 <- bridge_sampler(samples = jags_H1,
                                  log_posterior = log_posterior_H1,
                                  data = list(d = d[,case], n = n),
                                  lb = lb_H1, ub = ub_H1)
      bridge_H1.star<-list(NULL)

      bridge_H1.star[[1]] <- bridge_sampler(samples = jags_H1.star[[1]],
                                  log_posterior = log_posterior_H1.star,
                                  data = list(d = d[,case], n = n,
                                  r = 1 / sqrt(2)),
                                  lb = lb_H1, ub = ub_H1)
      bridge_H1.star[[2]] <- bridge_sampler(samples = jags_H1.star[[2]],
                                  log_posterior = log_posterior_H1.star,
                                  data = list(d = d[,case], n = n, r = 1),
                                  lb = lb_H1, ub = ub_H1)

      bridge_H1.star[[3]] <- bridge_sampler(samples = jags_H1.star[[3]],
                                  log_posterior = log_posterior_H1.star,
                                  data = list(d = d[,case], n = n,
                                  r = sqrt(2)),
                                  lb = lb_H1, ub = ub_H1)

      bridge_H0 <- bridge_sampler(samples = jags_H0,
                              log_posterior = log_posterior_H0,
                              data = list(d = d[,case], n = n),
                              lb = lb_H0, ub = ub_H0)

      #-----------------------------------------------------------------------
      # compute Bayes factor
      #-----------------------------------------------------------------------

      B01.1<-bf(bridge_H1, bridge_H0)
      B01.2<-bf(bridge_H1.star[[1]], bridge_H0)
      B01.3<-bf(bridge_H1.star[[2]], bridge_H0)
      B01.4<-bf(bridge_H1.star[[3]], bridge_H0)

      RES<-rbind(RES,c(n,case,B01.1[1],B01.2[1],B01.3[1],B01.4[1]))
    }
  }

  RES2<-data.frame(RES)
  names(RES2)<-c(''n'',''case'',''B01.1'',''B01.2'',''B01.3'',''B01.4'')
  RES2
```

Code for Bayesian Spearman's correlation test example (Normal distributions). (Adapted from van Doorn et al., 2020).

```
library(mixtools)  #for ellipse

###Gaussian

N <- 50 # Number of random samples
```

```
set.seed(123)
# Target parameters for univariate normal distributions
rho <- -0.6
mu1 <- 2; s1 <- 3
mu2 <- 4; s2 <- 4

# Parameters for bivariate normal distribution
mu <- c(mu1,mu2) # Mean
sigma <- matrix(c(s1^2, s1*s2*rho, s1*s2*rho, s2^2),
                2) # Covariance matrix

# Function to draw ellipse for bivariate normal data
ellipse_bvn <- function(bvn, alpha){
  Xbar <- apply(bvn,2,mean)
  S <- cov(bvn)
  ellipse(Xbar, S, alpha = alpha, col="red",lwd=1.5)
}

library(MASS)
bvn1 <- mvrnorm(N, mu = mu, Sigma = sigma )
colnames(bvn1) <- c("bvn1_X1","bvn1_X2")

plot(bvn1[,1],bvn1[,2],pch=16,xlab="X1",ylab="X2")
ellipse_bvn(bvn1,.2)
ellipse_bvn(bvn1,.5)

#Do the correlation test
#Spearman's rho
x <- bvn1[,1]
y <- bvn1[,2]

source('rankBasedCommonFunctions.R')   #From van Doorn et al. (2020)
source('spearmanSampler.R')# Spearman's rho function  #From van
Doorn et al. (2020)
# Default beta prior width is set to a = b = 1 for the sampler
rhoSamples <- spearmanGibbsSampler(xVals = x,
                                   yVals = y,
                                   nSamples = 5e3)

# Posterior distribution
hist(rhoSamples$rhoSamples, freq = FALSE)

# Give the posterior samples for rho to the function below to compute BF01
computeBayesFactorOneZero(rhoSamples$rhoSamples,
                          whichTest = "Spearman",
                          priorParameter = 1)


mean(rhoSamples.1$rhoSamples)  #Posterior mean of rho
```

References

Berger, J. (2008). A comparison of testing methodologies. In *Proceedings of the PHYSTAT-LHC Workshop on Statistical Issues for LHC Physics* (pp. 8–19). CERN 2008-001. https://doi.org/10.5170/CERN-2008-001.8

Berger, J. (2011). The Bayesian approach to discovery. In H. B. Prosper & L. Lyons (Eds.), *Proceedings of the PHYSTAT 2011 Workshop on Statistical Issues Related to Discovery Claims in Search Experiments and Unfolding* (pp. 17–26). https://doi.org/10.5170/CERN-2011-006.17

Gronau Q. F., Singmann H., & Wagenmakers E.-J. (2020). `bridgesampling`: An R package for estimating. Normalizing constants. *Journal of Statistical Software, 92*(10), 1–29. https://doi.org/10.18637/jss.v092.i10

Jeffreys, H. (1935). Some tests of significance, treated by the theory of probability. *Mathematical Proceedings of the Cambridge Philosophical Society, 31*, 203–222. https://doi.org/10.1017/S030500410001330X

Kass, R. E., & Raftery, A. E. (1995). Bayes factors. *Journal of the American Statistical Association, 90*(430), 773–795. https://doi.org/10.1080/01621459.1995.10476572

Li, Y., Zeng, T., & Yu, J. (2014). A new approach to Bayesian hypothesis testing. *Journal of Econometrics, 178*(3), 602–612.

Morey, R. D., Rouder, J. N., Pratte, M. S., & Speckman, P. L. (2011). Using MCMC chain outputs to efficiently estimate Bayes factors. *Journal of Mathematical Psychology, 55*, 368–378. https://doi.org/10.1016/j.jmp.2011.06.004

Plummer, M. (2003). JAGS: a program for analysis of Bayesian graphical models using gibbs sampling. In *Proceedings of the 3rd International Workshop on Distributed Statistical Computing (DSC 2003)* (pp. 1–10).

Robert, C. P. (2022). 50 shades of Bayesian testing of hypotheses. In S. R. Arni, G. Srinivasa Rao, A. Young, C. & R. Rao (Eds.), *Handbook of statistics—volume 47—advancements in Bayesian methods and implementation* (pp. 103–120). Elsevier.

Rouder, J. N., Speckman, P. L., Sun, D. et al. (2009). Bayesian t tests for accepting and rejecting the null hypothesis. *Psychonomic Bulletin & Review, 16*, 225–237 (2009). https://doi.org/10.3758/PBR.16.2.225

Tendeiro, J. N., & Kiers, H. A. L. (2019). A review of issues about null hypothesis Bayesian testing. *Psychological Methods, 24*(6), 774–795. https://doi.org/10.1037/met0000221

van Doorn J., Ly A., Marsman M., & Wagenmakers E.-J. (2020). Bayesian rank-based hypothesis testing for the rank sum test, the signed rank test, and Spearman's ρ. *Journal of Applied Statistics, 47*(16), 2984–3006. https://doi.org/10.1080/02664763.2019.1709053

Wasserstein, R. L., & Lazar, N. A. (2016). The ASA statement on p-values: Context, process, and purpose. *The American Statistician, 70*(2), 129–133. https://doi.org/10.1080/00031305.2016.1154108

Wei, Z., Yang, A., Rocha, L., Miranda, M. F., & Nathoo, F. S. (2022). A review of bayesian hypothesis testing and its practical implementations. *Entropy, 24*(2), 161. https://doi.org/10.3390/e24020161

Chapter 3
Regression Estimation for Length-Biased Data: A Review and Comparative Study

Mahboubeh Akbari, Najmeh Nakhaei Rad, Ding-Geng Chen, and Vahid Fakoor

3.1 Introduction

Prevalent cohort designs are commonly used in epidemiological research, especially when studying chronic diseases or conditions with a high prevalence in the population. This approach can become much more efficient than an incident cohort study, which focuses on individuals who are free of the condition or event at the beginning of the study. In this design, an individual qualifies to be sampled at recruitment only if their survival time exceeds the interval between disease incidence and sampling time, namely, the observed failure time is left-truncated. Left-truncation is well known to produce a biased sample, and a special case of left-truncated data is length-biased data when the initial event is constant over time. These incomplete data arise when the observed data are collected based on the lengths or durations of specific events (Cox & Miller, 1965; Zelen & Feinleib, 1969; Simon, 1980; Vardi, 1982, 1989; Zelen, 2004). In practice, the observation of failure time in the prevalent cohort is subject to right-censoring due to the study ending or loss to follow up during the study period. This scheme is referred to as a left-truncation

M. Akbari (✉) · N. Nakhaei Rad
Department of Statistics, University of Pretoria, Pretoria, South Africa
e-mail: mahboubeh.akbarilakeh@up.ac.za; najmeh.nakhaeirad@up.ac.za

D.-G. Chen
Department of Statistics, University of Pretoria, Pretoria, South Africa

College of Health Solution, Arizona State University, Phoenix, AZ, USA
e-mail: din.chen@up.ac.za

V. Fakoor
Department of Statistics, School of Mathematical Sciences, Ferdowsi University of Mashhad, Mashhad, Iran
e-mail: fakoor@um.ac.ir

D.-G. Chen, C. A. Coelho (eds.), *Biostatistics Modeling and Public Health Applications*, Emerging Topics in Statistics and Biostatistics,
https://doi.org/10.1007/978-3-031-69690-9_3

right-censoring (LTRC) model. It is important to note that, in scenarios with a constant incidence rate, right-censored survival data obtained from a prevalent study cohort are characterized as length-biased right-censored (LBRC). In this case, the left-truncation variable follows a uniform distribution that commonly referred to as the stationarity assumption (Asgharian et al., 2006). This type of data is encountered frequently in various fields, including epidemiology, survival analysis, marketing research, economics, industrial reliability, and observational studies. A substantial body of literature exists on the analysis of LBRC data, primarily focusing on nonparametric estimation for the unbiased distribution function (Vardi, 1982, 1989; Winter & Földes, 1988; Tsai et al., 1987; Wang, 1991; Asgharian et al., 2002; Asgharian & Wolfson, 2005; Huang & Qin, 2011; Wang et al., 2017) and density and hazard estimation (Akbari et al., 2024; Efromovich & Chu, 2018; Shariati et al., 2023).

In the literature, several examples of such data have been presented, providing valuable insights into the characteristics and complexities of this type of sampling. The Canadian Study of Health and Aging (CSHA), one of the largest epidemiology studies of dementia, is an example of this kind of data. From that cohort, the participants were screened for dementia in 1991. As indicated by Wolfson et al. (2001), the CSHA includes left-truncated observations, because survival data were collected from a prevalent cohort of dementia patients who had not experienced the failure event (death) at the time of recruitment. It has been shown that the disease incidence in the CSHA data is stable over time (Addona & Wolfson, 2006). Another example that is publicly available is the Channing house data which has been analyzed in Hyde (1980). The dataset was collected between 1964 and 1975 at Channing House, a retirement center in Palo Alto, California. The observed survival times are left-truncated because only individuals who have lived long enough to enter the retirement center will be included in the data. To accommodate the length-biased concept, only the elders aged 65 years or older as the target group of interest were considered.

In Fig. 3.1, a visual representation of a prevalent follow-up study is presented. It is evident that, at the time of recruitment, two individuals are considered ineligible to be included in the sample because they were not alive at that time. Censoring in this context happens when the outcome or event of interest for an individual is either

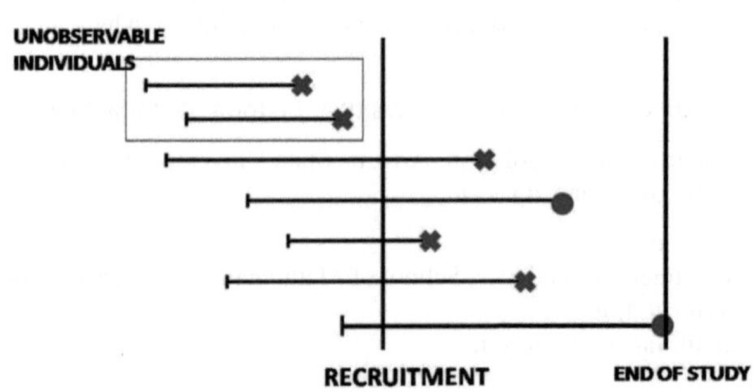

Fig. 3.1 A prevalent follow-up study

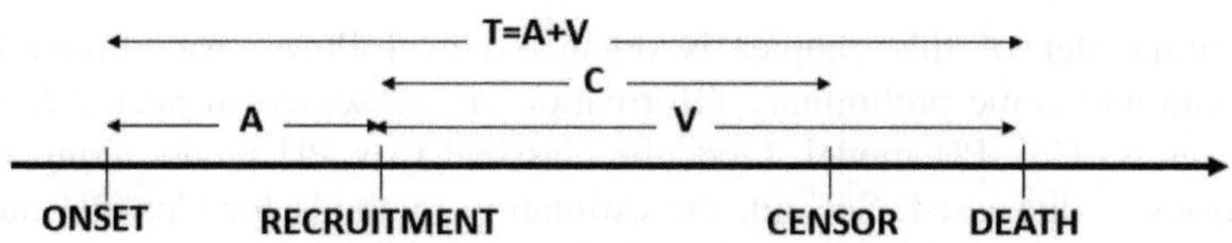

Fig. 3.2 A scheme of observed length-biased right-censored data

not observed or remains incomplete within the study period. The red circles indicate censored observations, and crosses show the failures.

Let $\tilde{T}$ represent the survival time of subjects in the target population (or unbiased population), $\tilde{A}$ denote the time between disease incidence and sampling time, and $\tilde{X}$ denote the covariate vector. In length-biased setting, $\tilde{A}$ distributed uniformly over $[0, \tau]$, where τ is the maximum support of unbiased survival time $\tilde{T}$ (Wang, 1991; Qin et al., 2011). The observed failure time has the conditional form $\tilde{T}|\tilde{T} > \tilde{A}$, denoted by T. We also use A and X to represent the observed truncation time and covariates, respectively. Consequently, (T, A, X) shares the same joint distribution as $(\tilde{T}, \tilde{A}, \tilde{X})$ conditional on $\tilde{T} \geq \tilde{A}$. Now, let (V, C) be random variables, where V represents the residual lifetime, i.e., the time from recruitment to death or censoring, and C denotes the residual censoring time, i.e., the time from enrollment to censoring occurrence. In Fig. 3.2, a schematic representation of a sample in a prevalent cohort study is shown using these notations.

In many studies, researchers are interested in exploring the relationships between covariates and a response variable. However, the presence of LBRC can make challenges. Firstly, the censoring is never noninformative because the censoring time $A + C$ and survival time $T = A + V$ share the same A. Secondly, the structures of the regression model for the target population and the observed length-biased data differ. As a result, the nonparametric and semiparametric estimation methods proposed for traditional survival data may not be appropriate for LBRC data. Given the non-invariance assumption of regression models under the length-biased sampling scheme, various approaches have been proposed in the literature (Ning et al., 2014b). These attempted to address the challenges provided by biased observations. Over the past two decades, there has been a growing interest in nonparametric and semiparametric estimation methods for regression coefficients in the context of LBRC data (see Shen et al., 2017).

In this chapter, we aim to present a chapter of the existing estimating approaches for Cox proportional hazard (PH) model and in accelerated failure time (AFT) model in the presence of LBRC data. The estimation methods for the Cox PH model with length-biased survival data can be classified into weighted estimating equations and likelihood-based approaches. In addition to frequentist methods, some research has been conducted in Bayesian framework. Existing estimating approaches for AFT model are based on estimating equation and hazard-based estimation methods using transformed survival observations.

The remainder of this chapter is organized as follows. An introduction to LBRC data and some preliminary information are presented in Sect. 3.2. Section 3.3 focuses on Cox PH model. First, the classical Cox PH model along with its assumptions is discussed. Second, the estimating methods for Cox PH model in the presence of LBRC data are explained. Then a simulation study is conducted to assess the performance of some estimating approaches. Section 3.4 follows a similar structure to Sect. 3.3 to explore and compare the existing estimating approaches for AFT model. To illustrate the performance of the estimating methods of Cox PH and AFT models for LBRC data, the Channing House dataset is used as an application in Sect. 3.5. Section 3.6 dedicates to various topics related to LBRC data including hazard proportional additive model, transformation model, managing missing data, and other relevant issues.

3.2 Preliminary and Notations

In a random sample of n independent subjects, the observed LBRC data are composed of $\{(A_i, Y_i, \Delta_i, \boldsymbol{X}_i),\ i{=}1, \ldots, n\}$, where $Y_i{=}A_i{+}\min(V_i, C_i) = A_i + \tilde{V}_i$ is the observed lifetime, $\Delta_i = I(V_i{\le}C_i)$ is censoring indicators, and $\boldsymbol{X}_i$ is the p-vector observed covariate for the individual i. Let $\tilde{F}(\cdot)$, $\tilde{f}(\cdot)$, and $\tilde{S}$ denote, respectively, the cumulative distribution, probability density, and survival function of $\tilde{T}$ in the unbiased population. In the rest of the chapter, we assume that f_q and S_q denote the density and survival function of a variable q, respectively. The joint distribution of (A, T) , as described in Lancaster (1992), is as follows:

$$f_{(A,T)}(a, t) = \frac{\tilde{f}(t)}{\mu}, \quad t > a > 0, \tag{3.1}$$

where $\mu = E(\tilde{T}) = \int_0^\infty t\tilde{f}(t)dt$. It is obvious that the observed length-biased survival time T given the covariates $\boldsymbol{X} = (\boldsymbol{X}_1, \ldots, \boldsymbol{X}_n)$ has the density function

$$f(t|\boldsymbol{X}) = \frac{t\tilde{f}(t|\boldsymbol{X})}{\mu(\boldsymbol{X})}, \quad t > 0.$$

Moreover, A and V share the same marginal density function

$$f_A(t|\boldsymbol{X}) = f_V(t|\boldsymbol{X}) = \frac{\tilde{S}(t|\boldsymbol{X})}{\mu(\boldsymbol{X})}, \quad t > 0. \tag{3.2}$$

Hence, from (3.1) and (3.2), the full likelihood function for the observed data $(A_i, Y_i, \Delta_i, \boldsymbol{X}_i)$ is proportional to

$$
\begin{aligned}
L_F &\propto \prod_{i=1}^{n} \frac{\tilde{f}(Y_i|\boldsymbol{X}_i)^{\Delta_i}\tilde{S}(Y_i|\boldsymbol{X}_i)^{1-\Delta_i}}{\mu(\boldsymbol{X}_i)} \\
&= \prod_{i=1}^{n} \frac{\tilde{f}(Y_i|\boldsymbol{X}_i)^{\Delta_i}\tilde{S}(Y_i|\boldsymbol{X}_i)^{1-\Delta_i}}{\tilde{S}(A_i|\boldsymbol{X}_i)} \times \prod_{i=1}^{n} \frac{\tilde{S}(A_i|\boldsymbol{X}_i)}{\mu(\boldsymbol{X}_i)} \\
&= L_T \times L_M,
\end{aligned}
\tag{3.3}
$$

where L_T is the truncation likelihood of Y conditioning on the truncation time A and L_M is the marginal likelihood of A.

3.3 The Semiparametric Cox Regression Model

This section is divided into three parts. The first part provides an explanation of the Cox PH model for traditional survival data. The second part discusses the estimation methods for the Cox PH model when dealing with LBRC data. The third part involves a simulation study to investigate the performance of different approaches for estimating regression coefficients under LBRC.

3.3.1 The Classical Cox PH Model

The Cox PH model is a popular statistical model used in survival analysis to examine the relationship between covariates and the time to an event, such as death or failure (Cox, 1972; Andersen & Gill, 1982; Kalbfleisch & Lawless, 1991; Andersen et al., 1993). In general, the underlying failure time $\tilde{T}$ follows a proportional hazards model for a given $\tilde{X}$

$$\lambda(t|\tilde{X}) = \lambda_0(t)\exp(\tilde{X}^{\mathsf{T}}\boldsymbol{\beta}), \tag{3.4}$$

where $\lambda_0(t)$ is an unspecified baseline hazard function and $\boldsymbol{\beta}$ is a $p \times 1$ vector of unknown regression coefficients for $\tilde{X}$. The probability of a particular failure at time Y_i, conditionally on the risk set $R_i = \{j : Y_i \leq Y_j\}$ for an uncensored individual, is

$$\frac{\exp(\tilde{X}_i^{\mathsf{T}}\boldsymbol{\beta})}{\sum_{j\in R_i}\exp(\tilde{X}_j^{\mathsf{T}}\boldsymbol{\beta})}.$$

Hence, the conditional log-likelihood and the score function are obtained as

$$L(\boldsymbol{\beta}) = \sum_{i=1}^{n} \Delta_i \left\{ \tilde{\boldsymbol{X}}_i^\top \boldsymbol{\beta} - \log \left(\sum_{j \in R_i} \exp(\tilde{\boldsymbol{X}}_j^\top \boldsymbol{\beta}) \right) \right\},$$

and

$$U_{\text{Cox}}(\boldsymbol{\beta}) = \sum_{i=1}^{n} \Delta_i \left\{ \tilde{\boldsymbol{X}}_i - \frac{\sum_{j \in R_i} \tilde{\boldsymbol{X}}_j \exp(\tilde{\boldsymbol{X}}_j^\top \boldsymbol{\beta})}{\sum_{j \in R_i} \exp(\tilde{\boldsymbol{X}}_j^\top \boldsymbol{\beta})} \right\}, \tag{3.5}$$

respectively. The literature on the Cox PH model is extensive, covering a wide range of topics such as different estimation techniques, model selection criteria, and diagnostic tools. Various approaches have been proposed to estimate coefficients of Cox PH model with traditional survival data, including likelihood-based, estimation equation, and Bayesian approaches (see Kalbfleisch & Schaubel, 2023).

3.3.2 The Length-Biased Cox PH Model

In a biased setting, it should be noted that the unbiased survival time $\tilde{T}$ follows (3.4), which may not hold for the observed survival time T. Let $\Lambda_0(t) = \int_0^t \lambda_0(u)du$ be the cumulative baseline hazard function. Then, $\tilde{S}(t|\boldsymbol{X}) = \exp\{-\Lambda_0(t)\exp(\boldsymbol{X}^\top\boldsymbol{\beta})\}$ and $\tilde{f}(t|\boldsymbol{X}) = \lambda(t|\boldsymbol{X})\tilde{S}(t|\boldsymbol{X})$. Therefore, using (3.3), the full likelihood function based on Cox PH model is proportional to the following expression:

$$L_F(\boldsymbol{\beta}, \Lambda_0) \propto \prod_{i=1}^{n} \frac{\{\lambda_0(Y_i)\exp(\boldsymbol{X}^\top\boldsymbol{\beta}_i)\}^{\Delta_i} \exp\{-\Lambda_0(Y_i)\exp(\boldsymbol{X}^\top\boldsymbol{\beta}_i)\}}{\int_0^\infty \exp\{-\Lambda_0(t)\exp(\boldsymbol{X}^\top\boldsymbol{\beta}_i)\}dt}.$$

The direct maximization of the objective function $L_F(\boldsymbol{\beta}, \Lambda_0)$ with respect to the parameters $(\boldsymbol{\beta}, \Lambda_0)$ is anticipated to produce estimators that are fully efficient. However, this approach is computationally intractable for two reasons. First, the inclusion of the nonparametric component Λ_0 in $L_F(\boldsymbol{\beta}, \Lambda_0)$ makes complexity in optimization process. Second, when the sample size is large, the maximization problem becomes more complex and computationally heavy due to the high-dimensional nature. As mentioned before, the full likelihood $L_F(\boldsymbol{\beta}, \Lambda_0)$ can be expressed as

$$
\begin{aligned}
L_F(\boldsymbol{\beta}, \Lambda_0) = & \prod_{i=1}^{n} \frac{\{\lambda_0(Y_i)\exp(\boldsymbol{X}^\top \boldsymbol{\beta}_i)\}^{\Delta_i}\exp\{-\Lambda_0(Y_i)\exp(\boldsymbol{X}^\top \boldsymbol{\beta}_i)\}}{\exp\{-\Lambda_0(A_i)\exp(\boldsymbol{X}^\top \boldsymbol{\beta}_i)\}} \\
& \times \prod_{i=1}^{n} \frac{\exp\{-\Lambda_0(A_i)\exp(\boldsymbol{X}^\top \boldsymbol{\beta}_i)\}}{\int_0^\infty \exp\{-\Lambda_0(t)\exp(\boldsymbol{X}^\top \boldsymbol{\beta}_i)\}dt} \\
= & L_T(\boldsymbol{\beta}, \Lambda_0) \times L_M(\boldsymbol{\beta}, \Lambda_0).
\end{aligned}
$$

Instead of maximizing the full likelihood function, the conditional likelihood approach focuses on maximizing the likelihood function $L_T(\boldsymbol{\beta}, \Lambda_0)$ under specific conditions or assumptions. The truncation likelihood, as described by Wang (1991) and Wang et al. (1993), can be expressed as the product of two components: the partial likelihood and the residual likelihood, $L_T(\boldsymbol{\beta}, \Lambda_0) = L_P(\boldsymbol{\beta}) \times L_R(\boldsymbol{\beta}, \Lambda_0)$, where the partial likelihood is defined as

$$
L_P(\boldsymbol{\beta}) = \prod_{i=1}^{n} \left\{ \frac{\exp\left(\boldsymbol{X}_i^\top \boldsymbol{\beta}\right)}{\sum_{j \in R_i^*} \exp\left(\boldsymbol{X}_j^\top \boldsymbol{\beta}\right)} \right\}^{\Delta_i},
$$

where $R_i^* = \{j : I(A_j \le Y_i \le Y_j)\}$ is the risk set at Y_i. Thus, the resulting score function is

$$
U_{PL}(\boldsymbol{\beta}) = \sum_{i=1}^{n} \Delta_i \left\{ \boldsymbol{X}_i - \frac{\sum_{j \in R_i^*} \boldsymbol{X}_j \exp\left(\boldsymbol{X}_j^\top \boldsymbol{\beta}\right)}{\sum_{j \in R_i^*} \exp\left(\boldsymbol{X}_j^\top \boldsymbol{\beta}\right)} \right\} \tag{3.6}
$$

Applying the partial likelihood method, proposed for the truncated data, is a straightforward approach to estimate covariate effects in length-biased data by solving (3.6) (Kalbfleisch & Lawless, 1991; Wang et al., 1993). However, it is important to note that the efficiency of these methods decreases when the truncation variable is specified. To address this issue, Wang (1996) proposed the construction of a pseudo-likelihood using a bias-adjusted risk set $R_i = \{j : I(Y_i \le Y_j)\}$ and obtained a score estimating equation to estimate $\boldsymbol{\beta}$ under length-biased sampling data as follows:

$$
U_W(\boldsymbol{\beta}) = \sum_{i=1}^{n} \left\{ \boldsymbol{X}_i - \frac{\sum_{j \in R_i} \boldsymbol{X}_j \exp\left(\boldsymbol{X}_j^\top \boldsymbol{\beta}\right) Y_j^{-1}}{\sum_{j \in R_i} \exp\left(\boldsymbol{X}_j^\top \boldsymbol{\beta}\right) Y_j^{-1}} \right\}. \tag{3.7}
$$

But this approach is applicable in situations where there is no censoring. To handle biased sampling with right-censoring, Tsai (2009) generalized the pseudo-partial likelihood approach of Wang (1996) by proposing the following estimating equation based on the score statistics:

$$U_T(\boldsymbol{\beta}) = \sum_{i=1}^{n} \Delta_i \left\{ \boldsymbol{X_i} - \frac{\sum_{j\in R_i} \boldsymbol{X}_j \exp\left(\boldsymbol{X}_j^\top \boldsymbol{\beta}\right) W(Y_i, Y_j)}{\sum_{j\in R_i} \exp\left(\boldsymbol{X}_j^\top \boldsymbol{\beta}\right) W(Y_i, Y_j)} \right\}, \tag{3.8}$$

where $W(Y_i, Y_j) = \Delta_j \frac{W_C(Y_j)-W_C(Y_j-Y_i)}{W_C(Y_j)} + (1-\Delta_j)\frac{S_C(Y_j-Y_i)-S_C(Yj)}{1-S_C(Y_j)}$ and $W_C(t) = \int_0^t S_C(s)ds$ in which S_C denotes the distribution of the residual censoring time C.

Under the assumption that C and (A, V) are independent given $\boldsymbol{X}$, Shen (2009) made an effort to extend Wang's (1996) estimating equation for LBRC data. Under the same condition, Qin and Shen (2010) proposed two inversely weighted estimating equations for the LBRC data with this

$$U_{QS}(\boldsymbol{\beta}) = \sum_{i=1}^{n} \Delta_i \left\{ \boldsymbol{X}_i - \frac{\sum_{j\in R_i} \Delta_j \boldsymbol{X}_j \exp\left(\boldsymbol{X}_j^\top \boldsymbol{\beta}\right) \left\{W_C(Y_j)\right\}^{-1}}{\sum_{j\in R_i} \Delta_j \exp\left(\boldsymbol{X}_j^\top \boldsymbol{\beta}\right) \left\{W_C(Y_j)\right\}^{-1}} \right\}, \tag{3.9}$$

where $W_C(Y_j)$ is considered as $W_1(Y_j) = Y_j S_C(Y_j - A_j)$ or $W_2(Y_j) = \int_0^{Y_j} S_C(t)dt$. The regression parameter $\boldsymbol{\beta}$ can be estimated by solving the estimation equation U_{QS}. When the exact form of S_C is unknown, it can be substituted with its consistent Kaplan-Meier estimator for the residual censoring time.

Although these methods, which are based on estimating equations, have computational advantages compared to likelihood-based approaches, they do not provide a straightforward way to analyze length-biased data when the censoring time depends on the covariates, and may not yield efficient estimators, Qin et al. (2011) considered the log-likelihood function and proposed an alternative computational approach based on EM algorithm. They jointly estimated the baseline hazards function and the covariate coefficients using the full likelihood function. Let $0 = t_0 < t_1 < t_2 < \cdots < t_k < \infty$ denote distinct observed time points, both censored and uncensored times, and Λ_0 has positive jumps $\lambda = (\lambda_1, \ldots, \lambda_k)$ at $\{t_1, \ldots, t_k\}$. In their approach, the EM algorithm is developed using the discretized version of $\Lambda_0(u) = \sum_{t_j \le u} \lambda_j$. For $i = 1, \ldots n$ and $j = 1, \ldots k$, let

$$\begin{aligned} w_{ij} &= \Delta_i I(Y_i = t_j) + (1-\Delta_i)\frac{p_{ij} I(Y_i \le t_j)}{\sum_{j=1}^{k} p_{ij} I(Y_i \le t_j)} \\ &\quad + \frac{\hat{\tau}}{\sum_{j=1}^{k} t_j p_{ij}} \left(1 - \frac{t_j}{\hat{\tau}}\right) p_{ij}, \end{aligned} \tag{3.10}$$

where $p_{ij} = \lambda_j \exp(\boldsymbol{X}_i^\top \boldsymbol{\beta}) \exp\left\{-\Lambda_0(t_j)\exp(\boldsymbol{X}_i^\top \boldsymbol{\beta})\right\}$ and $\hat{\tau} = \max_{i=1}^{n} Y_i$. Thus, in this case, $\boldsymbol{\beta}$ and λ_j can be solved from the following equations, respectively:

$$\sum_{i=1}^{n} w_{i+} \boldsymbol{X}_i - \sum_{l=1}^{k} w_{+l} \left\{ \frac{\sum_{i=1}^{n} \sum_{j=l}^{k} w_{ij} \boldsymbol{X}_i \exp\left(\boldsymbol{X}_i^\top \boldsymbol{\beta}\right)}{\sum_{i=1}^{n} \sum_{j=l}^{k} w_{ij} \exp\left(\boldsymbol{X}_i^\top \boldsymbol{\beta}\right)} \right\} = 0, \tag{3.11}$$

and

$$\lambda_j = \frac{w_{+j}}{\sum_{l=j}^{k} \sum_{i=1}^{n} w_{il} \exp\left(X_i^{\top} \boldsymbol{\beta}\right)}, \tag{3.12}$$

where $w_{i+} = \sum_{j=1}^{k} w_{ij}$ and $w_{+j} = \sum_{i=1}^{n} w_{ij}$. Using the obtained λ_j for $j = 1, \ldots, k$ and β from (3.11) and (3.12), one can update w_{ij} in (3.10) and repeat this loop until a convergence condition for $\boldsymbol{\beta}$ and λ_j is satisfied. This method provides more efficient estimators compared to the conditional likelihood approach and the estimating equation approaches.

The other idea proposed by Huang et al. (2012) is based on generalizing the profile likelihood method by replacing the nuisance parameters in the full likelihood (or the partial likelihood) with a consistent estimator that may depend on the parameter of interest. This approach is consistent under covariate-dependent censoring and can handle time-dependent covariates. In fact, Huang et al. (2012), instead of profiling out the nonparametric component Λ_0 in $L_F(\boldsymbol{\beta}, \Lambda_0)$, proposed to replace $\Lambda_0(t)$ with a simple estimate that is consistent. The resulting estimator of $\boldsymbol{\beta}$ is consistent even in the presence of censoring times depend on the covariates. By replacing the hazard function in the full likelihood with a Breslow-type estimator (denote $\hat{\Lambda}_{\boldsymbol{\beta}}$) which is the maximization of truncation likelihood $L_T(\boldsymbol{\beta}, \Lambda_0)$ for a fixed $\boldsymbol{\beta}$, they estimated the regression parameter $\boldsymbol{\beta}$ by maximizing the following pseudo-profile likelihood:

$$\begin{aligned} L_F(\boldsymbol{\beta}, \hat{\Lambda}_{\boldsymbol{\beta}}) &= L_T(\boldsymbol{\beta}, \hat{\Lambda}_{\boldsymbol{\beta}}) \times L_m(\boldsymbol{\beta}, \hat{\Lambda}_{\boldsymbol{\beta}}) \\ &= L_P(\boldsymbol{\beta}) \prod_{i=1}^{n} \frac{\exp\left\{-\hat{\Lambda}_{\boldsymbol{\beta}}(A_i) \exp\left(\boldsymbol{X}^{\top} \boldsymbol{\beta}_i\right)\right\}}{\int_0^{\infty} \exp\left\{-\hat{\Lambda}_{\boldsymbol{\beta}}(t) \exp\left(\boldsymbol{X}^{\top} \boldsymbol{\beta}_i\right)\right\} dt}. \end{aligned}$$

The next method has more simplicity for statistical practitioners. Huang and Qin (2012) developed a composite partial likelihood method for LBRC data. When there is no censoring, the composite conditional likelihood is given by the product of the conditional likelihood of V given A and the conditional likelihood A given V. In the presence of right-censoring, the composite conditional likelihood formulated as follows:

$$\begin{aligned} L_C(\boldsymbol{\beta}, \Lambda_0) &= \prod_{i=1}^{n} \left\{ \frac{f(Y_i|\boldsymbol{X}_i)}{S(A_i|\boldsymbol{X}_i)} \times \frac{f(Y_i|\boldsymbol{X}_i)}{S(\tilde{V}_i|\boldsymbol{X}_i)} \right\}^{\Delta_i} \left\{ \frac{S(Y_i|\boldsymbol{X}_i)}{S(A_i|\boldsymbol{X}_i)} \right\}^{1-\Delta_i} \qquad (3.13) \\ &= \prod_{i=1}^{n} \frac{f(Y_i|\boldsymbol{X}_i)^{\Delta_i} S(Y_i|\boldsymbol{X}_i)^{1-\Delta_i}}{S(A_i|\boldsymbol{X}_i)} \left\{ \frac{f(Y_i|\boldsymbol{X}_i)}{S(\tilde{V}_i|\boldsymbol{X}_i)} \right\}^{1-\Delta_i} \\ &= \prod_{i=1}^{n} \frac{\left\{\lambda_0(Y_i) \exp\left(\boldsymbol{X}^{\top} \boldsymbol{\beta}_i\right)\right\}^{2\Delta_i} \exp\left\{-(1+\Delta_i)\Lambda_0(Y_i) \exp\left(\boldsymbol{X}^{\top} \boldsymbol{\beta}_i\right)\right\}}{\exp\left\{-\left(\Lambda_0(A_i) + \Delta_i \Lambda_0(\tilde{V}_i)\right) \exp\left(\boldsymbol{X}^{\top} \boldsymbol{\beta}_i\right)\right\}}, \end{aligned}$$

which is the product of the conditional likelihood of Y given A for all survival times and that of Y given V for uncensored survival times. For any fixed $\boldsymbol{\beta}$, it can be observed that the composite conditional likelihood function is maximized by the consistent Breslow-type estimator given below:

$$\hat{\Lambda}_{\boldsymbol{\beta}}(t) = \sum_{i=1}^{n} \frac{2\Delta_i I(Y_i \le t)}{\sum_{j=1}^{n} \exp\left(\boldsymbol{X}_j^{\top}\boldsymbol{\beta}\right)\left\{I(A_j \le Y_i \le Y_j) + \Delta_j I(\tilde{V}_j \le Y_i \le Y_j)\right\}}.$$

Thus, profiling out the nonparametric component Λ_0 in $L_C(\boldsymbol{\beta}, \Lambda_0)$, the maximum composite partial likelihood estimator is obtained by solving

$$U_C(\beta) = \sum_{i=1}^{n} \Delta_i \times \left\{ X_i - \frac{\sum_{j=1}^{n} \boldsymbol{X}_j \exp\left(\boldsymbol{X}_j^{\top}\boldsymbol{\beta}\right)\left\{I(A_j \le Y_i \le Y_j) + \Delta_j I(\tilde{V}_j \le Y_i \le Y_j)\right\}}{\sum_{j=1}^{n} \exp\left(\boldsymbol{X}_j^{\top}\boldsymbol{\beta}\right)\left\{I(A_j \le Y_i \le Y_j) + \Delta_j I(\tilde{V}_j \le Y_i \le Y_j)\right\}} \right\}. \quad (3.14)$$

Liu et al. (2016) proposed a maximum likelihood estimator for censored survival data with a selection biased in which the selection process is modeled parametrically. Therefore, this method is applicable not only for LBRC data but also for general left-truncation data with a known truncation distribution. In LBRC context, their method offers computational advantages compared to the EM approach suggested by Qin et al. (2011) and performs better in terms of bias, particularly in scenarios with a high censoring rate.

Wang and Zhou (2018) addressed the computational difficulties encountered in Huang et al.'s (2012) work and the theoretical issues raised in semiparametric maximum likelihood estimation proposed by Huang and Qin (2012). Using the discretized version of $\Lambda_0(u)$, Wang and Zhou (2018) proposed the following modified log-likelihood function to estimate $\boldsymbol{\beta}$ and Λ_0:

$$\begin{aligned} L_{WZ}(\boldsymbol{\beta}, \Lambda_0) = \sum_{i=1}^{n} \Bigg\{ & \Delta_i \log(\Lambda_0(Y_i)) I(Y_i \le \tau) + \tilde{\boldsymbol{X}} I(Y_i \le \tau) \\ & - \int_0^{\tau} I(Y_i \ge t) \exp(\boldsymbol{X}_i^{\top}\boldsymbol{\beta}) d\Lambda_0(t) \\ & - \log\left(\int_0^{\infty} \exp\left(-\int_0^{t} \exp(\boldsymbol{X}_i^{\top}\boldsymbol{\beta}) d\Lambda_0(s)\right) dt\right) \Bigg\}. \end{aligned}$$

Another likelihood-based approach for estimating parameters in the Cox PH model has been proposed by Jazi (2024). This method adjusts the bias of sample risk sets following the idea of Wang (1996). His method is applied for any truncation time that should be modeled parametrically. He showed when the truncation time has exponential distribution, his proposed method outperforms the left-truncation method of Gijbels and Wang (1993) and maximum likelihood approach of Liu et al. (2015). Despite the computational advantages of Jazi's method, it is not applicable when the censoring distribution depends on covariates.

In addition to these frequentist methods, Harun et al. (2021) proposed an estimator within the Bayesian framework. They considered monotone integrated splines in order to estimate the unknown nondecreasing baseline cumulative hazard function flexibly.

3.3.3 Simulation Study for Cox Model

In this section, a simulation study was conducted to evaluate the performance of some common estimating approaches mentioned in the previous section. In addition, we aim to assess the impact of length-biased sampling on the analysis and evaluate the necessity of taking it into account in the modeling process. We generated unbiased failure times $\tilde{T}$ from the following Cox PH model:

$$\lambda(t|X) = \lambda_0(t)\exp\left(\boldsymbol{\beta}_1\tilde{X}_1 + \boldsymbol{\beta}_2\tilde{X}_2\right),$$

based on the fact that $S(t) = \exp\left\{-\Lambda_0(t)\exp\left(\tilde{\boldsymbol{X}}^{\top}\boldsymbol{\beta}\right)\right\}$. We assumed $\boldsymbol{\beta} = (\boldsymbol{\beta}_1, \boldsymbol{\beta}_2) = (0.5, 1)$ and $(1, 1)$, the binary covariate $\tilde{X}_1 \sim \text{Bernoulli}(1, 0.5)$, the continuous covariate $\tilde{X}_2 \sim \text{uniform}(-0.5, 0.5)$, and constant and increasing baseline hazard functions as $\lambda_0(t) = 2$ or $2t$. Following Huang and Qin (2011), the enrollment time was set to be 100, and the truncation times were considered as $100 - U$, where U has a uniform distribution $(0, 100)$. The residual censoring variable was generated from a uniform distribution on interval $(0, \tau_c)$, where τ_c was chosen so that the overall censoring rate was approximately 10%, 30%, and 50%. Therefore, the censoring indicator was $\delta_i = I(T_i \leq C_i + A_i)$. For each scenario, we repeated the simulation 1000 times with cohorts of size $n = 100, 200$.

We considered the following approaches for estimating Cox regression coefficients in the presence of length-biased data: (i) the traditional estimating equation (Classic) method (Cox, 1972), (ii) the partial likelihood (PL) method (Wang et al., 1993), (iii) the two estimating equation (QSI, QSII) approaches (Qin & Shen, 2010), and (iv) the composite partial likelihood (CPL) method (Huang & Qin, 2012). The traditional estimator proposed by Cox (1972) can be obtained using the "coxph" function in the "Survival" package in R software. In the presence of LBRC data, to obtain QSI and QSII estimators, we can use "coxph" function with a "offset" option to add a linear predictor in the Cox model as follows (Qin & Shen, 2010):

$$> \text{coxph(Surv(Y,rep(1,m))} \sim X_1 + X_2 + \text{offset}(-\log(\hat{W}_C))), \text{data=fdata}),$$

where "fdata" is the subset of the whole data matrix among subjects with only observed failure times and m is the number of observed times. When $W_C = W_2$, as an alternative way, we can utilize the "CoxPhLb" package. This package explores the assumptions of the Cox model including the functional form of a continuous covariate and the proportional hazards assumption. Finally, we employed the Newton–Raphson method to obtain PL and CPL estimators, which can also be used to solve the corresponding estimating equation.

Tables 3.1 and 3.2 provide the simulation results considering $\lambda_0 = 2$ and $\lambda_0 = 2t$ including empirical bias (Bias), empirical standard error (SE), and 95% confidence

Table 3.1 Simulation results for Cox PH model with $\lambda_0(t) = 2$

			$n = 100$			$n = 200$		
$\boldsymbol{\beta}$	C%	Methods	Bias	SE	Coef 95% CIs	Bias	SE	Coef 95% CIs
(0.5,1)	10%	Classic	0.2432	0.2511	(0.25,1.24)	0.2410	0.1616	(0.42,1.06)
			0.5051	0.4361	(0.65,2.36)	0.4840	0.3021	(0.89,2.08)
		PL	−0.0018	0.2486	(0.01,0.99)	0.0097	0.1644	(0.19,0.83)
			0.0359	0.4133	(0.23,1.85)	0.0137	0.2858	(0.45,1.57)
		QSI	0.0009	0.1947	(0.12,0.88)	0.0048	0.1269	(0.26,0.75)
			0.0160	0.3300	(0.37,1.66)	0.0093	0.2255	(0.57,1.45)
		QSII	0.0202	0.1971	(0.13,0.91)	0.0128	0.1247	(0.27,0.76)
			0.0462	0.3350	(0.39,1.70)	0.0279	0.2274	(0.58,1.47)
		CPL	0.0047	0.1799	(0.15,0.86)	0.0059	0.1190	(0.27,0.74)
			0.0238	0.3140	(0.41,1.64)	0.0127	0.2143	(0.59,1.43)
	30%	Classic	0.2788	0.265	(0.26,1.3)	0.2630	0.1846	(0.40,1.12)
			0.5563	0.4871	(0.60,2.51)	0.5343	0.3240	(0.90,2.17)
		PL	0.0167	0.2550	(0.02,1.02)	−0.0011	0.1840	(0.14,0.86)
			0.0314	0.4880	(0.08,1.99)	0.0030	0.3246	(0.37,1.64)
		QSI	−0.0174	0.2543	(−0.02, 0.98)	−0.0186	0.1837	(0.12,0.84)
			−0.0354	0.4446	(0.09,1.84)	−0.0467	0.3289	(0.31,1.60)
		QSII	0.0211	0.2355	(0.06,0.98)	0.0178	0.1617	(0.20,0.83)
			0.0580	0.4179	(0.24,1.88)	0.0298	0.2948	(0.45,1.61)
		CPL	0.0084	0.1929	(0.13,0.89)	0.0033	0.1324	(0.24,0.76)
			0.0288	0.3668	(0.31,1.75)	0.0083	0.2422	(0.53,1.48)
	50%	Classic	0.3001	0.3029	(0.21,1.39)	0.2966	0.1960	(0.41,1.18)
			0.6102	0.4969	(0.64,2.58)	0.6030	0.3405	(0.94,2.27)
		PL	0.0080	0.3013	(−0.08, 1.10)	0.0079	0.2002	(0.12,0.90)
			0.0168	0.5178	(0.00,2.03)	0.0147	0.3288	(0.37,1.66)
		QSI	−0.0476	0.3124	(−0.16, 1.06)	−0.0683	0.2180	(0.00,0.86)
			−0.1057	0.5396	(−0.16, 1.95)	−0.1243	0.3922	(0.11,1.64)
		QSII	0.0224	0.2740	(−0.01, 1.06)	0.0074	0.1787	(0.16,0.86)
			0.0594	0.5059	(0.07,2.05)	0.0311	0.3236	(0.40,1.67)
		CPL	0.0019	0.2161	(0.08,0.93)	0.0019	0.1439	(0.22,0.78)
			0.0156	0.3829	(0.27,1.77)	0.0147	0.2482	(0.53,1.50)

(continued)

Table 3.1 (continued)

			$n = 100$			$n = 200$		
$\boldsymbol{\beta}$	C%	Methods	Bias	SE	Coef 95% CIs	Bias	SE	Coef 95% CIs
(1,1)	10%	Classic	0.520	0.2940	(0.94, 2.10)	0.5187	0.2075	(1.11,1.93)
			0.5064	0.4508	(0.62, 2.39)	0.4986	0.3003	(0.91,2.09)
		PL	0.0161	0.2793	(0.47, 1.56)	0.0230	0.2030	(0.63,1.42)
			0.0149	0.4312	(0.17, 1.86)	0.0191	0.2963	(0.44,1.60)
		QSI	0.0084	0.2237	(0.57, 1.45)	0.0172	0.1508	(0.72,1.31)
			0.0031	0.3335	(0.35, 1.66)	0.0069	0.2237	(0.57,1.45)
		QSII	0.0324	0.2238	(0.59, 1.47)	0.0313	0.1498	(0.74,1.33)
			0.0432	0.3463	(0.36, 1.72)	0.0308	0.2240	(0.59,1.47)
		CPL	0.0124	0.2137	(0.59, 1.43)	0.0203	0.1517	(0.72,1.32)
			0.0095	0.3246	(0.37, 1.65)	0.0168	0.2153	(0.59,1.44)
	30%	Classic	0.5482	0.3021	(0.96, 2.14)	0.5361	0.2163	(1.11,1.96)
			0.5392	0.4472	(0.66, 2.42)	0.5355	0.3183	(0.91,2.16)
		PL	0.0194	0.3095	(0.41, 1.63)	0.0059	0.2121	(0.59,1.42)
			0.0187	0.4557	(0.13, 1.91)	0.0033	0.3134	(0.39,1.62)
		QSI	−0.0293	0.2671	(0.45, 1.49)	−0.027	0.1872	(0.61,1.34)
			−0.0642	0.4260	(0.10, 1.77)	−0.0759	0.3015	(0.33,1.52)
		QSII	0.0376	0.2490	(0.55, 1.53)	0.0269	0.1744	(0.69,1.37)
			0.0110	0.4003	(0.23, 1.80)	0.0030	0.2735	(0.47,1.54)
		CPL	0.0073	0.2294	(0.56, 1.46)	0.0079	0.1618	(0.69,1.32)
			−0.0050	0.3296	(0.35, 1.64)	−0.0056	0.2338	(0.54,1.45)
	50%	Classic	0.5896	0.3413	(0.92, 2.26)	0.5841	0.2255	(1.14,2.03)
			0.6069	0.5371	(0.55, 2.66)	0.5998	0.3644	(0.89,2.31)
		PL	0.0110	0.3195	(0.38, 1.64)	0.0201	0.2167	(0.60,1.44)
			0.0358	0.5373	(−0.02, 2.09)	0.0348	0.3563	(0.34,1.73)
		QSI	−0.0691	0.3199	(0.30, 1.56)	−0.0847	0.2313	(0.46,1.37)
			−0.0881	0.5044	(−0.08, 1.90)	−0.1195	0.3630	(0.17,1.59)
		QSII	0.0478	0.2958	(0.47, 1.63)	0.0254	0.2059	(0.62,1.43)
			0.0292	0.4630	(0.12, 1.94)	0.0115	0.3227	(0.38,1.64)
		CPL	0.0121	0.2468	(0.53, 1.50)	0.0124	0.1712	(0.68,1.35)
			0.0107	0.4017	(0.22, 1.80)	0.0112	0.2658	(0.49,1.53)

interval (Coef 95% CIs) of the estimates. The empirical bias is an average of 1000 biases obtained in each repetition. The empirical SE is the standard error of 1000 estimates obtained from 1000 repetitions, and the Coef 95% CIs are the normal approximation confidence intervals for coefficients.

Based on the findings presented in Tables 3.1 and 3.2, the following conclusions can be drawn:

- The traditional Cox PH approach suffers from bias due to the ignorance of truncation.
- The QSI, QSII, and CPL methods proposed to address LBRC exhibit better performance than the PL method in most cases, as the PL method ignores the

Table 3.2 Simulation results for Cox PH model with $\lambda_0(t) = 2t$

			$n = 100$			$n = 200$		
$\boldsymbol{\beta}$	C%	Methods	Bias	SE	Coef 95% CIs	Bias	SE	Coef 95% CIs
(0.5,1)	10%	Classic	0.1426	0.2297	(0.19, 1.09)	0.1336	0.1559	(0.33,0.94)
			0.2649	0.4192	(0.44, 2.09)	0.2602	0.2657	(0.74,1.78)
		PL	0.0197	0.2310	(0.07, 0.97)	0.0046	0.1587	(0.19,0.82)
			0.0209	0.4150	(0.21, 1.83)	0.0004	0.2741	(0.46,1.54)
		QSI	0.0142	0.1979	(0.13, 0.90)	0.0011	0.1353	(0.24,0.77)
			0.0058	0.3589	(0.30, 1.71)	0.0026	0.2288	(0.55,1.45)
		QSII	0.0207	0.1970	(0.13, 0.91)	0.0072	0.1335	(0.25,0.77)
			0.0168	0.3594	(0.31, 1.72)	0.0164	0.2295	(0.57,1.47)
		CPL	0.0139	0.1899	(0.14, 0.89)	0.0029	0.1288	(0.25,0.76)
			0.0101	0.3503	(0.32, 1.70)	0.0056	0.2227	(0.57,1.44)
	30%	Classic	0.1609	0.2678	(0.14, 1.19)	0.1662	0.1856	(0.30,1.03)
			0.3411	0.4773	(0.41, 2.28)	0.3168	0.3308	(0.67,1.97)
		PL	0.0061	0.2693	(−0.02, 1.03)	0.0158	0.1829	(0.16,0.87)
			0.0365	0.4670	(0.12, 1.95)	0.0154	0.3216	(0.39,1.65)
		QSI	−0.0045	0.2805	(−0.05, 1.05)	−0.0047	0.1962	(0.11,0.88)
			0.0103	0.4895	(0.05, 1.97)	−0.0272	0.3394	(0.31,1.64)
		QSII	0.0214	0.2540	(0.02, 1.02)	0.0211	0.1745	(0.18,0.86)
			0.0595	0.4458	(0.19, 1.93)	0.0242	0.3082	(0.42,1.63)
		CPL	0.0073	0.2224	(0.07, 0.94)	0.0148	0.1528	(0.22,0.81)
			0.0334	0.3855	(0.28, 1.79)	0.0112	0.2699	(0.48,1.54)
	50%	Classic	0.1806	0.2896	(0.11, 1.25)	0.1931	0.2053	(0.29,1.10)
			0.3672	0.5373	(0.31, 2.42)	0.3876	0.3677	(0.67,2.11)
		PL	0.0099	0.2934	(−0.07, 1.08)	0.0101	0.2057	(0.11,0.91)
			0.0041	0.5182	(−0.01, 2.02)	0.0302	0.3736	(0.30,1.76)
		QSI	−0.0582	0.3636	(−0.27, 1.15)	−0.0375	0.2599	(−0.05,0.97)
			−0.0846	0.6175	(−0.30, 2.13)	−0.0957	0.4584	(0.01,1.80)
		QSII	0.0083	0.3078	(−0.10, 1.11)	0.0198	0.2118	(0.10,0.93)
			0.0294	0.5527	(−0.05, 2.11)	0.0213	0.3652	(0.31,1.74)
		CPL	0.0029	0.2365	(0.04, 0.97)	0.0121	0.1670	(0.18,0.84)
			0.0089	0.4350	(0.16, 1.86)	0.0206	0.2980	(0.44,1.60)
(1,1)	10%	Classic	0.2938	0.2606	(0.78, 1.80)	0.2762	0.1773	(0.93,1.62)
			0.3029	0.4307	(0.46, 2.15)	0.2784	0.2764	(0.74,1.82)
		PL	0.0287	0.2571	(0.52, 1.53)	0.0166	0.1749	(0.67,1.36)
			0.0366	0.4153	(0.22, 1.85)	0.0172	0.2787	(0.47,1.56)
		QSI	0.0226	0.2239	(0.58, 1.46)	0.0127	0.1503	(0.72,1.31)
			0.0355	0.3660	(0.32, 1.75)	0.0193	0.2369	(0.56,1.48)
		QSII	0.0353	0.2254	(0.59, 1.48)	0.0229	0.1500	(0.73,1.32)
			0.0488	0.3700	(0.32, 1.77)	0.0291	0.2388	(0.56,1.50)
		CPL	0.0227	0.2179	(0.60, 1.45)	0.0136	0.1488	(0.72,1.31)
			0.0330	0.3545	(0.34, 1.73)	0.0138	0.2293	(0.56,1.46)

(continued)

Table 3.2 (continued)

β	C%	Methods	$n = 100$			$n = 200$		
			Bias	SE	Coef 95% CIs	Bias	SE	Coef 95% CIs
	30%	Classic	0.3353	0.2880	(0.77, 1.90)	0.3051	0.1960	(0.92,1.69)
			0.3243	0.4682	(0.41, 2.24)	0.3191	0.3218	(0.69,1.95)
		PL	0.0453	0.2920	(0.47, 1.62)	0.0022	0.1975	(0.62,1.39)
			0.0292	0.4840	(0.08, 1.98)	0.0117	0.3256	(0.37,1.65)
		QSI	0.0112	0.2938	(0.44, 1.59)	−0.0229	0.2053	(0.57,1.38)
			−0.0187	0.4776	(0.05, 1.92)	−0.0362	0.3510	(0.28,1.65)
		QSII	0.0450	0.2667	(0.52, 1.57)	0.0188	0.1800	(0.67,1.37)
			0.0231	0.4429	(0.16, 1.89)	0.0194	0.3009	(0.43,1.61)
		CPL	0.0261	0.2407	(0.55, 1.50)	0.0020	0.1609	(0.69,1.32)
			0.0109	0.3882	(0.25, 1.77)	0.0108	0.2669	(0.49,1.53)
	50%	Classic	0.3947	0.3252	(0.76, 2.03)	0.3785	0.2337	(0.92,1.84)
			0.3981	0.5517	(0.32, 2.48)	0.3754	0.3687	(0.65,2.10)
		PL	0.0422	0.3167	(0.42, 1.66)	0.0247	0.2295	(0.57,1.47)
			0.0411	0.5336	(0.00, 2.09)	0.0252	0.3810	(0.28,1.77)
		QSI	−0.0708	0.3908	(0.16, 1.70)	−0.0807	0.2652	(0.40,1.44)
			−0.0650	0.6262	(−0.29, 2.16)	−0.1007	0.4371	(0.04,1.76)
		QSII	0.0452	0.3317	(0.40, 1.70)	0.0402	0.2227	(0.60,1.48)
			0.0502	0.5562	(−0.04, 2.14)	0.0235	0.3452	(0.35,1.70)
		CPL	0.0313	0.2723	(0.50, 1.57)	0.0258	0.1918	(0.65,1.40)
			0.0276	0.4460	(0.15, 1.90)	0.0169	0.3005	(0.43,1.61)

stationary assumption. In addition, for high censoring rate, QSII outperforms QSI.

- The CPL provides unbiased estimator with the lowest standard error values. Therefore, this method has the best performance in all the cases. However, the results of QSI estimator are close to CPL under light censoring rate.
- It is obvious that by increasing n, the bias and standard error of estimates decrease.
- As expected, by increasing the censoring rate, the bias and standard error of estimates increase.
- It is worth knowing that the shape of baseline hazard function, whether constant or increasing, does not impact the results.

3.4 The Semiparametric AFT Model

In this section, first, we explain the AFT model for the traditional survival data. Second, the estimation methods for the AFT model in the presence of LBRC data are explored. Finally, a simulation study is conducted to assess the performance of various approaches.

3.4.1 The Classical AFT Model

The AFT model is a useful alternative to the Cox PH model when the PH assumption is not valid. This model relates the logarithm of the failure time linearly to the covariates (Cox & Oakes, 1984; Kalbfleisch & Prentice, 2002) and also referred to as log-linear model. Mathematically, the AFT model can be represented as

$$\log(\tilde{T}) = \tilde{\boldsymbol{X}}^{\mathsf{T}}\boldsymbol{\beta} + \tilde{\epsilon}, \tag{3.15}$$

where $\boldsymbol{\beta}$ is a $p \times 1$ vector of unknown regression coefficients and $\tilde{\epsilon}$ is the random error independent of $\tilde{\boldsymbol{X}}$ with an unspecified probability density function $f_{\tilde{\epsilon}}$. Let $\lambda_{\tilde{\xi}}(\cdot)$ and $\Lambda_{\tilde{\xi}}(\cdot)$ denote the hazard and cumulative hazard functions of $\tilde{\xi} = \exp(\tilde{\epsilon})$, respectively. Then, the survival and hazard functions of $\tilde{T}$, given $\tilde{X}$, are

$$\tilde{S}(t|\tilde{\boldsymbol{X}}) = \exp\left\{-\Lambda_{\tilde{\xi}}\left(te^{-\tilde{\boldsymbol{X}}^{\mathsf{T}}\boldsymbol{\beta}}\right)\right\}, \quad \lambda(t|\tilde{\boldsymbol{X}}) = \lambda_{\tilde{\xi}}\left(te^{-\tilde{\boldsymbol{X}}^{\mathsf{T}}\boldsymbol{\beta}}\right)e^{-\tilde{\boldsymbol{X}}^{\mathsf{T}}\boldsymbol{\beta}}, \tag{3.16}$$

respectively. From (3.16), it is concluded that, in general, the two assumptions of Cox PH model and AFT model cannot be reconciled. Therefore, the model of interest is typically either an AFT model or a Cox PH model, except when the distribution of error is Weibull. Several approaches have been proposed in the literature for estimating the coefficients of AFT model for traditional survival data including rank-based estimating equations, least squares estimators, and the kernel-smoothed profile likelihood method (see Prentice, 1978; Buckley & James, 1979; Miller & Halpern, 1982; Ritov, 1990; Tsiatis, 1990; Lai & Ying, 1991a; Ying, 1993; Lin & Ying, 1995; Kalbfleisch & Prentice, 2002; Jin et al., 2003; Zeng & Lin, 2007). Prentice (1978) proposed the following naive estimator for $\boldsymbol{\beta}$ ignoring the biased sampling:

$$\hat{\boldsymbol{\beta}} = \left\{\sum_{i=1}^{n}\frac{\Delta_i\boldsymbol{X}_i\boldsymbol{X}_i^{\mathsf{T}}}{\hat{S}_C(Y_i)}\right\}^{-1}\sum_{i=1}^{n}\frac{\Delta_i\boldsymbol{X}_i\log(Y_i)}{\hat{S}_C(Y_i)}, \tag{3.17}$$

where $\hat{S}_C(\cdot)$ is the Kaplan-Meier estimator for censoring variable C.

3.4.2 The Length-Biased AFT Model

In the presence of LBRC data, we assume that the unbiased survival time $\tilde{T}$ follows Eq. (3.15). A challenge here is that the conditional distribution of $\tilde{T}$ given the covariate $\tilde{\boldsymbol{X}}$ under biased sampling does not conform to the same AFT model for $\tilde{T}$. Therefore, in the presence of left-truncated right-censored (LTRC) data, certain methods such as the rank-based estimating equation estimator proposed by Lai and Ying (1991b) and the M-estimators by Lai and Ying (1994) did not take into account the truncation information. As a result, these methods may be less efficient when applying for LTRC data. The rank-based estimating equation proposed by Lai and Ying (1991a) for left-truncated data is as follows:

$$U_{LT}(\boldsymbol{\beta}) = \sum_{i=1}^{n} \Delta_i \left\{ \boldsymbol{X}_i - \frac{\sum_{j=1}^{n} \boldsymbol{X}_j I\left(A_j e^{-\boldsymbol{X}_j^\top \boldsymbol{\beta}} \leq Y_i e^{-\boldsymbol{X}_i^\top \boldsymbol{\beta}} \leq Y_j e^{-\boldsymbol{X}_j^\top \boldsymbol{\beta}}\right)}{\sum_{j=1}^{n} I\left(A_j e^{-\boldsymbol{X}_j^\top \boldsymbol{\beta}} \leq Y_i e^{-\boldsymbol{X}_i^\top \boldsymbol{\beta}} \leq Y_j e^{-\boldsymbol{X}_j^\top \boldsymbol{\beta}}\right)} \right\}. \tag{3.18}$$

By solving equation (3.18), the vector of regression parameters denoted by $\tilde{\boldsymbol{\beta}}$ is obtained, excluding the intercept term. In this case, the intercept can be estimated using the weighted average given as

$$\beta_0 = \left\{ \sum_{i=1}^{n} \frac{\Delta_i}{\int_0^{Y_{i0}} \hat{S}_{C_0}(t)dt} \right\}^{-1} \sum_{i=1}^{n} \frac{\Delta_i \left(\log(Y_i) - \boldsymbol{X}_i^\top \tilde{\boldsymbol{\beta}} \right)}{\int_0^{Y_{i0}} \hat{S}_{C_0}(t)dt},$$

where $Y_{i0} = Y_i \exp\{-\boldsymbol{X}_i^\top \tilde{\boldsymbol{\beta}}\}$ and $\hat{S}_{C_0}(\cdot)$ is the Kaplan-Meier estimator for censoring variable $C_i \exp\{-\boldsymbol{X}_i^\top \tilde{\boldsymbol{\beta}}\}$. Due to the limitations of existing methods for handling LBRC data, researchers have made efforts to develop more efficient and accurate estimators. Shen et al. (2009) proposed an inverse weighted estimating equation (IWEE) for AFT model under LBRC data. Under the assumption that the censoring time is independent of the covariates, they showed that

$$E\left(\frac{\Delta(\log(Y) - \boldsymbol{X}^\top \boldsymbol{\beta})}{W_C(Y)} \middle| \boldsymbol{X} \right) = 0,$$

where $W_C(t)$ is defined similarly to the one used in Eq. (3.8). Thus, the regression coefficients $\boldsymbol{\beta}$ are estimated by setting the following unbiased estimating equation equal to zero:

$$U_S(\boldsymbol{\beta}) = \sum_{i=1}^{n} Q(\boldsymbol{X}_i) \Delta_i \boldsymbol{X}_i \frac{\log(Y_i) - \boldsymbol{X}_i^\top \boldsymbol{\beta}}{W_C(Y_i)},$$

where $Q(\cdot)$ is a positive, scalar weight function. Therefore, their proposed consistent and asymptotically normal estimator has a closed-form expression as follows:

$$\hat{\boldsymbol{\beta}} = \left\{ \sum_{i=1}^{n} \frac{\Delta_i \boldsymbol{X}_i \boldsymbol{X}_i^\top}{\int_0^{Y_i} \hat{S}_C(t)dt} \right\}^{-1} \sum_{i=1}^{n} \frac{\Delta_i \boldsymbol{X}_i \log(Y_i)}{\int_0^{Y_i} \hat{S}_C(t)dt}. \tag{3.19}$$

As previously mentioned, if unbiased survival time $\tilde{T}$ follows the AFT model in (3.15), then under biased sampling, T may not fall into the same family. When length-biased failure times are not subject to right-censoring, Chen (2010) and Mandel and Ritov (2010) investigated a special model of AFT. This model exhibits an invariance property under biased sampling. In fact, this property implies that T follows the same AFT model, with a particular density assumption for the error variable. They assumed $\xi = \exp(\epsilon)$, where ϵ is a random error in the biased AFT model. The density function of ξ, denoted as $f_\xi(\cdot)$, follows the length-biased density $f_\xi(y) = y f_{\tilde{\xi}}(y)/\mu_{\tilde{\xi}}$. Under this assumption and in the presence of the length-biased data (T, X), the logarithm of the biased failure time T is also expressed as $\log(T) = \boldsymbol{X}^\top \boldsymbol{\beta} + \epsilon$. It should be noted that the biased covariate $\boldsymbol{X}$ has a weighted density function given as $f_X(\boldsymbol{X}) = \exp\{\boldsymbol{X}^\top \boldsymbol{\beta}\} f_{\tilde{X}}(X)/E(\exp\{\tilde{\boldsymbol{X}}^\top \boldsymbol{\beta}\})$. Mandel and Ritov (2010) found that the least squares estimator outperformed the estimator proposed by Chen (2010) in terms of standard errors. However, neither of these methods is applicable to LBRC data.

An estimator proposed by Shen et al. (2009) has a restriction that the censoring variable is independent of the covariates. To address this limitation of their work for analyzing LBRC data, Ning et al. (2011) proposed a solution. They suggested a Buckley–James-type estimating equation as an alternative approach. The Buckley–James-type estimator is the root of the following estimating equation:

$$U_{BJ}(\beta) = \sum_{i=1}^{n} \boldsymbol{X}_i \left\{ \Delta_i \frac{\log(Y_i) - \boldsymbol{X}_i^\top \boldsymbol{\beta}}{Y_i \exp\left(-\boldsymbol{X}_i^\top \boldsymbol{\beta}\right)} + (1 - \Delta_i) \frac{\int_{Y_{i0}}^{\infty} u^{-1} \log(u) d\hat{F}_0(u; \boldsymbol{\beta})}{1 - \hat{F}_0(Y_{i0}; \boldsymbol{\beta})} \right\}, \tag{3.20}$$

where $\hat{F}_0(\cdot; \boldsymbol{\beta})$ is the nonparametric maximum likelihood estimator proposed by Vardi (1989) using transformed data $(A_{i0}, Y_{i0}) = (A_i e^{-\boldsymbol{X}_i^\top \boldsymbol{\beta}}, Y_i e^{-\boldsymbol{X}_i^\top \boldsymbol{\beta}})$.

It is worth noting that the Buckley–James method may exhibit low efficiency when random errors do not follow a normal distribution or when there is heavy censoring. Note that in AFT model the observed failure times can be transformed to identically independent distributed random variables without covariate effects. Using this property, to accommodate length-biased data Ning et al. (2014b) modified the rank-based estimating equation that was initially proposed by Lai and Ying (1991b) for general left-truncated and right-censored data as follows:

$$U_{N_I}(\boldsymbol{\beta}) = \sum_{i=1}^{n} \Delta_i \left\{ \boldsymbol{X}_i - \frac{\sum_{j=1}^{n} \boldsymbol{X}_j R\left(Y_j e^{-\boldsymbol{X}_j^\top \boldsymbol{\beta}}, Y_i e^{-\boldsymbol{X}_i^\top \boldsymbol{\beta}}\right)}{\sum_{j=1}^{n} R\left(Y_j e^{-\boldsymbol{X}_j^\top \boldsymbol{\beta}}, Y_i e^{-\boldsymbol{X}_i^\top \boldsymbol{\beta}}\right)} \right\},$$

with the at-risk set for $t_j \geq t_i$,

$$R(t_j, t_i) = \Delta_j \frac{W_C(t_j) - W_C(t_j - t_i)}{W_C(t_j)} + (1 - \Delta_j) \frac{S_C(t_j) - S_C(t_j - t_i)}{S_C(t_j)}, \tag{3.21}$$

which is similar to the at-risk set proposed by Tsai (2009) for Cox PH model under LBRC. Consistent estimators are used to substitute the unknown quantities in (3.21).

Another estimator for LBRC AFT model is based on inverse weighting and ranking estimation equation and the transformed length-biased data $\tilde{T}_0 = \tilde{T} e^{-\boldsymbol{X}^\top \boldsymbol{\beta}}$.

This estimator is an extension of Wang's (1996) work for Cox PH model. In fact under the AFT model assumption for $\tilde{T}$ and based on the Eq. (3.16), the hazard function of $\tilde{T}_0$ has the form $\lambda_{\tilde{T}_0}(t) = \lambda_{\xi}(t) = \lambda_0(t)$, which is independent of the covariates $\boldsymbol{X}$ ($\boldsymbol{\beta} = 0$). Thus, using a technique similar to that of Qin and Shen (2010) for Cox PH model, they constructed an estimating equation under AFT model for LBRC data as follows:

$$U_{N_{II}}(\boldsymbol{\beta}) = \sum_{i=1}^{n} \Delta_i \times \left\{ \boldsymbol{X}_i - \frac{\sum_{j=1}^{n} \Delta_j \boldsymbol{X}_j I\left(Y_j e^{-\boldsymbol{X}_j^{\top}\boldsymbol{\beta}} \geq Y_i e^{-\boldsymbol{X}_i^{\top}\boldsymbol{\beta}}\right) \left\{W_C(Y_j e^{-\boldsymbol{X}_j^{\top}\boldsymbol{\beta}})\right\}^{-1}}{\sum_{j=1}^{n} \Delta_j I\left(Y_j e^{-\boldsymbol{X}_j^{\top}\boldsymbol{\beta}} \geq Y_i e^{-\boldsymbol{X}_i^{\top}\boldsymbol{\beta}}\right) \left\{W_C(Y_j e^{-\boldsymbol{X}_j^{\top}\boldsymbol{\beta}})\right\}^{-1}} \right\}.$$

It should be noted that their method still needs the assumption that the censoring distribution is independent of covariates. Using transformed data and by embedding the transformed AFT model into a Cox PH model, Ning et al. (2014a) derived full likelihood function for the transformed observed data $\{Y_i e^{-\boldsymbol{X}_i^{\top}\boldsymbol{\beta}}, A_i e^{-\boldsymbol{X}_i^{\top}\boldsymbol{\beta}}, \Delta_i\}$. Their unbiased estimating equation to obtain $\boldsymbol{\beta}$ based on the Cox PH model is as follows:

$$U_{PH}(\Lambda_0, \boldsymbol{\beta}) = \sum_{i=1}^{n} \boldsymbol{X}_i \left\{ \Delta_i - \Lambda_0\left(y_i e^{-\boldsymbol{X}^{\top}\boldsymbol{\beta}_i}\right) + \frac{\int \Lambda_0(s) \exp\{-\Lambda_0(s)\}\, ds}{\int \exp\{-\Lambda_0(s)\}\, ds} \right\}. \tag{3.22}$$

The unknown baseline hazard function Λ_0 can be estimated in (3.22).

Qiu et al. (2016) suggested a rank-based estimation approach for AFT model in the presence of length-biased data, inspired by the composite partial likelihood method introduced by Huang and Qin (2012). They considered the transformed data $\log(\tilde{T}_i) - \boldsymbol{X}_i^{\top}\boldsymbol{\beta}$ and embedded the transformed AFT model into a Cox PH model to construct an estimation equation. Let $K(\cdot)$ be a cumulative distribution function on the real line such that it is nondecreasing and satisfies $\lim_{u \to +\infty} K(u)du \to 1$ and $\lim_{u \to -\infty} K(u)du \to 0$. In order to find a consistent solution in practice, they obtained a smoothed composite estimating equation as follows:

$$U_n(\boldsymbol{\beta}) = \sum_{i=1}^{n} \Delta_i \left\{ \boldsymbol{X}_i - \frac{\sum_{j=1}^{n} \boldsymbol{X}_j a_{ij}}{\sum_{j=1}^{n} a_{ij}} \right\},$$

where

$$a_{ij} = \left\{ K\left(\frac{Y_j^* - Y_i^*}{h_n}\right) - K\left(\frac{A_j^* - Y_i^*}{h_n}\right) \right\} + \Delta_j \left\{ K\left(\frac{Y_j^* - Y_i^*}{h_n}\right) - K\left(\frac{\tilde{V}_j^* - Y_i^*}{h_n}\right) \right\},$$

with the transformed data

$$\left(A_i^*, Y_i^*, \tilde{V}_i^*\right) = \left(\log(A_i) - \boldsymbol{X}_i^\top \boldsymbol{\beta}, \log(Y_i) - \boldsymbol{X}_i^\top \boldsymbol{\beta}, \log(\tilde{V}_i) - \boldsymbol{X}_i^\top \boldsymbol{\beta}\right).$$

Their suggested approach exhibits a straightforward structure and demonstrates robustness even when the censoring times and covariates are dependent.

By following Huang and Qin (2012), Chen et al. (2017) proposed a kernel-smoothed composite likelihood method for $\boldsymbol{\beta}$. The resulting approach is more efficient and has computational simplicity because the optimization of the log composite likelihood function can be easily implemented by existing procedures. According to (3.13) and (3.16), the composite conditional likelihood under AFT model takes form

$$L_C(\boldsymbol{\beta}, \Lambda_{\tilde{\xi}}) = \frac{1}{n}\prod_{i=1}^{n} \frac{\left[\lambda_{\tilde{\xi}}\left(Y_i e^{-\boldsymbol{\beta}^\top \tilde{X}}\right) e^{-\boldsymbol{\beta}^\top \tilde{X}}\right]^{2\Delta_i} \exp\left\{-(1+\Delta_i)\Lambda_{\tilde{\xi}}\left(Y_i e^{-\boldsymbol{\beta}^\top \tilde{X}}\right)\right\}}{\exp\left\{-\Lambda_{\tilde{\xi}}\left(A_i e^{-\boldsymbol{\beta}^\top \tilde{X}}\right) - \Delta_i \Lambda_{\tilde{\xi}}\left(\tilde{V}_i e^{-\boldsymbol{\beta}^\top \tilde{X}}\right)\right\}}.$$

3.4.3 Simulation Study for AFT Model

In this section, we assessed the performance of various estimators for AFT model and compared them with the estimator obtained from the estimating equation for the traditional survival data in (3.17). To conduct a simulation study, we considered AFT model in (3.15) with two independent covariates: X_1 was generated from a Bernoulli distribution with $P(X_1 = 1) = 0.5$ and X_2 from a uniform distribution (0, 1). The distribution of random error, $\tilde{\epsilon}$, was assumed to be Uniform $(-0.5, 0.5)$ and a normal distribution with mean zero and standard deviation 0.3. The true values of $\boldsymbol{\beta}$ were considered $(1, 0.5, 1)$ and $(1, 1, 1)$. To generate length-biased simulation data, we followed the instruction provided in Sect. 3.3.3. The residual censoring variables measured from the examination time (C_i) were generated from uniform distribution for various censoring percentages 10%, 30%, and 50%. The cohort sample sizes of 100 and 200 were considered with 1000 repetitions.

We considered the following approaches for estimating AFT regression coefficients in the presence of length-biased data: (i) the classical estimating equation (Classic) (Prentice, 1978), (ii) the rank-based estimator for left-truncated data (LT) (Lai & Ying, 1991b), (iii) IWEE estimator (Shen et al., 2009), (iv) Buckley–James (BJ) estimator Ning et al. (2011), And (v) the two estimators of Ning et al. (2014b,a) (N_I and N_{II}).

The results include the empirical bias, the empirical standard deviation, and 95% confidence interval for obtained estimates. Based on the results presented in Tables 3.3, 3.4, 3.5 and 3.6, the following conclusions can be drawn:

- The estimator LT that considers left-truncation time has been found to have better performance compared to the classic estimator.

Table 3.3 Simulation results for AFT model for true coefficients $\beta = (1, 0.5, 1)$ and uniform error distribution

			$n = 100$			$n = 200$		
β	C%	Methods	Bias	SE	Coef 95% CIs	Bias	SE	Coef 95% CIs
(1,0.5,1)	10%	Classic	0.0881	0.0481	(0.99, 1.18)	0.0884	0.0347	(1.02, 1.16)
			0.0015	0.0619	(0.38, 0.62)	0.0026	0.0442	(0.42, 0.59)
			−0.0007	0.1082	(0.79, 1.21)	0.0067	0.0811	(0.85, 1.17)
		LT	0.0027	0.0502	(0.90, 1.10)	−0.0005	0.0366	(0.93, 1.07)
			0.0015	0.0619	(0.38, 0.62)	0.0026	0.0442	(0.42, 0.59)
			−0.0007	0.1082	(0.79, 1.21)	0.0067	0.0811	(0.85, 1.17)
		IWEE	0.0033	0.0529	(0.90, 1.11)	0.0015	0.0383	(0.93, 1.08)
			0.0006	0.0681	(0.37, 0.63)	0.0002	0.0478	(0.41, 0.59)
			−0.0002	0.1210	(0.76, 1.24)	0.0013	0.0871	(0.83, 1.17)
		BJ	0.0015	0.0518	(0.90, 1.10)	−0.0001	0.0486	(0.90, 1.10)
			−0.0021	0.0707	(0.36, 0.64)	−0.0015	0.0464	(0.41, 0.59)
			−0.0031	0.1310	(0.74, 1.25)	−0.0009	0.0832	(0.84, 1.16)
		NI	−0.4903	8.3633	(−15.88, 16.9)	−0.1435	5.3186	(−9.57, 11.28)
			0.0016	0.0623	(0.38, 0.62)	0.0026	0.0444	(0.42, 0.59)
			−0.0005	0.1084	(0.79, 1.21)	0.0068	0.0812	(0.85, 1.17)
		NII	0.3783	4.5156	(−7.47, 10.23)	0.3028	4.9264	(−8.35, 10.96)
			0.0014	0.0624	(0.38, 0.62)	0.0027	0.0445	(0.42, 0.59)
			−0.0005	0.1084	(0.79, 1.21)	0.0067	0.0812	(0.85, 1.17)
	30%	Classic	0.1265	0.0601	(1.01, 1.24)	0.1334	0.0445	(1.05, 1.22)
			−0.0126	0.0767	(0.34, 0.64)	0.0065	0.0553	(0.40, 0.62)
			−0.0401	0.1333	(0.70, 1.22)	−0.0051	0.0945	(0.81, 1.18)
		LT	0.0126	0.0585	(0.90, 1.13)	0.0009	0.0429	(0.92, 1.09)
			−0.0126	0.0767	(0.34, 0.64)	0.0065	0.0553	(0.40, 0.62)
			−0.0401	0.1333	(0.70, 1.22)	−0.0051	0.0945	(0.81, 1.18)
		IWEE	0.0052	0.0588	(0.89, 1.12)	0.0030	0.0400	(0.92, 1.08)
			−0.0053	0.0767	(0.34, 0.65)	0.0004	0.0506	(0.40, 0.60)
			−0.0157	0.1325	(0.72, 1.24)	−0.0042	0.0916	(0.82, 1.18)
		BJ	−0.0284	0.8192	(−0.63, 2.58)	−0.0026	0.0719	(0.86, 1.14)
			−0.0187	0.5565	(−0.61, 1.57)	0.0009	0.0483	(0.41, 0.60)
			−0.0072	0.1489	(0.70, 1.28)	−0.0009	0.0879	(0.83, 1.17)
		NI	−0.4188	9.9386	(−18.9, 20.06)	−0.1166	4.4218	(−7.78, 9.55)
			−0.0126	0.0797	(0.33, 0.64)	0.0074	0.0584	(0.39, 0.62)
			−0.0395	0.1360	(0.69, 1.23)	−0.0043	0.0961	(0.81, 1.18)
		NII	0.6270	6.4368	(−10.99, 14.24)	0.8475	8.3164	(−14.45, 18.15)
			−0.0129	0.0770	(0.34, 0.64)	0.0067	0.0552	(0.40, 0.62)
			−0.0405	0.1341	(0.70, 1.22)	−0.0050	0.0955	(0.81, 1.18)

(continued)

Table 3.3 (continued)

$\boldsymbol{\beta}$	C%	Methods	$n = 100$			$n = 200$		
			Bias	SE	Coef 95% CIs	Bias	SE	Coef 95% CIs
	50%	Classic	0.2127	0.0760	(1.06, 1.36)	0.2753	0.0609	(1.16, 1.39)
			−0.0963	0.0862	(0.23, 0.57)	−0.1172	0.0613	(0.26, 0.50)
			−0.1927	0.1562	(0.50, 1.11)	−0.2290	0.1217	(0.53, 1.01)
		LT	0.0575	0.0637	(0.93, 1.18)	0.0723	0.0449	(0.98, 1.16)
			−0.0963	0.0862	(0.23, 0.57)	−0.1172	0.0613	(0.26, 0.5)
			−0.1927	0.1562	(0.50, 1.11)	−0.2290	0.1217	(0.53, 1.01)
		IWEE	0.0036	0.0611	(0.88, 1.12)	0.0024	0.0430	(0.92, 1.09)
			−0.0112	0.0834	(0.33, 0.65)	−0.0055	0.0585	(0.38, 0.61)
			−0.0198	0.1419	(0.70, 1.26)	−0.0074	0.1065	(0.78, 1.2)
		BJ	−0.0688	0.6843	(−0.41, 2.27)	−0.0484	0.1642	(0.63, 1.27)
			−0.0571	0.5077	(−0.55, 1.44)	−0.0833	0.2283	(−0.03, 0.86)
			−0.0621	0.4074	(0.14, 1.74)	−0.1348	0.3842	(0.11, 1.62)
		NI	0.2061	23.5415	(−44.94, 47.35)	0.1721	2.7072	(−4.13, 6.48)
			−0.0616	1.2252	(−1.96, 2.84)	−0.1234	0.1347	(0.11, 0.64)
			0.4640	19.9014	(−37.54, 40.47)	−0.2436	0.1518	(0.46, 1.05)
		NII	0.7186	17.0357	(−31.67, 35.11)	1.8401	10.6543	(−18.04, 23.72)
			−0.0972	0.0868	(0.23, 0.57)	−0.1165	0.0622	(0.26, 0.51)
			−0.1925	0.1588	(0.50, 1.12)	−0.2310	0.1236	(0.53, 1.01)

Table 3.4 Simulation results for AFT model for true coefficients $\beta = (1, 1, 1)$ and uniform error distribution

β	C%	Methods	$n = 100$			$n = 200$		
			Bias	SE	Coef 95% CIs	Bias	SE	Coef 95% CIs
(1,1,1)	10%	Classic	0.0858	0.0563	(0.98, 1.20)	0.0888	0.0391	(1.01, 1.17)
			0.0058	0.0668	(0.87, 1.14)	0.0052	0.0468	(0.91, 1.10)
			0.0022	0.1116	(0.78, 1.22)	0.0023	0.0808	(0.84, 1.16)
		LT	0.0003	0.0589	(0.88, 1.12)	0.0008	0.0413	(0.92, 1.08)
			0.0058	0.0668	(0.87, 1.14)	0.0052	0.0468	(0.91, 1.10)
			0.0022	0.1116	(0.78, 1.22)	0.0023	0.0808	(0.84, 1.16)
		IWEE	0.0059	0.0618	(0.88, 1.13)	0.0067	0.0440	(0.92, 1.09)
			−0.0014	0.0719	(0.86, 1.14)	−0.0025	0.0521	(0.90, 1.10)
			−0.0003	0.1315	(0.74, 1.26)	−0.0038	0.0936	(0.81, 1.18)
		BJ	−0.0239	0.8877	(−0.76, 2.72)	0.0048	0.0515	(0.90, 1.11)
			−0.0248	0.7156	(−0.43, 2.38)	−0.0048	0.0551	(0.89, 1.10)
			0.0011	0.1457	(0.72, 1.29)	−0.0020	0.0889	(0.82, 1.17)
		NI	0.0858	0.0563	(0.98, 1.20)	−0.1429	7.3263	(−13.5, 15.22)
			0.0060	0.0674	(0.87, 1.14)	0.0053	0.0471	(0.91, 1.10)
			0.0022	0.1119	(0.78, 1.22)	0.0024	0.0809	(0.84, 1.16)
		NII	0.2112	3.0440	(−4.76, 7.18)	0.4056	8.2692	(−14.8, 17.61)
			0.0059	0.0673	(0.87, 1.14)	0.0052	0.0470	(0.91, 1.10)
			0.0022	0.1120	(0.78, 1.22)	0.0024	0.0810	(0.84, 1.16)

(continued)

Table 3.4 (continued)

			$n = 100$			$n = 200$		
β	C%	Methods	Bias	SE	Coef 95% CIs	Bias	SE	Coef 95% CIs
	30%	Classic	0.1045	0.0631	(0.98,1.23)	0.0997	0.0427	(1.02, 1.18)
			0.0223	0.0802	(0.87,1.18)	0.0508	0.0613	(0.93, 1.17)
			−0.0691	0.1388	(0.66,1.20)	−0.0294	0.1025	(0.77, 1.17)
		LT	−0.0069	0.0691	(0.86,1.13)	−0.0306	0.0504	(0.87, 1.07)
			0.0223	0.0802	(0.87,1.18)	0.0508	0.0613	(0.93, 1.17)
			−0.0691	0.1388	(0.66,1.20)	−0.0294	0.1025	(0.77, 1.17)
		IWEE	0.0057	0.0676	(0.87,1.14)	0.0016	0.0458	(0.91, 1.09)
			−0.0042	0.0796	(0.84,1.15)	−0.0005	0.056	(0.89, 1.11)
			−0.0132	0.1377	(0.72,1.26)	−0.0054	0.1016	(0.80, 1.19)
		BJ	−0.3347	10.6455	(-20.2,21.53)	−0.0846	2.2138	(−3.42, 5.25)
			−0.2432	7.6803	(-14.3,15.81)	−0.0550	1.4381	(−1.87, 3.76)
			−0.0195	0.5086	(-0.02,1.98)	−0.0043	0.1684	(0.67, 1.33)
		NI	−1.2732	20.6536	(-40.75,40.21)	−1.3035	17.0627	(−33.75, 33.14)
			0.0229	0.0810	(0.86,1.18)	0.0532	0.0698	(0.92, 1.19)
			−0.0695	0.1398	(0.66,1.20)	−0.0287	0.1055	(0.76, 1.18)
		NII	0.4876	15.5904	(-29.07,32.04)	0.7146	8.024	(−14.01, 17.44)
			0.0251	0.1151	(0.80,1.25)	0.0512	0.0615	(0.93, 1.17)
			−0.0689	0.1399	(0.66,1.21)	−0.0299	0.1029	(0.77, 1.17)
	50%	Classic	0.1671	0.0837	(1.00,1.33)	0.1874	0.0672	(1.06, 1.32)
			−0.0418	0.1019	(0.76,1.16)	−0.0212	0.0796	(0.82, 1.13)
			−0.2395	0.1730	(0.42,1.10)	−0.3111	0.1225	(0.45, 0.93)
		LT	0.0342	0.0787	(0.88,1.19)	0.0249	0.0628	(0.90, 1.15)
			−0.0418	0.1019	(0.76,1.16)	−0.0212	0.0796	(0.82, 1.13)
			−0.2395	0.1730	(0.42,1.10)	−0.3111	0.1225	(0.45, 0.93)
		IWEE	0.0076	0.0685	(0.87,1.14)	0.0044	0.0487	(0.91, 1.10)
			−0.0136	0.0863	(0.82,1.16)	−0.0076	0.0598	(0.88, 1.11)
			−0.0219	0.1533	(0.68,1.28)	−0.0075	0.1073	(0.78, 1.20)
		BJ	−0.0520	0.2276	(0.50,1.39)	−0.0157	0.1250	(0.74, 1.23)
			−0.0484	0.2555	(0.45,1.45)	−0.0378	0.2147	(0.54, 1.38)
			−0.0511	0.3794	(0.21,1.69)	−0.0488	0.3301	(0.30, 1.60)
		NI	−0.8160	11.5691	(−22.49,22.86)	−0.3965	6.4394	(−12.02, 13.22)
			0.3429	10.1086	(−18.47,21.16)	0.5159	16.9633	(−31.73, 34.76)
			0.1422	10.2247	(−18.9,21.18)	0.2802	18.8301	(−35.63, 38.19)
		NII	1.4426	25.7344	(−48,52.88)	2.2503	15.1541	(−26.45, 32.95)
			−0.0355	0.2199	(0.53,1.40)	−0.0211	0.0794	(0.82, 1.13)
			−0.2396	0.1734	(0.42,1.10)	−0.3101	0.1253	(0.44, 0.94)

Table 3.5 Simulation results for AFT model with true coefficients $\beta = (1, 0.5, 1)$ and normal error distribution

			$n = 100$			$n = 200$		
β	C%	Methods	Bias	SE	Coef 95% CIs	Bias	SE	Coef 95% CIs
(1,0.5,1)	10%	Classic	0.0986	0.0534	(0.99, 1.20)	0.0984	0.0381	(1.02, 1.17)
			0.0012	0.0656	(0.37, 0.63)	0.0005	0.0482	(0.41, 0.60)
			−0.0078	0.1190	(0.76, 1.23)	0.0054	0.0820	(0.84, 1.17)
		LT	0.0060	0.0552	(0.90, 1.11)	0.0016	0.0394	(0.92, 1.08)
			0.0012	0.0656	(0.37, 0.63)	0.0005	0.0482	(0.41, 0.60)
			−0.0078	0.1190	(0.76, 1.23)	0.0054	0.0820	(0.84, 1.17)
		IWEE	0.0067	0.0569	(0.9, 1.12)	0.0042	0.0408	(0.92, 1.08)
			−0.0001	0.0698	(0.36, 0.64)	−0.0033	0.0511	(0.40, 0.60)
			−0.0086	0.1284	(0.74, 1.24)	−0.0009	0.0870	(0.83, 1.17)
		BJ	0.0034	0.0658	(0.87, 1.13)	0.0029	0.0395	(0.93, 1.08)
			0.0001	0.0676	(0.37, 0.63)	−0.0035	0.0487	(0.40, 0.59)
			−0.0035	0.1227	(0.76, 1.24)	0.0003	0.0823	(0.84, 1.16)
		NI	0.0168	2.4016	(−3.69, 5.72)	0.0771	1.8090	(−2.47, 4.62)
			0.0013	0.0657	(0.37, 0.63)	0.0006	0.0483	(0.41, 0.60)
			−0.0076	0.1191	(0.76, 1.23)	0.0055	0.0820	(0.84, 1.17)
		NII	0.2493	3.0006	(−4.63, 7.13)	0.1864	1.9845	(−2.7, 5.08)
			0.0013	0.0657	(0.37, 0.63)	0.0005	0.0484	(0.41, 0.60)
			−0.0076	0.1189	(0.76, 1.23)	0.0055	0.0820	(0.84, 1.17)
	30%	Classic	0.1483	0.0733	(1.00, 1.29)	0.1566	0.0605	(1.04, 1.28)
			−0.0219	0.0865	(0.31, 0.65)	−0.0087	0.0699	(0.35, 0.63)
			−0.0513	0.1485	(0.66, 1.24)	−0.0290	0.1097	(0.76, 1.19)
		LT	0.0224	0.0667	(0.89, 1.15)	0.0083	0.0514	(0.91, 1.11)
			−0.0219	0.0865	(0.31, 0.65)	−0.0087	0.0699	(0.35, 0.63)
			−0.0513	0.1485	(0.66, 1.24)	−0.0290	0.1097	(0.76, 1.19)
		IWEE	0.0088	0.0641	(0.88, 1.13)	0.0022	0.0435	(0.92, 1.09)
			−0.0051	0.0826	(0.33, 0.66)	−0.0022	0.0550	(0.39, 0.61)
			−0.0044	0.1438	(0.71, 1.28)	−0.0058	0.0944	(0.81, 1.18)
		BJ	0.0037	0.0872	(0.83, 1.17)	−0.0031	0.0791	(0.84, 1.15)
			−0.0031	0.0773	(0.35, 0.65)	0.0003	0.0526	(0.40, 0.60)
			0.0027	0.1343	(0.74, 1.27)	0.0024	0.0889	(0.83, 1.18)
		NI	0.1448	7.9973	(−14.53, 16.82)	0.0879	5.4406	(−9.58, 11.75)
			−0.0113	0.3395	(−0.18, 1.15)	−0.0016	1.6197	(−2.68, 3.67)
			−0.0639	0.4187	(0.12, 1.76)	−0.0107	2.2075	(−3.34, 5.32)
		NII	0.3794	3.7077	(−5.89, 8.65)	0.1979	0.9553	(−0.67, 3.07)
			−0.0220	0.0867	(0.31, 0.65)	−0.0085	0.0702	(0.35, 0.63)
			−0.0511	0.1487	(0.66, 1.24)	−0.0290	0.1097	(0.76, 1.19)

(continued)

Table 3.5 (continued)

β	C%	Methods	$n = 100$ Bias	SE	Coef 95% CIs	$n = 200$ Bias	SE	Coef 95% CIs
	50%	Classic	0.2300	0.0896	(1.05, 1.41)	0.2936	0.0752	(1.15, 1.44)
			−0.1021	0.0972	(0.21, 0.59)	−0.1297	0.0732	(0.23, 0.51)
			−0.2096	0.1785	(0.44, 1.14)	−0.2548	0.1430	(0.46, 1.03)
		LT	0.0631	0.0703	(0.93, 1.20)	0.0795	0.0521	(0.98, 1.18)
			−0.1021	0.0972	(0.21, 0.59)	−0.1297	0.0732	(0.23, 0.51)
			−0.2096	0.1785	(0.44, 1.14)	−0.2548	0.1430	(0.46, 1.03)
		IWEE	0.0065	0.0640	(0.88, 1.13)	0.0036	0.0453	(0.91, 1.09)
			−0.0106	0.0886	(0.32, 0.66)	−0.0060	0.0604	(0.38, 0.61)
			−0.0245	0.1535	(0.67, 1.28)	−0.0078	0.1110	(0.77, 1.21)
		BJ	−0.0473	0.2271	(0.51, 1.40)	−0.0055	0.0965	(0.81, 1.18)
			−0.0406	0.2088	(0.05, 0.87)	−0.0110	0.1278	(0.24, 0.74)
			−0.0690	0.3979	(0.15, 1.71)	−0.0184	0.2455	(0.50, 1.46)
		NI	−1.0799	28.0014	(−54.96, 54.8)	−0.1992	9.2719	(−17.37, 18.97)
			0.0047	1.7551	(−2.94, 3.94)	−0.1578	2.4776	(−4.51, 5.20)
			−0.0434	4.0893	(−7.06, 8.97)	−0.1697	5.4085	(−9.77, 11.43)
		NII	1.1381	6.6702	(−10.94, 15.21)	1.6155	10.5817	(−18.12, 23.36)
			−0.1027	0.0985	(0.20, 0.59)	−0.1289	0.0739	(0.23, 0.52)
			−0.2109	0.1812	(0.43, 1.14)	−0.2543	0.1449	(0.46, 1.03)

Table 3.6 Simulation results for AFT model with true coefficients $\beta = (1, 1, 1)$ and normal error distribution

β	C%	Methods	$n = 100$ Bias	SE	Coef 95% CIs	$n = 200$ Bias	SE	Coef 95% CIs
(1,1,1)	10%	Classic	0.0920	0.0600	(0.97, 1.21)	0.0931	0.0432	(1.01, 1.18)
			0.0083	0.0729	(0.87, 1.15)	0.0088	0.0534	(0.90, 1.11)
			−0.0026	0.1173	(0.77, 1.23)	0.0002	0.0873	(0.83, 1.17)
		LT	−0.0019	0.0619	(0.88, 1.12)	−0.0031	0.0452	(0.91, 1.08)
			0.0083	0.0729	(0.87, 1.15)	0.0088	0.0533	(0.90, 1.11)
			−0.0026	0.1173	(0.77, 1.23)	−0.0002	0.0872	(0.83, 1.17)
		IWEE	0.0049	0.0650	(0.88, 1.13)	0.0011	0.0473	(0.91, 1.09)
			−0.0013	0.0782	(0.85, 1.15)	0.0027	0.0574	(0.89, 1.12)
			−0.0057	0.1325	(0.73, 1.25)	0.0006	0.0971	(0.81, 1.19)
		BJ	0.0007	0.0711	(0.86, 1.14)	−0.0001	0.0562	(0.89, 1.11)
			0.0001	0.0760	(0.85, 1.15)	0.0009	0.0500	(0.89, 1.11)
			0.0004	0.1190	(0.77, 1.23)	−0.0005	0.0870	(0.83, 1.17)
		NI	−0.2513	7.9938	(−14.92, 16.42)	−0.0007	2.9691	(−4.82, 6.82)
			0.0085	0.0730	(0.87, 1.15)	0.0090	0.0530	(0.90, 1.11)
			−0.0026	0.1173	(0.77, 1.23)	−0.0002	0.0872	(0.83, 1.17)
		NII	0.0151	3.1637	(−5.19, 7.22)	0.0931	0.0431	(1.01, 1.18)
			0.0085	0.0730	(0.87, 1.15)	0.0090	0.0530	(0.90, 1.11)
			−0.0026	0.1173	(0.77, 1.23)	−0.0002	0.0870	(0.83, 1.17)

(continued)

Table 3.6 (continued)

			$n = 100$			$n = 200$		
β	C%	Methods	Bias	SE	$Coef95\%CIs$	Bias	SE	$Coef95\%CIs$
	30%	Classic	0.1228	0.0744	(0.98, 1.27)	0.1209	0.0562	(1.01, 1.23)
			0.0099	0.0930	(0.83, 1.19)	0.0427	0.0733	(0.90, 1.19)
			-0.0802	0.1459	(0.63, 1.21)	-0.0701	0.1191	(0.70, 1.16)
		LT	0.0014	0.0756	(0.85, 1.15)	-0.0247	0.0593	(0.86, 1.09)
			0.0099	0.0930	(0.83, 1.19)	0.0427	0.0734	(0.90, 1.19)
			-0.0802	0.1459	(0.63, 1.21)	-0.0701	0.1194	(0.70, 1.16)
		IWEE	0.0078	0.0692	(0.87, 1.14)	0.0031	0.0492	(0.91, 1.1)
			-0.0068	0.0830	(0.83, 1.16)	-0.0039	0.0600	(0.88, 1.11)
			-0.0113	0.1439	(0.71, 1.27)	-0.0078	0.1011	(0.79, 1.19)
		BJ	0.0061	0.0680	(0.87, 1.14)	0.0019	0.0583	(0.89, 1.11)
			-0.0052	0.0804	(0.84, 1.15)	-0.0045	0.0581	(0.88, 1.11)
			0.0011	0.1329	(0.74, 1.26)	-0.0016	0.0952	(0.81, 1.18)
		NI	-1.1736	15.267	(−30.1, 29.75)	-0.7318	10.514	(−20.34, 20.88)
			0.0116	0.0961	(0.82, 1.20)	0.0432	0.0730	(0.90, 1.19)
			-0.0799	0.1463	(0.63, 1.21)	-0.0701	0.1200	(0.70, 1.16)
		NII	0.5556	10.3403	(−18.71, 21.82)	0.7501	7.9910	(−13.91, 17.41)
			0.0102	0.0936	(0.83, 1.19)	0.0428	0.0740	(0.90, 1.19)
			-0.0804	0.1457	(0.63, 1.21)	-0.0699	0.1200	(0.70, 1.16)
	50%	Classic	0.1972	0.1133	(0.98, 1.42)	0.2427	0.1163	(1.01, 1.47)
			−0.0730	0.1216	(0.69, 1.17)	−0.0736	0.1232	(0.69, 1.17)
			−0.2228	0.1814	(0.42, 1.13)	−0.2946	0.1424	(0.43, 0.98)
		LT	0.0530	0.0901	(0.88, 1.23)	0.0559	0.0892	(0.88, 1.23)
			−0.0730	0.1216	(0.69, 1.17)	−0.0736	0.1231	(0.69, 1.17)
			−0.2228	0.1814	(0.42, 1.13)	−0.2946	0.1424	(0.43, 0.98)
		IWEE	0.0064	0.0676	(0.87, 1.14)	0.0018	0.0540	(0.9, 1.11)
			−0.0110	0.0835	(0.83, 1.15)	−0.0038	0.0670	(0.87, 1.13)
			−0.0230	0.1620	(0.66, 1.29)	−0.0037	0.1112	(0.78, 1.21)
		BJ	−0.0408	0.2039	(0.56, 1.36)	−0.0157	0.1310	(0.73, 1.24)
			−0.0581	0.2592	(0.43, 1.45)	−0.0167	0.2043	(0.58, 1.38)
			−0.0792	0.3847	(0.17, 1.67)	−0.0211	0.3263	(0.34, 1.62)
		NI	−1.2266	17.6903	(−34.9, 34.45)	0.3371	11.204	(−20.61, 23.28)
			0.5072	12.8461	(−23.67, 26.69)	−0.2020	2.8131	(−4.72, 6.31)
			0.4004	14.6918	(−27.4, 30.2)	−0.6171	5.9630	(−11.3, 12.07)
		NII	0.6812	17.1098	(−31.85, 35.22)	2.2663	21.822	(−39.51, 46.04)
			−0.0889	0.5350	(−0.14, 1.96)	−0.0741	0.1231	(0.68, 1.17)
			−0.2690	1.6758	(−2.55, 4.02)	−0.2943	0.1431	(0.43, 0.99)

- For the sample size of 100, the results are different according to the assumed error distribution. In this case, when the error has uniform distribution, IWEE estimator has the best performance in terms of bias and SE. When the error distribution is normal, BJ is the best.
- The two estimators, N_I and N_{II}, do not offer a reliable estimate for the intercept term.
- In general, without any knowledge about the error distribution, when the sample size increases, the BJ has the best performance in the presence of moderate censoring. When the censoring rate is heavy, IWEE estimator outperforms others.
- It is obvious that by increasing n, the bias and standard error of estimates decrease.
- As expected, by increasing the censoring rate, the bias and standard error of estimates increase.

3.5 Real Data Analysis

In this section, we analyze the Channing House data (Hyde, 1980) with the proposed methods. The Channing House is a retirement center in Palo Alto, California, which includes ages of 462 retirees (97 men and 365 women) at entry and at the termination of the study, from January 1964 to July 1975. To accommodate the length-biased concept, only the elders aged 65 years or older as the target group of interest were considered. Based on a formal test proposed by Addona and Wolfson (2006) (which is available in "CoxPhLB" package in R), it can be found that a subset includes the people older than 65 years at entry and is a length-biased dataset (p-value = 0.794). There are 450 people included in this subset. According to the record, there were 44 men and 128 women who died at Channing House; therefore the censoring rate is 62%.

To investigate whether the gender affects the risk of survival of retirees in the length biased subset, we assumed both Cox PH and AFT models to find the best regression model. In this dataset, the covariate is a binary variable in which $X = 1$ indicates a male subject as the reference. To compute the standard error for this dataset, we employed a bootstrap sample with a size of B = 200.

Table 3.7 shows the results for different estimating approaches for Cox PH and AFT models. According to the obtained results from simulation studies for Cox PH model, we consider the CPL results as the best. Therefore, the coefficient estimate value is −0.194 with standard error 0.145, which shows the risk of survival for men is greater than women, namely women survived longer than men in Channing House. Moreover, due to the obtained confidence interval (−0.477,0.09) which contains zero, the above conclusion is nonsignificant.

For the AFT model, as mentioned in Sect. 3.4.3, Shen's estimators outperform the others under high censoring. The corresponding results are reported here, providing coefficient estimates of 2.791 for the intercept and 0.003 for the gender covariate. The standard error of the second estimator is 0.081. Utilizing the bootstrap method,

Table 3.7 Comparison the implementation of traditional and length-biased methods for the Channing House dataset

	Cox PH model			
	Coef	exp(coef)	SE(coef)	Coef 95%CIs
Classic	−0.166	0.847	0.176	(−0.511,0.179)
PL	−0.265	0.767	0.188	(−0.634,0.104)
QSI	−0.147	0.864	0.156	(−0.451,0.158)
QSII	−0.111	0.895	0.167	(−0.444,0.221)
CPL	−0.194	0.824	0.145	(−0.477,0.090)
	AFT model			
	Intercept	Coef	SE(coef)	Coef 95%CIs
Classic	2.798	0.035	0.060	(−0.061,0.175)
LY	2.735	0.035	0.063	(−0.066,0.180)
IWEE	2.791	0.003	0.081	(−0.100,0.147)
BJ	2.846	0.014	0.089	(−0.128,0.219)
NI	2.798	0.035	0.094	(−0.118,0.239)
NII	2.799	0.040	0.091	(−0.108,0.237)

the 95% confidence interval is $(-0.1, 0.147)$. These results suggest that gender does not significantly impact survival time in the Channing House.

3.6 Miscellaneous

In addition to Cox PH and AFT models, other regression models have been proposed in the literature for LBRC data. Moreover, in analyzing LBRC data, one can face some challenges such as missing data, time-varying covariates, and varying coefficient. In this section, first, we briefly introduce the other regression models of LBRC data including additive hazard and linear transformation models. Second, we address the possible challenges in analyzing LBRC data.

3.6.1 *Other Regression Models*

Additive Hazards Model

The additive hazards model is a useful alternative to Cox PH model, which focuses on modeling the difference in the risk (Aalen, 1980; Cox & Oakes, 1984; Thomas, 1986). It is also known as Aalen's additive model. The formulation of the additive hazards model is given by

$$\lambda(t|\boldsymbol{X}) = \lambda_0(t) + \tilde{\boldsymbol{X}}^{\mathsf{T}}\boldsymbol{\beta},$$

where $\tilde{\boldsymbol{X}}$ is a vector of the covariates, $\lambda_0(t)$ is the unspecified baseline hazard function, and β is a p-dimensional vector of parameters. In the presence of left-truncation and right-censoring, a few methods are available in the literature to estimate the parameters of additive hazards model including the conditional estimating equation (Huang & Qin, 2013) and the pseudo-likelihood inference (Chen, 2019). For LBRC data, Ma et al. (2015) proposed composite estimators for the additive risk model under length-biased sampling. For the other references, see Shen (2009), Zhao et al. (2017), Zhang et al. (2018), and Yang et al. (2023).

Linear Transformation Model

Under the transformation model, it is assumed that the survival time $\tilde{T}$ is linearly related to the covariates with a specified error distribution (Cheng et al., 1995), namely

$$H(\tilde{T}) = -\tilde{\boldsymbol{X}}^{\mathsf{T}}\boldsymbol{\beta} + \epsilon,$$

where $H(\cdot)$ is an unknown increasing transformation function, $\tilde{\boldsymbol{X}}$ represents the vector of covariates, $\boldsymbol{\beta}$ is the vector of regression coefficients, and ϵ is the error term following a specified distribution and is independent of $\tilde{\boldsymbol{X}}$. Unlike the AFT models, the transformation model does explicitly specify the distribution of ϵ (Dabrowska & Doksum, 1988; Cheng et al., 1995; Fine, 1999). The most commonly used forms of $H(\cdot)$ are the log transformation, the identity transformation, and the Box-Cox transformation. This model also reduces to Cox PH model and the proportional odds model when ϵ has an extreme value distribution and a logistic distribution, respectively.

Shen et al. (2009) proposed an unbiased estimating equation for LBRC data based on the ranks of observed failure times. They assumed that the censoring variable C is independent of the covariates. Wang and Wang (2015) proposed a new estimator obtained from counting process-based unbiased estimating equations. The proposed method is robust when the censoring time depends on covariates. Ma et al. (2016) developed a weighted estimating equation for the case-cohort design with length-biased and right-censored data. Their approach estimates the regression parameters and the transformation function H simultaneously, which can be used even when the censoring variable and covariates are dependent.

3.6.2 *Challenges*

Missing Covariates

In clinical and epidemiological studies, missing data in some components of the covariate vector can pose challenges when applying regression models, directly. There are several studies in the literature which have addressed the problem of coefficient estimation in traditional Cox PH model with missing covariates (see Paik

& Tsai, 1997; Lipsitz & Ibrahim, 1998; Rathouz, 2007). However, these estimating methods are not applicable in the presence of LBRC data. Hu et al. (2015) extended the composite partial likelihood approach of Huang and Qin (2012) for LBRC data to accommodate missing covariates.

Varying Coefficient

Sometimes an exposure variable is included in the regression model to assess its impact on the outcome and to control the potential confounding factors. The duration of treatment, the level of environmental pollution, and the amount of time spent engaging in a specific behavior are some examples of exposure variables.

Effects of confounding factors and exposure variables on the hazard function can change with the grade of an exposure variable represented by W. Fan et al. (2006) proposed the following Cox PH model with varying coefficients for traditional survival data:

$$\lambda(t|\tilde{\boldsymbol{X}}, W) = \lambda_0(t) \exp\{\tilde{\boldsymbol{X}}^{\mathsf{T}} \boldsymbol{\beta}(W) + g(W)\}, \tag{3.23}$$

where $\boldsymbol{\beta}(\cdot)$ and $g(\cdot)$ are unknown coefficient functions, describing the extent to which the association varies with the continuous exposure variable W. In the presence of LBRC data, Zhang et al. (2014) considered this model and proposed a local estimating equation approach using the method proposed by Qin and Shen (2010). Xu and Zhou (2019) proposed a local composite likelihood procedure to estimate unknown coefficient functions in this model.

Lin and Zhou (2014) considered the following varying-coefficient transformation model:

$$H(\tilde{T}) = \tilde{\boldsymbol{X}}^{\mathsf{T}} \boldsymbol{\beta}(W) + \epsilon,$$

where $H(\cdot)$ is a known transformation function, $\boldsymbol{\beta}(\cdot)$ is unknown coefficient functions, and $\tilde{\boldsymbol{X}}$ is a vector of p-dimensional covariates. They proposed an estimation method for varying coefficients by constructing a local inverse probability weighted estimating equation for LBRC data.

Wei et al. (2018) developed a local linear fitting technique to estimate varying coefficients for the partially linear transformation model in the presence of LBRC data. The partially linear transformation model is given by

$$H(\tilde{T}) = -\tilde{\boldsymbol{X}}^{\mathsf{T}} \boldsymbol{\beta} - g(W) + \epsilon,$$

where $H(\cdot)$ is an unknown monotonic increasing transformation function, $\tilde{\boldsymbol{X}}$ is a $p \times 1$ dimensional time-independent covariate, $\boldsymbol{\beta}$ is an unknown $p \times 1$ vector of regression coefficients, W is a scalar covariate, $g(\cdot)$ is an unspecified smooth function (with $g(0) = 0$ for identifiability purpose), and ϵ is an error term with a completely specified distribution and independent of $\tilde{\boldsymbol{X}}$ and W.

Acknowledgments This work was based upon research supported in part by the National Research Foundation (NRF) of South Africa, Ref.: RA210106581084, Grant No. 150170, and the South African DST-NRF-MRC SARChI Research Chair in Biostatistics (Grant No. 114613). The opinions expressed and conclusions arrived at are those of the authors and are not necessarily to be attributed to the NRF.

References

Aalen, O. (1980) A model for nonparametric regression analysis of counting processes. In *Mathematical Statistics and Probability Theory: Proceedings, Sixth International Conference, Wisła (Poland), 1978* (pp. 1–25). Springer.

Addona, V., & Wolfson, D. B. (2006). A formal test for the stationarity of the incidence rate using data from a prevalent cohort study with follow-up. *Lifetime Data Analysis, 12*, 267–284.

Akbari, M., Akbari, M., & Fakoor, V. (2024). Some asymptotic properties of kernel density estimation under length-biased and right-censored data. In H. Doosti (Ed.), *Book title: Flexible nonparametric curve estimation.*

Andersen, P. K., Borgan, O., Gill, R. D., & Keiding, N. (1993). *Statistical models based on counting processes*. Springer Science & Business Media.

Andersen, P. K., & Gill, R. D. (1982). Cox's regression model for counting processes: A large sample study. *The Annals of Statistics, 10*, 1100–1120.

Asgharian, M., M'Lan, C. E., & Wolfson, D. B. (2002). Length-biased sampling with right censoring: an unconditional approach. *Journal of the American Statistical Association, 97*, 201–209.

Asgharian, M., & Wolfson, D. B. (2005). Asymptotic behavior of the unconditional NPMLE of the length-biased survivor function from right censored prevalent cohort data. *The Annals of Statistics, 33*, 2109–2131.

Asgharian, M., Wolfson, D. B., & Zhang, X. (2006). Checking stationarity of the incidence rate using prevalent cohort survival data. *Statistics in Medicine, 25*, 1751–1767.

Buckley, J., & James, I. (1979). Linear regression with censored data. *Biometrika, 66*, 429–436.

Chen, L.-P. (2019). Pseudo likelihood estimation for the additive hazards model with data subject to left-truncation and right-censoring. *Statistics and Its Interface, 12*, 135–148.

Chen, X., Hu, N., & Sun, J. (2017). Smooth composite likelihood analysis of length-biased and right-censored data with aft model. *Statistica Sinica, 27*, 229–242.

Chen, Y. Q. (2010). Semiparametric regression in size-biased sampling. *Biometrics, 66*, 149–158.

Cheng, S., Wei, L. J., & Ying, Z. (1995). Analysis of transformation models with censored data. *Biometrika, 82*, 835–845.

Cox, D. R. (1972). Regression models and life-tables. *Journal of the Royal Statistical Society: Series B (Methodological), 34*, 187–202.

Cox, D. R., & Miller, H. D. (1965). *The theory of stochastic processes* (Vol. 134). CRC Press.

Cox, D. R., & Oakes, D. (1984). *Analysis of survival data* (Vol. 21). CRC Press.

Dabrowska, D. M., & Doksum, K. A. (1988). Partial likelihood in transformation models with censored data. *Scandinavian Journal of Statistics, 15*, 1–23.

Efromovich, S., & Chu, J. (2018). Hazard rate estimation for left truncated and right censored data. *Annals of the Institute of Statistical Mathematics, 70*, 889–917.

Fan, J., Lin, H., & Zhou, Y. (2006). Local partial-likelihood estimation for lifetime data. *Annals of Statistics, 34*(1), 290–325.

Fine, J. P. (1999). Analysing competing risks data with transformation models. *Journal of the Royal Statistical Society: Series B (Statistical Methodology), 16*(4), 817–830.

Gijbels, I., & Wang, J. L. (1993). Strong representations of the survival function estimator for truncated and censored data with applications. *Journal of Multivariate Analysis, 47*, 210–229.

Harun, N., Cai, B., & Shen, Y. (2021). A Bayesian semiparametric method for analyzing length-biased data. *Journal of Applied Statistics, 48*, 977–992.
Hu, N., Chen, X., & Sun, J. (2015). Regression analysis of length-biased and right-censored failure time data with missing covariates. *Scandinavian Journal of Statistics, 42*, 438–452.
Huang, C.-Y., & Qin, J. (2011). Nonparametric estimation for length-biased and right-censored data. *Biometrika, 98*, 177–186.
Huang, C.-Y., & Qin, J. (2012). Composite partial likelihood estimation under length-biased sampling, with application to a prevalent cohort study of dementia. *Journal of the American Statistical Association, 107*, 946–957.
Huang, C.-Y., & Qin, J. (2013). Semiparametric estimation for the additive hazards model with left-truncated and right-censored data. *Biometrika, 100*, 877–888.
Huang, C.-Y., Qin, J., & Follmann, D. A. (2012). A maximum pseudo-profile likelihood estimator for the cox model under length-biased sampling. *Biometrika, 99*, 199–210.
Hyde, J. (1980) *Testing survival with incomplete observations*. (pp. 31–46). Wiley.
Jazi, O. A. (2024). Estimation for the cox model with biased sampling data via risk set sampling. *Journal of Statistical Planning and Inference, 228*, 1–10.
Jin, Z., Lin, D., Wei, L., & Ying, Z. (2003). Rank-based inference for the accelerated failure time model. *Biometrika, 90*, 341–353.
Kalbfleisch, J., & Lawless, J. (1991). Regression models for right truncated data with applications to aids incubation times and reporting lags. *Statistica Sinica, 1*, 19–32.
Kalbfleisch, J. D., & Prentice, R. L. (2002). *The statistical analysis of failure time data*. Wiley.
Kalbfleisch, J. D., & Schaubel, D. E. (2023). Fifty years of the cox model. *Annual Review of Statistics and its Application, 10*, 1–23.
Lai, T. L., & Ying, Z. (1991a). Large sample theory of a modified Buckley-James estimator for regression analysis with censored data. *The Annals of Statistics, 19*, 1370–1402.
Lai, T. L., & Ying, Z. (1991b). Rank regression methods for left-truncated and right-censored data. *The Annals of Statistics, 19*, 531–556.
Lai, T. L., & Ying, Z. (1994). A missing information principle and m-estimators in regression analysis with censored and truncated data. *The Annals of Statistics, 22*, 1222–1255.
Lancaster, T. (1992). *The econometric analysis of transition data*. Cambridge University Press.
Lin, C., & Zhou, Y. (2014). Analyzing right-censored and length-biased data with varying-coefficient transformation model. *Journal of Multivariate Analysis, 130*, 45–63.
Lin, D., & Ying, Z. (1995). Semiparametric inference for the accelerated life model with time-dependent covariates. *Journal of Statistical Planning and Inference, 44*, 47–63.
Lipsitz, S. R., & Ibrahim, J. G. (1998). Estimating equations with incomplete categorical covariates in the cox model. *Biometrics, 54*, 1002–1013.
Liu, H., Ning, J., Qin, J., & Shen, Y. (2016). Semiparametric maximum likelihood inference for truncated or biased-sampling data. *Statistica Sinica, 26*, 1087–1115.
Liu, P., Wang, Y., & Zhou, Y. (2015). Quantile residual lifetime with right-censored and length-biased data. *Annals of the Institute of Statistical Mathematics, 67*, 999–1028.
Ma, H., Qiu, Z., & Zhou, Y. (2016). Semiparametric transformation models with length-biased and right-censored data under the case-cohort design. *Statistics and Its Interface, 9*, 213–222.
Ma, H., Zhang, F., & Zhou, Y. (2015). Composite estimating equation approach for additive risk model with length-biased and right-censored data. *Statistics & Probability Letters, 96*, 45–53.
Mandel, M., & Ritov, Y. (2010). The accelerated failure time model under biased sampling. *Biometrics, 66*, 1306–1308.
Miller, R., & Halpern, J. (1982). Regression with censored data. *Biometrika, 69*, 521–531.
Ning, J., Qin, J., & Shen, Y. (2011). Buckley-James-type estimator with right-censored and length-biased data. *Biometrics, 67*, 1369–1378.
Ning, J., Qin, J., & Shen, Y. (2014a). Score estimating equations from embedded likelihood functions under accelerated failure time model. *Journal of the American Statistical Association, 109*, 1625–1635.
Ning, J., Qin, J., & Shen, Y. (2014b). Semiparametric accelerated failure time model for length-biased data with application to dementia study. *Statistica Sinica, 24*, 313.

Paik, M. C., & Tsai, W.-Y. (1997). On using the cox proportional hazards model with missing covariates. *Biometrika, 84*, 579–593.

Prentice, R. L. (1978). Linear rank tests with right censored data. *Biometrika, 65*, 167–179.

Qin, J., Ning, J., Liu, H., & Shen, Y. (2011). Maximum likelihood estimations and EM algorithms with length-biased data. *Journal of the American Statistical Association, 106*, 1434–1449.

Qin, J., & Shen, Y. (2010). Statistical methods for analyzing right-censored length-biased data under cox model. *Biometrics, 66*, 382–392.

Qiu, Z., Qin, J., & Zhou, Y. (2016). Composite estimating equation method for the accelerated failure time model with length-biased sampling data. *Scandinavian Journal of Statistics, 43*, 396–415.

Rathouz, P. J. (2007). Identifiability assumptions for missing covariate data in failure time regression models. *Biostatistics, 8*, 345–356.

Ritov, Y. (1990) Estimation in a linear regression model with censored data. *The Annals of Statistics, 18*, 303–328.

Shariati, A., Doosti, H., Fakoor, V., & Asgharian, M. (2023). Uniform confidence bands for hazard functions from censored prevalent cohort survival data. *Electronic Journal of Statistics, 17*, 1807–1847.

Shen, P.-S. (2009). Hazards regression for length-biased and right-censored data. *Statistics & Probability Letters, 79*, 457–465.

Shen, Y., Ning, J., & Qin, J. (2009). Analyzing length-biased data with semiparametric transformation and accelerated failure time models. *Journal of the American Statistical Association, 104*, 1192–1202.

Shen, Y., Ning, J., & Qin, J. (2017). Nonparametric and semiparametric regression estimation for length-biased survival data. *Lifetime Data Analysis, 23*, 3–24.

Simon, R. (1980). Length biased sampling in etiologic studies. *American Journal of Epidemiology, 111*, 444–452.

Thomas, D. (1986). Use of auxiliary information in fitting nonproportional hazards models. In *Modern statistical methods in chronic disease epidemiology* (p. 197210).

Tsai, W. Y. (2009). Pseudo-partial likelihood for proportional hazards models with biased-sampling data. *Biometrika, 96*, 601–615.

Tsai, W.-Y., Jewell, N. P., & Wang, M.-C. (1987). A note on the product-limit estimator under right censoring and left truncation. *Biometrika, 74*, 883–886.

Tsiatis, A. A. (1990) Estimating regression parameters using linear rank tests for censored data. *The Annals of Statistics, 18*, 354–372.

Vardi, Y. (1982). Nonparametric estimation in the presence of length bias. *The Annals of Statistics, 10*, 616–620.

Vardi, Y. (1989). Multiplicative censoring, renewal processes, deconvolution and decreasing density: nonparametric estimation. *Biometrika, 76*, 751–761.

Wang, M.-C. (1991). Nonparametric estimation from cross-sectional survival data. *Journal of the American Statistical Association, 86*, 130–143.

Wang, M.-C. (1996). Hazards regression analysis for length-biased data. *Biometrika, 83*, 343–354.

Wang, M.-C., Brookmeyer, R. and Jewell, N. P. (1993) Statistical models for prevalent cohort data. *Biometrics*, 1–11.

Wang, X., & Wang, Q. (2015). Estimation for semiparametric transformation models with length-biased sampling. *Journal of Statistical Planning and Inference, 156*, 80–89.

Wang, X., & Zhou, X.-H. (2018). Semiparametric maximum likelihood estimation for the cox model with length-biased survival data. *Journal of statistical planning and inference, 196*, 163–173.

Wang, Y., Zhou, Z., Zhou, X.-H., & Zhou, Y. (2017). Nonparametric and semiparametric estimation of quantile residual lifetime for length-biased and right-censored data. *Canadian Journal of Statistics, 45*, 220–250.

Wei, W., Wan, A. T., & Zhou, Y. (2018). Partially linear transformation model for length-biased and right-censored data. *Journal of Nonparametric Statistics, 30*, 332–367.

Winter, B., & Földes, A. (1988). A product-limit estimator for use with length-biased data. *Canadian Journal of Statistics, 16*, 337–355.

Wolfson, C., Wolfson, D. B., Asgharian, M., M'Lan, C. E., Østbye, T., Rockwood, K., & Hogan, D. F. (2001). A reevaluation of the duration of survival after the onset of dementia. *New England Journal of Medicine, 344*, 1111–1116.

Xu, D., & Zhou, Y. (2019). Local composite partial likelihood estimation for length-biased and right-censored data. *Journal of Statistical Computation and Simulation, 89*, 2661–2677.

Yang, Q., Wang, C., He, H., Zhou, X., & Song, X. (2023). Additive hazards model with time-varying coefficients and imaging predictors. *Statistical Methods in Medical Research, 32*, 353–372.

Ying, Z. (1993) A large sample study of rank estimation for censored regression data. *The Annals of Statistics, 21*, 76–99.

Zelen, M. (2004). Forward and backward recurrence times and length biased sampling: age specific models. *Lifetime Data Analysis, 10*, 325–334.

Zelen, M., & Feinleib, M. (1969). On the theory of screening for chronic diseases. *Biometrika, 56*, 601–614.

Zeng, D., & Lin, D. (2007). Efficient estimation for the accelerated failure time model. *Journal of the American Statistical Association, 102*, 1387–1396.

Zhang, F., Chen, X., & Zhou, Y. (2014). Proportional hazards model with varying coefficients for length-biased data. *Lifetime Data Analysis, 20*, 132–157.

Zhang, F., Zhao, X., & Zhou, Y. (2018). An embedded estimating equation for the additive risk model with biased-sampling data. *Science China Mathematics, 61*, 1495–1518.

Zhao, M., Lin, C.-J., & Zhou, Y. (2017). Analyzing right-censored length-biased data with additive hazards model. *Acta Mathematicae Applicatae Sinica, English Series, 33*, 893–908.

Chapter 4
Nonparametric Methods for Incomplete Multivariate Data: Applications to Quality of Life Outcomes

Yue Cui and Solomon W. Harrar

4.1 Introduction

Multivariate data commonly arise in medical, sociological, and behavioral research. For example, in clinical trials the primary outcome is typically assessed at multiple time points and compared across treatment groups. Multivariate data also arise when the experimental units are subjected to multiple treatments and outcome of interest is measured by multiple variables. Such data are usually analyzed by parametric MANOVA tests such as Wilks' Λ. However, the corresponding assumptions such as multivariate normality and homoscedasticity are hard to meet in practice and therefore may lead to wrong results. Moreover, if data are nonmetric, such as ordinal or ordered categorical, the classic parametric models are not applicable since means no longer provide meaningful measures of effect size. To overcome these limitations, some progress has been made with rank-based methods for classical multivariate problems, e.g., (Sen & Puri, 1971). However, the body of research documented in this book assumes a continuous location family for data distributions.

A fully nonparametric univariate model was proposed by Brunner and Munzel (2000) for two independent samples. This nonparametric model abandons the assumptions of continuity or normality of distribution functions and provides a nonparametric measure of effect size. This model was further extended by Konietschke et al. (2012) to the matched-pair data under the assumption of missing

Y. Cui (✉)
Department of Mathematics, Missouri State University, Springfield, MO, USA
e-mail: YueCui@MissouriState.edu

S. W. Harrar
Dr. Bing Zhang Department of Statistics, University of Kentucky, Lexington, KY, USA
e-mail: Solomon.Harrar@uky.edu

D.-G. Chen, C. A. Coelho (eds.), *Biostatistics Modeling and Public Health Applications*, Emerging Topics in Statistics and Biostatistics,
https://doi.org/10.1007/978-3-031-69690-9_4

completely at random and, thus, observations in two samples are allowed to be dependent.

In the multivariate setting, let observations be modeled by independent random vectors $\boldsymbol{X}_{ij} = (X_{ij}^{(1)}, \cdots, X_{ij}^{(d)})^\top \sim \boldsymbol{F}_{ij}$, $i = 1, \cdots, a$, $j = 1, \cdots, n_i$, with possibly dependent components and marginal distributions given by $X_{ij}^{(k)} \sim F_i^{(k)}$. Munzel and Brunner (2000a, 2000b) developed a nonparametric approach to the analysis of multivariate data. Their results were derived using the asymptotic theory for rank statistics developed in, e.g., Akritas and Arnold (1994), Brunner and Denker (1994), and Akritas et al. (1997). Specifically, based on the assumption that the sample size per treatment tends to infinity, whereas the number of treatments (factor levels, cells) remains fixed (large n_i small a case), they derived asymptotic results to test both the multivariate null hypothesis $H_0^F : \boldsymbol{F}_1 = \cdots = \boldsymbol{F}_a$ and the marginal null hypothesis $\overline{H}_0^F : F_1^{(l)} = \cdots = F_a^{(l)}$ for $l = 1, \cdots, d$. This problem has also been investigated by Bathke and Harrar (2008) and Harrar and Bathke (2008) in the asymptotic setting where the number of treatments tends to infinity, whereas the sample size per treatment is fixed (large a small n_i case). In these two papers, multivariate factorial structures were considered in the balanced and unbalanced designs, respectively. Different from the aforementioned nonparametric tests on multivariate null hypothesis or marginal null hypothesis, Brunner et al. (2002) generalized Brunner and Munzel (2000) to the fully nonparametric model and developed inferential methods for the so-called nonparametric effect sizes, $\boldsymbol{p} = (p_1, \cdots, p_d)^\top$, where p_l is the nonparametric effect size on the lth response variable.

The aim of this chapter is to generalize (Brunner et al., 2002) to complex multivariate data structures. In (Brunner et al., 2002), each subject can receive only one of the treatments so that the two samples are independent. In this chapter, we relax this condition by allowing some subjects to receive both treatments and, therefore, the two samples to be dependent. The resulting data structure may be regarded as missing data problem in the sense that subjects that received only one treatment are considered as having missing data on the other treatment. Existing methods or strategies for handing missing data in multivariate models assume unrealistic missing patterns, e.g., monotone missing pattern. It is also the aim of this chapter to derive inferential methods for multivariate data in the presence of missing data that occur at component (variable) level rather than treatment level. In addition to asymptotic solution for the above two problems, we also propose approximations for small samples along the ideas of Brunner et al. (1997) and Brunner et al. (2002).

This chapter is organized as follows. Section 4.2 describes *Asthma Randomized Trial of Indoor Wood Smoke* (ARTIS), which is the motivation for methods developed in this chapter. A precise formulation of the statistical model, nonparametric measure of effect size, and hypothesis of no treatment effect are introduced in Sect. 4.3. The asymptotic theory is developed in Sect. 4.4. More specifically, the asymptotic multivariate normal distribution of the estimator of nonparametric effect size is derived in a closed form. Estimator of the covariance matrix of the limiting distribution is also derived. The covariance matrix is estimated by manipulating the so-called overall and internal rankings, and it is proved to be L_2 consistent. Based on the main results in Sect. 4.4, two tests of treatment effects are proposed in Sect. 4.5. These tests are the rank versions of the Wald-type and ANOVA-type tests. In Sect. 4.6, extensions to general missing patterns are presented. The numerical accuracy of both statistics under the two missing patterns are investigated in a simulation study in Sect. 4.7. Application of the new methods is illustrated with the ARTIS data set in Sect. 4.8. Discussion and some concluding remarks are provided in Sect. 4.9. All proofs and technical details are placed in the Appendix.

4.2 Motivating Examples

The research in this chapter is motivated by the *Asthma Randomized Trial of Indoor Wood Smoke* (ARTIS) (Noonan et al., 2017), which investigates the impact of home heating sources on quality of life for children with asthma. The study is a randomized placebo-controlled intervention trial with two intervention strategies for reducing in-home woodsmoke particulate matter (PM). Eligible participants included children with asthma, age 6–8 years old, residing in a nontobacco-smoking household that used older-model wood stoves as primary heating source. All children with asthma in a household were included in the study. ARTIS was conducted over 5 years, and each household participated in two consecutive winter periods during which they experienced household interventions. The households were assigned randomly to three treatments: placebo group receiving sham air-filtration devices, air-filter group receiving air-filtration devices, and wood stove group receiving improved-technology wood-burning appliances.

The primary health outcome was the score on Pediatric Asthma Quality of Life Questionnaire (PAQLQ) administered directly to children at each visit. PAQLQ is a 23-item asthma-specific battery that provides an overall score as well as domain scores for activity limitations (5 items), symptoms (10 items), and emotional function (8 items), with each item rated in a 7-point scale. The higher the score, the better the clinical record. The design in the ARTIS has multiple levels of nesting (clustering). Data are collected from each child multiple times in the pre- and post-intervention winters. In some houses, multiple children are enrolled. In (Cui et al., 2021), the authors avoided clustering effect of children in the same house by randomly selecting one of the children from each household that has multiple participating children. For each selected child, multiple measurements from multiple visits are regarded as dependent replicates. However, the methods in (Cui et al., 2021) can only analyze one item or domain variable at a time. For multiple items or domain variables, multiplicity adjustment is needed to correct the p-values.

The ideas of the nonparametric test proposed in (Cui et al., 2021) can be extended to the multivariate data so that the response variables can be tested jointly. Here, to facilitate a smooth development, all clustering effects are ignored. Therefore, we confine attention to one visit per child and one child per home. Details on

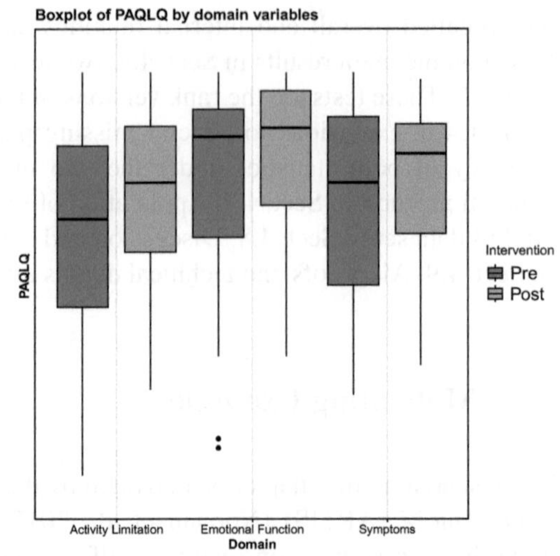

Fig. 4.1 Box plot of the Quality of Life scores for each domain

missing patterns and sample size allocations based on the randomly chosen sample are provided in Sect. 4.8.

Boxplots for domain variables at each intervention period in the air-filter group are shown in Fig. 4.1. The objective of the study is to monitor the pattern of change in the domain scores before and after the air-filter intervention. Note that the outcomes are ordered categorical, and, therefore, analyzing them using mean-based or other parametric effect size measures would be inappropriate. Also, it can be readily seen from the boxplots that the scores in post-intervention period tend to be greater than those in the pre-intervention period for all domains. Of major interest is estimating appropriate intervention effects and testing whether the air-filter intervention effect is significant, i.e., PAQLQ scores of post-intervention group are higher than those in pre-intervention group on at least one domain variable.

4.3 Statistical Model and Hypothesis

We consider multivariate data from n independent random vectors. Each vector contains observations of a subject on d response variables and for two treatment groups, i.e., subjects may receive both treatments. This situation may arise by design or as a result of missing values. Define a subject as a *complete* case on the lth component (variable) if it has measurements on the lth component for both treatment groups, and an *incomplete* case if he/she has measurement on the lth component in the gth group only.

Denote $X_{gj}^{(c)(l)}$ as observation on the lth component of the jth complete case in the gth treatment group and $X_{gk}^{(i)(l)}$ as observation on the lth component of the kth incomplete case in the gth treatment group. Further denote $n_c^{(l)}$ as the number of complete cases on the lth component and $n_g^{(l)}$ as the number of incomplete cases on the lth component within the gth group, $g = 1, 2$.

To facilitate ease of presentation, we first focus on a simple structure, where a subject will have no data in a group if there are no data on any component within that group. Under this structure, $n_c^{(l)}$, $n_1^{(l)}$, and $n_2^{(l)}$ do not depend on l, and, hence, we refer to n_c, n_1 and n_2, respectively. Later in Sect. 4.6, we present the generalizations to arbitrary structures (missing patterns).

Then data for complete cases are collected in vectors as

$$\mathbf{X}_j^{(c)} = (\mathbf{X}_{1j}^{(c)}, \mathbf{X}_{2j}^{(c)}) \text{ where } \mathbf{X}_{gj}^{(c)} = (X_{gj}^{(c)(1)}, \cdots, X_{gj}^{(c)(d)}), g = 1, 2, j = 1, \cdots, n_c,$$

and data for incomplete cases are similarly collected in vectors as

$$\mathbf{X}_{gk}^{(i)} = (X_{gk}^{(i)(1)}, \cdots, X_{gk}^{(i)(d)}), g = 1, 2, k = 1, \cdots, n_g.$$

Assume the joint distribution of data in the same treatment group to be identical for all subjects, i.e., $\boldsymbol{X}_{gj}^{(c)}$, $j = 1, \cdots, n_c$, and $\boldsymbol{X}_{gj'}^{(i)}$, $j' = 1, \cdots, n_g$, are *i.i.d.* within treatment group $g = 1, 2$. Also, marginal distributions for complete and incomplete cases on the same component and in the same treatment group are assumed to be the same, i.e., $X_{gk}^{(A)(l)} \sim F_g^{(l)}$ for $A \in \{c, i\}$. The data scheme of the above model is displayed in Table 4.1 where each row contains observations of a subject and * indicates that data are not available for the subject in that group.

In order to accommodate metric, discrete, dichotomous as well as ordinal data in a unified way, we use the normalized distribution function (Ruymgaart, 1980),

Table 4.1 Schematic representation of the data. Stars denote missing observations

Subject	TX=1	TX=2
1	$\mathbf{X}_{11}^{(c)} = (X_{11}^{(c)(1)}, \cdots, X_{11}^{(c)(d)})$	$\mathbf{X}_{21}^{(c)} = (X_{21}^{(c)(1)}, \cdots, X_{21}^{(c)(d)})$
2	$\mathbf{X}_{12}^{(c)} = (X_{12}^{(c)(1)}, \cdots, X_{12}^{(c)(d)})$	$\mathbf{X}_{22}^{(c)} = (X_{22}^{(c)(1)}, \cdots, X_{22}^{(c)(d)})$
$\vdots$	$\vdots$	$\vdots$
n_c	$\mathbf{X}_{1n_c}^{(c)} = (X_{1n_c}^{(c)(1)}, \cdots, X_{1n_c}^{(c)(d)})$	$\mathbf{X}_{2n_c}^{(c)} = (X_{2n_c}^{(c)(1)}, \cdots, X_{2n_c}^{(c)(d)})$
$n_c + 1$	$\mathbf{X}_{11}^{(i)} = (X_{11}^{(i)(1)}, \cdots, X_{11}^{(i)(d)})$	*
$\vdots$	$\vdots$	$\vdots$
$n_c + n_1$	$\mathbf{X}_{1n_1}^{(i)} = (X_{1n_1}^{(i)(1)}, \cdots, X_{1n_1}^{(i)(d)})$	*
$n_c + n_1 + 1$	*	$\mathbf{X}_{21}^{(i)} = (X_{21}^{(i)(1)}, \cdots, X_{21}^{(i)(d)})$
$\vdots$	$\vdots$	$\vdots$
$n_c + n_1 + n_2$	*	$\mathbf{X}_{2n_2}^{(i)} = (X_{2n_2}^{(i)(1)}, \cdots, X_{2n_2}^{(i)(d)})$

i.e., $F_g^{(l)}(x) = \frac{1}{2}[F_g^{(l)+}(x) + F_g^{(l)-}(x)]$, which is the average of left-continuous and right-continuous distribution functions. That is,

$$F_g^{(l)}(x) = \frac{1}{2}[P(X_{gk}^{(A)(l)} \leq x) + P(X_{gk}^{(A)(l)} < x)]$$

$$\text{for} \quad g = 1, 2, l = 1, \cdots, d \quad \text{and} \quad A \in \{c, i\}.$$

Note that $F_g^{(l)}(x)$ is an arbitrary distribution function except the trivial case of one-point distribution.

The statistical model considered here does not entail any parameter by which adequate treatment effects can be described. Therefore, treatment effects are defined via marginal distributions $F_1^{(l)}(x)$ and $F_2^{(l)}(x)$ as

$$p^{(l)} = \int F_1^{(l)} dF_2^{(l)} = p(X_{11}^{(c)(l)} < X_{21}^{(c)(l)}) + \frac{1}{2} P(X_{11}^{(c)(l)} = X_{21}^{(c)(l)}),$$
$$l = 1, \cdots, d, \tag{4.1}$$

which is the so-called nonparametric relative treatment effect for the lth response, $l = 1, \cdots, d$. Actually, $p^{(l)}$ is the generalized Wilcoxon–Mann–Whitney (WMW) effect introduced in (Brunner & Munzel, 2000). The tendency of observations from $F_1^{(l)}$ being smaller or larger than $F_2^{(l)}$ can be assessed by the comparisons $p^{(l)} > \frac{1}{2}$ or $p^{(l)} < \frac{1}{2}$. Especially, when $p^{(l)} = \frac{1}{2}$, observations from $F_1^{(l)}$ do not tend to be smaller or larger than observations from $F_2^{(l)}$, and this situation is regarded as "no treatment effect" for the lth component. In this respect, we can characterize the case of "no treatment effect" in the general multivariate model by the condition that $p^{(l)} = \frac{1}{2}$ for all $l = 1, \cdots, d$. Now, let $\boldsymbol{p} = (p^{(1)}, \cdots, p^{(d)})^\top$ be the vector of relative treatment effects. Then the hypothesis of no treatment effect in the multivariate model can be expressed as

$$H_0 : \boldsymbol{p} = \frac{1}{2}\mathbb{1}_d,$$

where $\mathbb{1}_d = (1, \cdots, 1)^\top$ is a vector of all 1's. Equivalently, $H_0 : p^{(l)} = \frac{1}{2}$ for all $l = 1, \cdots, d$.

One can easily show that $F_1^{(l)} = F_2^{(l)}$ implies $p^{(l)} = \frac{1}{2}$, but the converse is not necessarily true. Indeed, the inference method for $\boldsymbol{p}$ allows for heteroscedastic variances, skewness, and higher moments of distributions in the two groups.

To construct an appropriate inference procedure, we need to come up with a consistent estimator for the effect size vector and derive its asymptotic distribution. In the next section, we will derive an (asymptotically) unbiased and consistent estimator of $\boldsymbol{p}$ and establish its asymptotic normality. In order to derive the results, we need the following regularity assumption:

Assumption 4.3.1 $n_c + n_g \to \infty$ such that $\frac{n}{n_c+n_g} \leq N_0 < \infty$, $g = 1, 2$. □

This assumption guarantees that either the number of complete cases or both of the incomplete cases are large. In particular, we do not want either n_1 or n_2 alone to dominate the total sample size. Therefore, it includes the most common practice-oriental sample size allocations:

(a) $n_c \to \infty, n_1, n_2 \leq M < \infty$, or
(b) $n_c \to \infty, n_1 \to \infty, n_2 \leq M < \infty$, or
(c) $n_c \to \infty, n_1 \to \infty, n_2 \to \infty$, or
(d) $n_c \leq N_c, n_1 \to \infty, n_2 \to \infty$

where M and N_c are constants.

4.4 Asymptotic Theory

4.4.1 Effect Size Estimator

To get the asymptotically unbiased and consistent estimator of the relative treatment effect $p^{(l)}$, we replace $F_1^{(l)}$ and $F_2^{(l)}$ with their empirical counterparts $\widehat{F}_1^{(l)}$ and $\widehat{F}_2^{(l)}$. For the lth component, let $\theta_g^{(l)} = \frac{n_c^{(l)}}{n_c^{(l)}+n_g^{(l)}} = \frac{n_c^{(l)}}{m_g^{(l)}}$ be the relative sample size of complete and incomplete data in the gth group. Notice that under the data structure shown in Table 4.1, $\theta_g^{(l)}$'s are identical for all components within the same group. For simplicity, we drop the superscript (l) in the subsequence section. Using relative sample size as weights, define the weighted empirical distribution function by

$$\widehat{F}_g^{(l)}(x) = \theta_g \widehat{F}_g^{(c)(l)}(x) + (1-\theta_g)\widehat{F}_g^{(i)(l)}(x), \quad g = 1, 2, \quad \text{where} \tag{4.2}$$

$$\widehat{F}_g^{(c)(l)}(x) = \frac{1}{n_c}\sum_{k=1}^{n_c} c(x - X_{gk}^{(c)(l)}) \quad \text{and} \quad \widehat{F}_g^{(i)(l)}(x) = \frac{1}{n_g}\sum_{k=1}^{n_g} c(x - X_{gk}^{(i)(l)})$$

denote the empirical distribution functions of complete and incomplete cases, respectively. Here, the function $c(x) = 0, \frac{1}{2}, 1$ according to $x < 0, = 0, > 0$ is the normalized count function.

A weighted estimator $\widehat{p}^{(l)}$ of $p^{(l)}$ can then be achieved by plugging in $\widehat{F}_1^{(l)}$ and $\widehat{F}_2^{(l)}$ into the integral representation in (4.1), and the resulting estimator is

$$
\begin{aligned}
\widehat{p}^{(l)} &= \int \widehat{F}_1^{(l)} d\widehat{F}_2^{(l)} \\
&= \frac{1}{m_1 m_2}[n_c^2 \int \widehat{F}_1^{(c)(l)} d\widehat{F}_2^{(c)(l)} + n_c n_2 \int \widehat{F}_1^{(c)(l)} d\widehat{F}_2^{(i)(l)} \\
&\quad + n_c n_1 \int \widehat{F}_1^{(i)(l)} d\widehat{F}_2^{(c)(l)} + n_1 n_2 \int \widehat{F}_1^{(i)(l)} d\widehat{F}_2^{(i)(l)}].
\end{aligned} \tag{4.3}
$$

One can verify that

$$
\widehat{p}^{(l)} = \frac{1}{N}(\theta_2 \overline{R}_{2\cdot}^{(c)(l)} - \theta_1 \overline{R}_{1\cdot}^{(c)(l)} + (1-\theta_2)\overline{R}_{2\cdot}^{(i)(l)} - (1-\theta_1)\overline{R}_{1\cdot}^{(i)(l)}) + \frac{1}{2}, \tag{4.4}
$$

where $\overline{R}_{g\cdot}^{(c)(l)} = \frac{1}{n_c}\sum_{k=1}^{n_c} R_{gk}^{(c)(l)}$ and $\overline{R}_{g\cdot}^{(i)(l)} = \frac{1}{n_g}\sum_{k=1}^{n_g} R_{gk}^{(i)(l)}$ are the means of ranks $R_{gk}^{(c)(l)}$ and $R_{gk}^{(i)(l)}$ of $X_{gk}^{(c)(l)}$ and $X_{gk}^{(i)(l)}$ among all $N = 2n_c + n_1 + n_2$ observations on the lth component among both groups.

Proposition 4.4.1 *Let $\widehat{\boldsymbol{p}} = (\widehat{p}^{(1)}, \cdots, \widehat{p}^{(d)})^\top$ be as defined in (4.4). Then, under Assumption 4.3.1:*

(1) $E(\widehat{\boldsymbol{p}}) \to \boldsymbol{p}$.
(2) $\widehat{\boldsymbol{p}} \overset{a.s.}{\to} \boldsymbol{p}$.

□

Proof Since d is finite, it suffices to show asymptotic unbiasedness and strong consistency of the relative effect size on each component, i.e., $E(\widehat{p}^{(l)}) \to p^{(l)}$ and $\widehat{p}^{(l)} \overset{a.s.}{\to} p^{(l)}$. Proof of these statements is provided in Proposition 4.1 of (Konietschke et al., 2012) and is therefore omitted. □

4.4.2 Asymptotic Distribution

It is shown in Theorem 4.4.1 that $\sqrt{n}(\widehat{\boldsymbol{p}} - \boldsymbol{p})$ is asymptotically equivalent to a random vector, whose components are sums of independent random variables. Define $Y_{gk}^{(A)(l)} = F_s^{(l)}(X_{gk}^{(A)(l)})$, $g, s \in \{1, 2\}$, $g \neq s$, $A \in \{c, i\}$, and denote $Z_k^{(c)(l)} = \theta_2 Y_{2k}^{(c)(l)} - \theta_1 Y_{1k}^{(c)(l)}$. Then define

$$
\sqrt{n}U^{(l)} = \sqrt{n}(\frac{1}{n_c}\sum_{k=1}^{n_c} Z_k^{(c)(l)} + \frac{1}{m_2}\sum_{k=1}^{n_2} Y_{2k}^{(i)(l)} - \frac{1}{m_1}\sum_{k=1}^{n_1} Y_{1k}^{(i)(l)}) + \sqrt{n}(1 - 2p^{(l)}). \tag{4.5}
$$

Theorem 4.4.1 *Let $\sqrt{n}\boldsymbol{U} = \sqrt{n}(U^{(1)}, \cdots, U^{(d)})^\top$. Then under Assumptions 4.3.1,*

$$
\| \sqrt{n}(\widehat{\boldsymbol{p}} - \boldsymbol{p}) - \sqrt{n}\boldsymbol{U} \|_2^2 \to 0,
$$

where $\| \cdot \|_2$ *is* L_2*-norm of vector, i.e., for a* q*-dimensional vector,* $\| \boldsymbol{x} \|_2 = (\sum_{i=1}^{q} x_i^2)^{\frac{1}{2}}$.

Proof This statement can be proved by showing $E[\sqrt{n}(\widehat{p}^{(l)} - p^{(l)}) - \sqrt{n}U^{(l)}]^2 \rightarrow 0$ for all $l = 1, \cdots, d$. The proof is similar to Theorem 4.4.1 in (Konietschke & Brunner, 2009) and is therefore omitted. □

Based on Theorem 4.4.1, it suffices to consider the distribution of vector $\sqrt{n}\boldsymbol{U}$. Let $\lambda_1, \cdots, \lambda_d$ denote the eigenvalues of $\boldsymbol{V} = Cov(\sqrt{n}\boldsymbol{U})$ and let $\min_{1 \le l \le d} \{\lambda_l\}$ be the smallest eigenvalue. To derive the asymptotic distribution of $\sqrt{n}\boldsymbol{U}$, we need the regularity condition below:

Assumption 4.4.1 Let $\min_{1 \le l \le d} \{\lambda_l\} \ge \lambda_0 > 0$, where λ_0 is some constant. □

Theorem 4.4.2 *Under Assumptions 4.3.1 and 4.4.1, the statistic* $\sqrt{n}(\widehat{\boldsymbol{p}} - \boldsymbol{p})$ *has asymptotically a multivariate normal distribution with mean* $\boldsymbol{0}$ *and covariance matrix* $\boldsymbol{V}$.

Proof The asymptotic normality of $\sqrt{n}(\widehat{\boldsymbol{p}} - \boldsymbol{p})$ can be established from the asymptotic distribution of random vector $\sqrt{n}\boldsymbol{U}$. Apart from some constants, $\sqrt{n}U^{(l)}$ is the sum of three independent random variables. Since the random variables $Z_k^{(c)(l)}$ and $Y_{gk}^{(i)(l)}$, $g \in \{1, 2\}$ are uniformly bounded by Assumption 4.3.1, asymptotic normality of $\sqrt{n}U^{(l)}$ can be completed by verifying the Lindeberg's condition. Furthermore, the joint normality is verified by the Cramér–Wold device. □

4.4.3 Estimation of the Asymptotic Covariance Matrix

To apply the results in Theorem 4.4.2, a L_2-consistent estimator of $\boldsymbol{V}$ is derived in this section. Denote by $v^{(l,r)}$ as the (l, r)th entry of $\boldsymbol{V}$. Then, by independence of $Z_k^{(c)(l)}$, $Y_{1k}^{(i)(l)}$ and $Y_{2k}^{(i)(l)}$ and also independence between subjects,

$$
\begin{aligned}
v^{(l,r)} &= n\mathrm{Cov}(U^{(l)}, U^{(r)}) \\
&= n\big[\mathrm{Cov}(\frac{1}{m_1}\sum_{k=1}^{n_1} Y_{1k}^{(i)(l)}, \frac{1}{m_1}\sum_{k=1}^{n_1} Y_{1k}^{(i)(r)}) \\
&\quad + \mathrm{Cov}(\frac{1}{m_2}\sum_{k=1}^{n_2} Y_{2k}^{(i)(l)}, \frac{1}{m_2}\sum_{k=1}^{n_2,} Y_{2k}^{(i)(r)}) + \\
&\quad \mathrm{Cov}(\frac{1}{n_c}\sum_{k=1}^{n_c} Z_k^{(c)(l)}, \frac{1}{n_c}\sum_{k=1}^{n_c} Z_k^{(c)(r)})]
\end{aligned}
$$

$$= n[\frac{n_1}{m_1^2}\mathrm{Cov}(Y_{11}^{(i)(l)}, Y_{11}^{(i)(r)}) + \frac{n_2}{m_2^2}\mathrm{Cov}(Y_{21}^{(i)(l)}, Y_{21}^{(i)(r)})$$

$$+ \frac{1}{n_c}\mathrm{Cov}(Z_1^{(c)(l)}, Z_1^{(c)(r)})]$$

$$= n(\frac{n_1}{m_1^2}c_1^{(l,r)} + \frac{n_2}{m_2^2}c_2^{(l,r)} + \frac{1}{n_c}c_3^{(l,r)}), \tag{4.6}$$

where $c_g^{(l,r)} = \mathrm{Cov}(Y_{g1}^{(i)(l)}, Y_{g1}^{(i)(r)})$ for $g = 1, 2$ and $c_3^{(l,r)} = \mathrm{Cov}(Z_1^{(c)(l)}, Z_1^{(c)(r)})$. Suppose the random variables $Y_{gk}^{(A)(l)}$ were observable, and then natural estimators of $c_g^{(l,r)}$ are the empirical covariance

$$\tilde{c}_g^{(l,r)} = \frac{1}{n_g - 1}\sum_{k=1}^{n_g}(Y_{gk}^{(i)(l)} - \overline{Y}_{g\cdot}^{(i)(l)})(Y_{gk}^{(i)(r)} - \overline{Y}_{g\cdot}^{(i)(r)}), \quad g = 1, 2,$$

and

$$\tilde{c}_3^{(l,r)} = \frac{1}{n_c - 1}\sum_{k=1}^{n_c}(Z_k^{(c)(l)} - \overline{Z}_{\cdot}^{(c)(l)})(Z_k^{(c)(r)} - \overline{Z}_{\cdot}^{(c)(r)}),$$

where $\overline{Y}_{g\cdot}^{(c)(l)} = \frac{1}{n_c}\sum_{k=1}^{n_c} Y_{gk}^{(c)(l)}$, $\overline{Y}_{g\cdot}^{(i)(l)} = \frac{1}{n_g}\sum_{k=1}^{n_g} Y_{gk}^{(i)(l)}$, and $\overline{Z}_{\cdot}^{(c)(l)} = \frac{1}{n_c}\sum_{k=1}^{n_c} Z_k^{(c)(l)}$. Consequently, an estimator of $v^{(l,r)}$ is given by

$$\tilde{v}^{(l,r)} = n(\frac{n_1}{m_1^2}\tilde{c}_1^{(l,r)} + \frac{n_2}{m_2^2}\tilde{c}_2^{(l,r)} + \frac{1}{n_c}\tilde{c}_3^{(l,r)}). \tag{4.7}$$

Now, let $\boldsymbol{Y}_{gk}^{(A)} = (Y_{gk}^{(A)(1)}, \cdots, Y_{gk}^{(A)(d)})^\top$, $\overline{\boldsymbol{Y}}_{g\cdot}^{(A)} = (\overline{Y}_{g\cdot}^{(A)(1)}, \cdots, \overline{Y}_{g\cdot}^{(A)(d)})^\top$, $\boldsymbol{Z}_k^{(c)} = (Z_k^{(c)(1)} \cdots, Z_k^{(c)(d)})^\top$, and $\overline{\boldsymbol{Z}}_{\cdot}^{(c)} = (\overline{Z}_{\cdot}^{(c)(1)}, \cdots, \overline{Z}_{\cdot}^{(c)(d)})^\top$. Then a natural estimator of $\boldsymbol{V}$ is given by $\widetilde{\boldsymbol{V}} = \widetilde{\boldsymbol{V}}_c + \widetilde{\boldsymbol{V}}_1 + \widetilde{\boldsymbol{V}}_2$, where

$$\widetilde{\boldsymbol{V}}_c = \frac{n}{n_c(n_c - 1)}\sum_{k=1}^{n_c}(\boldsymbol{Z}_k^{(c)} - \overline{\boldsymbol{Z}}_{\cdot}^{(c)})(\boldsymbol{Z}_k^{(c)} - \overline{\boldsymbol{Z}}_{\cdot}^{(c)})^\top \quad \text{and}$$

$$\widetilde{\boldsymbol{V}}_g = n\frac{n_g}{m_g^2(n_g - 1)}\sum_{k=1}^{n_g}(\boldsymbol{Y}_{gk}^{(i)} - \overline{\boldsymbol{Y}}_{g\cdot}^{(i)})(\boldsymbol{Y}_{gk}^{(i)} - \overline{\boldsymbol{Y}}_{g\cdot}^{(i)})^\top, \quad g = 1, 2.$$

However, the random variables $Y_{gk}^{(A)(l)}$ are not observable and must be replaced by observable ones, which are "close enough" in probability. One can verify that $\widehat{F}_g^{(l)}$ defined in (4.2) can be represented as

$$\widehat{F}_g^{(l)} = \frac{1}{n_c + n_g}[\sum_{k=1}^{n_c} c(x - X_{gk}^{(c)(l)}) + \sum_{k=1}^{n_g} c(x - X_{gk}^{(i)(l)})], \quad g = 1, 2.$$

Hence, the empirical counterparts $\widehat{Y}_{gk}^{(A)(l)} = \widehat{F}_s^{(l)}(X_{gk}^{(A)(l)})$, $s \neq g \in \{1, 2\}$, $A \in \{c, i\}$ can be expressed in terms of the overall ranks $R_{gk}^{(A)(l)}$ from $X_{gk}^{(A)(l)}$ among all N observations on the lth component, and the internal ranks $R_{gk}^{(A,g)(l)}$ of $X_{gk}^{(A)(l)}$ among all $n_c + n_g$ observations on the lth component in the gth treatment group. Specifically,

$$\widehat{Y}_{gk}^{(A)(l)} = \frac{1}{n_c + n_s}(R_{gk}^{(A)(l)} - R_{gk}^{(A,g)(l)}), g \neq s \in \{1, 2\}, A \in \{c, i\} \text{ and } l = 1, \cdots, d.$$

Further, let $\boldsymbol{R}_{gk}^{(A)} = (R_{gk}^{(A)(1)}, \cdots, R_{gk}^{(A)(d)})^\top$ and $\boldsymbol{R}_{gk}^{(A,g)} = (R_{gk}^{(A,g)(1)}, \cdots, R_{gk}^{(A,g)(d)})^\top$ denote the vector of the ranks $R_{gk}^{(A)(l)}$ and $R_{gk}^{(A,g)(l)}$, respectively, for $g = 1, 2$ and $l = 1, \cdots, d$. Also, define

$$\overline{\boldsymbol{R}}_{g\cdot}^{(c)} = \frac{1}{n_c}\sum_{k=1}^{n_c} \boldsymbol{R}_{gk}^{(c)}, \quad \overline{\boldsymbol{R}}_{g\cdot}^{(i)} = \frac{1}{n_g}\sum_{k=1}^{n_g} \boldsymbol{R}_{gk}^{(i)},$$

$$\overline{\boldsymbol{R}}_{g\cdot}^{(c,g)} = \frac{1}{n_c}\sum_{k=1}^{n_c} \boldsymbol{R}_{gk}^{(c,g)} \text{ and } \overline{\boldsymbol{R}}_{g\cdot}^{(i,g)} = \frac{1}{n_g}\sum_{k=1}^{n_g} \boldsymbol{R}_{gk}^{(i,g)} = \frac{n_g + 1}{2}\mathbb{1}_d, \quad g = 1, 2.$$

Let $\boldsymbol{B}_{gk}^{(A)} = \boldsymbol{R}_{gk}^{(A)} - \boldsymbol{R}_{gk}^{(A,g)}$, $\overline{\boldsymbol{B}}_{g\cdot}^{(A)} = \overline{\boldsymbol{R}}_{g\cdot}^{(A)} - \overline{\boldsymbol{R}}_{g\cdot}^{(A,g)}$ for $A \in \{c, i\}$. As proposed before, an estimator of $\boldsymbol{V}$ is given by $\widehat{\boldsymbol{V}} = \widehat{\boldsymbol{V}}_c + \widehat{\boldsymbol{V}}_1 + \widehat{\boldsymbol{V}}_2$, where

$$\widehat{\boldsymbol{V}}_g = n\frac{n_g}{m_1^2 m_2^2 (n_g - 1)}\sum_{k=1}^{n_g}(\boldsymbol{B}_{gk}^{(i)} - \overline{\boldsymbol{B}}_{g\cdot}^{(i)})(\boldsymbol{B}_{gk}^{(i)} - \overline{\boldsymbol{B}}_{g\cdot}^{(i)})^\top, g = 1, 2 \text{ and} \tag{4.8}$$

$$\widehat{\boldsymbol{V}}_c = n\frac{n_c}{m_1^2 m_2^2 (n_c - 1)}\sum_{k=1}^{n_c}[\boldsymbol{B}_{2k}^{(c)} - \overline{\boldsymbol{B}}_{2\cdot}^{(c)} - (\boldsymbol{B}_{1k}^{(c)} - \overline{\boldsymbol{B}}_{1\cdot}^{(c)})][\boldsymbol{B}_{2k}^{(c)} - \overline{\boldsymbol{B}}_{2\cdot}^{(c)} - (\boldsymbol{B}_{1k}^{(c)} - \overline{\boldsymbol{B}}_{1\cdot}^{(c)})]^\top. \tag{4.9}$$

The consistency of the estimator $\widehat{\boldsymbol{V}}$ is established in Theorem 4.4.3.

Theorem 4.4.3 *Under Assumption 4.3.1 and 4.4.1,*

$$\parallel \widehat{\boldsymbol{V}} - \boldsymbol{V} \parallel_2^2 \to 0,$$

where $\parallel \cdot \parallel_2$ *is* L_2*-norm of matrix, i.e., for any* $s \times t$ *matrix* A, $\parallel A \parallel_2 = (\sum_{i=1}^s \sum_{j=1}^t |a_{ij}|^2)^{1/2}$.

Proof In Appendix. □

4.5 Test Statistics

In this section, we will introduce two test statistics for $H_0 : \widehat{\boldsymbol{p}} = \frac{1}{2}\mathbb{1}_d$. The first one is Wald-type statistic, which is commonly used for nonparametric model in the multivariate structure. The second one is ANOVA-type statistic, which is first introduced in (Brunner et al., 1997) for univariate factorial designs and further extended to the multivariate structure in (Brunner et al., 2002).

4.5.1 Wald-Type Statistic

From Theorem 4.4.2, it follows under $H_0 : \boldsymbol{p} = \frac{1}{2}\mathbb{1}_d$ that the statistic $\sqrt{n}\boldsymbol{V}^{-1/2}(\widehat{\boldsymbol{p}} - \frac{1}{2}\mathbb{1}_d)$ has asymptotic multivariate standard normal distribution $\mathbf{N}_d(\mathbf{0}, \boldsymbol{I}_d)$. By the Continuous Mapping Theorem, distribution of the quadratic form

$$Q_n^* = n \cdot (\widehat{\boldsymbol{p}} - \frac{1}{2}\mathbb{1}_d)^\top \boldsymbol{V}^{-1}(\widehat{\boldsymbol{p}} - \frac{1}{2}\mathbb{1}_d) \tag{4.10}$$

tends to a central χ^2-distribution with d degrees of freedom. However, the covariance matrix $\boldsymbol{V}$ is unknown and must be replaced by a consistent estimator. From Theorem 4.4.3, it follows that $\| \widehat{\boldsymbol{V}}^{-1} - \boldsymbol{V}^{-1} \|_2^2 \rightarrow 0$ under Assumption 4.4.1. Therefore, under H_0, the quadratic form

$$Q_n = n \cdot (\widehat{\boldsymbol{p}} - \frac{1}{2}\mathbb{1}_d)^\top \widehat{\boldsymbol{V}}^{-1}(\widehat{\boldsymbol{p}} - \frac{1}{2}\mathbb{1}_d) \tag{4.11}$$

has the same asymptotic distribution as Q_n^*, which is also a χ^2-distribution with d degrees of freedom. This can be verified by

$$\| Q_n^* - Q_n \|_2^2 \leq n \cdot \| \widehat{\boldsymbol{p}} - \frac{1}{2}\mathbb{1}_d \|_2^2 \cdot \| \boldsymbol{V}^{-1} - \widehat{\boldsymbol{V}}^{-1} \|_2^2 \rightarrow 0,$$

which follows by Proposition 4.4.1 (2). Therefore, the null hypothesis $H_0 : \boldsymbol{p} = \frac{1}{2}\mathbb{1}_d$ will be rejected at significance level α if $Q_n \geq \chi^2_\alpha$.

The quadratic form Q_n is called the nonparametric Wald-type statistic. It is well known that this statistic has slow convergence to the limiting χ^2-distribution. Thus Q_n may become extremely liberal unless a very large sample size is available. Hence, Wald-type statistics should only be applied in the case of large sample sizes.

4.5.2 ANOVA-Type Statistic

In practice, data sets may not have large enough sample size, and the Wald-type statistic may not provide accurate results. Therefore, it is necessary to develop a test with small sample approximation which maintains the preassigned level with satisfactory accuracy. The idea for developing such a procedure is to replace the inverse $\widehat{\boldsymbol{V}}^{-1}$ of the estimated covariance matrix in (4.11) with $1/tr(\widehat{\boldsymbol{V}})$ much in the same way the ANOVA tests do and consider the asymptotic distribution of the resulting quadratic form.

Details of the approximation process can be found in (Brunner et al., 2002) and are summarized below.

Approximation Procedure Under Assumptions 4.3.1 and 4.4.1, the statistic

$$F_n = \frac{n}{tr(\widehat{\boldsymbol{V}})}(\widehat{\boldsymbol{p}} - \frac{1}{2}\mathbb{1}_d)^\top(\widehat{\boldsymbol{p}} - \frac{1}{2}\mathbb{1}_d) = \frac{n}{tr(\widehat{\boldsymbol{V}})} \cdot \sum_{l=1}^{d}(\widehat{p}^{(l)} - \frac{1}{2})^2 \tag{4.12}$$

has, approximately, a central $F(\hat{\nu}, \infty)$ distribution under $H_0 : \boldsymbol{p} = \frac{1}{2}\mathbb{1}_d$, where $\hat{\nu} = \frac{[tr(\widehat{\boldsymbol{V}})]^2}{tr(\widehat{\boldsymbol{V}}^2)}$.

Test statistic F_n is called ANOVA-type statistic. For small sample sizes, the null hypothesis $H_0 : \boldsymbol{p} = \frac{1}{2}\mathbb{1}_d$ will be rejected at significance level α if $F_n \geq F_\alpha(\hat{\nu}, \infty)$.

4.6 Extension to General Missing Pattern

In Sects. 4.3–4.5, we assumed that incomplete data occur at treatment level as, for example, a subject not showing up for a scheduled treatment. That means this subject will have no observation on all variables for that treatment group. However, in practical applications, missing data may occur for any component (variable) within a treatment group. In this situation, the total number of possible missing patterns is $2^{2d} - 1$, not counting completely missing cases. Also note that the order of the missing patterns is completely arbitrary and is irrelevant to the methodology to be developed. The central idea of our approach is to combine estimates from cases with different missing patterns by weighing them appropriately. Let the $2d \times n$ data matrix be denoted as $\boldsymbol{X} = (\boldsymbol{X}_1, \cdots, \boldsymbol{X}_n)$, where the first d rows are measurements on the d variables in the first group and the remaining d rows are measurements on the d variables in the second group. The columns represent subjects. Suppose there are K missing patterns in the data set and let $\boldsymbol{X}$ be partitioned as $(\boldsymbol{X}^{(1)}, \cdots, \boldsymbol{X}^{(K)})$ where $K \leq 2^{2d} - 1$ and $\boldsymbol{X}^{(k)}$ is a $2d \times n_k$ matrix of observations for the kth missing pattern. That is, $\boldsymbol{X}^{(k)}$ contains data from n_k subjects for whom there are observations on the same p_k components, say $(j_1, \cdots, j_{p_k})$, among all $2d$ components, and no observations for the remaining $2d - p_k$ components. For the sake of brevity, we assume that all possible patterns are represented in the data matrix, i.e., $K = 1, 2, \cdots, 2^{2d} - 1$. To further display missing patterns by means of component allocations, we define a $2d \times 2d$ matrix B_k such that for $s = 1, \cdots, 2d$, the sth row of B_k has unity at the j_sth position and zero elsewhere. With the assumption that at least one subject has complete data on all components in both groups (i.e., $n_1 \geq 1$), $B_1 = I_{2d}$.

Based on the notations defined above, complete and incomplete sample sizes on the lth component can be represented as

$$n_c^{(l)} = \sum_{k=1}^{K} n_k I_{\{B_{k,l}=B_{k,l+d}=1\}}, \quad n_1^{(l)} = \sum_{k=1}^{K} n_k I_{\{B_{k,l}=1, B_{k,l+d}=0\}}$$

$$\text{and} \quad n_2^{(l)} = \sum_{k=1}^{K} n_k I_{\{B_{k,l}=0, B_{k,l+d}=1\}},$$

where $B_{k,l}$ refers to the lth diagonal entry of matrix B_k. In addition, denote $m_g^{(l)} = n_c^{(l)} + n_g^{(l)}$ and $n = \sum_{k=1}^{K} n_k$. Similar to Assumption 4.3.1, we need an assumption on the sample size allocations.

Assumption 4.6.1 $\min_{g,l}\{n_c^{(l)} + n_g^{(l)}\} \to \infty$ such that $\max_{g,l}\{\frac{n}{n_c^{(l)}+n_g^{(l)}}\} \leq N_0 < \infty$ for $l = 1, \cdots, d$ and $g = 1, 2$. □

Let $\Delta_{gk}^{(A)(l)} = 1$ if $X_{gk}^{(A)(l)}$ is observed, and $\Delta_{gk}^{(A)(l)} = 0$ otherwise. Define the index set $S^{(c,l)} = \{k : \Delta_{1k}^{(c)(l)} \cdot \Delta_{2k}^{(c)(l)} = 1\}$ of all complete cases on the lth component. Similarly, define $S^{(g,l)} = \{k : \Delta_{gk}^{(i)(l)} = 1 \wedge \Delta_{g'k}^{(i)(l)} = 0\}$, $g \neq g' \in \{1, 2\}$ as the index set of all incomplete cases on the lth component in the gth group. In this setup, we define

$$\widehat{F}_g^{(c)(l)}(x) = \frac{1}{n_c^{(l)}} \sum_{k=1}^{n_c^{(l)}} c(x - X_{gk}^{(c)(l)}) \quad \text{and} \quad \widehat{F}_g^{(i)(l)}(x) = \frac{1}{n_g^{(l)}} \sum_{k=1}^{n_g^{(l)}} c(x - X_{gk}^{(i)(l)})$$

and plug them in Eq. (4.2) to define the empirical distribution functions $\widehat{F}_g^{(l)}(x)$, $g = 1, 2$. This estimate will be used in Eq. (4.3) to define an estimator $\widehat{\boldsymbol{p}}$ of the vector of relative treatment effects $\boldsymbol{p}$. Furthermore, write

$$\sqrt{n}U^{(l)} = \sqrt{n}\Big[\frac{1}{m_2^{(l)}} \sum_{k \in S^{(c,l)}} F_1^{(l)}(X_{2k}^{(c)(l)}) - \frac{1}{m_1^{(l)}} \sum_{k \in S^{(c,l)}} F_2^{(l)}(X_{1k}^{(c)(l)})$$
$$+ \frac{1}{m_2^{(l)}} \sum_{k \in S^{(2,l)}} F_1^{(l)}(X_{2k}^{(i)(l)}) - \frac{1}{m_1^{(l)}} \sum_{k \in S^{(1,l)}} F_2^{(l)}(X_{1k}^{(i)(l)})\Big] + \sqrt{n}(1 - 2p^{(l)})$$

$$= \sqrt{n}\Big(\frac{1}{n_c^{(l)}}\sum_{k\in S^{(c,l)}} Z_k^{(c)(l)} + \frac{1}{m_2^{(l)}}\sum_{k\in S^{(2,l)}} Y_{2k}^{(i)(l)} - \frac{1}{m_1^{(l)}}\sum_{k\in S^{(1,l)}} Y_{1k}^{(i)(l)}\Big)$$
$$+ \sqrt{n}(1-2p^{(l)}),$$

where $Z_k^{(c)(l)} = \theta_2^{(l)} Y_{2k}^{(c)(l)} - \theta_1^{(l)} Y_{1k}^{(c)(l)}$. Let $\sqrt{n}\boldsymbol{U} = \sqrt{n}(U^{(1)}, \cdots, U^{(d)})^\top$ and $\boldsymbol{V} = Cov(\sqrt{n}\boldsymbol{U})$. At this point, we can prove that Theorem 4.4.1 still holds by verifying $\mathrm{E}[\sqrt{n}(\widehat{p}^{(l)} - p^{(l)}) - \sqrt{n}U^{(l)}]^2 \to 0$ for all $l = 1, \cdots, d$. Therefore, under Assumptions 4.4.1 and 4.6.1, $\sqrt{n}(\widehat{\boldsymbol{p}} - \boldsymbol{p})$ has asymptotically a multivariate normal distribution with mean $\boldsymbol{0}$ and covariance $\boldsymbol{V}$, as proved in Theorem 4.4.2. The (l, r)th entry of the covariance matrix $\boldsymbol{V}$ can be computed as

$$v^{(l,r)} = n\mathrm{Cov}(U^{(l)}, U^{(r)})$$
$$= n\mathrm{Cov}\Big(\frac{1}{n_c^{(l)}}\sum_{k\in S^{(c,l)}} Z_k^{(c)(l)} + \frac{1}{m_2^{(l)}}\sum_{k\in S^{(2,l)}} Y_{2k}^{(i)(l)} - \frac{1}{m_1^{(l)}}\sum_{k\in S^{(1,l)}} Y_{1k}^{(i)(l)},$$
$$\frac{1}{n_c^{(r)}}\sum_{k\in S^{(c,r)}} Z_k^{(c)(r)} + \frac{1}{m_2^{(r)}}\sum_{k\in S^{(2,r)}} Y_{2k}^{(i)(r)} - \frac{1}{m_1^{(r)}}\sum_{k\in S^{(1,r)}} Y_{1k}^{(i)(r)}\Big)$$
$$= n\Big[\frac{1}{n_c^{(l)} n_c^{(r)}}\underbrace{\mathrm{Cov}\Big(\sum_{k\in S^{(c,l)}} Z_k^{(c)(l)}, \sum_{k\in S^{(c,r)}} Z_k^{(c)(r)}\Big)}_{C_1} \tag{4.13}$$
$$+ \frac{1}{n_c^{(l)} m_2^{(r)}}\underbrace{\mathrm{Cov}\Big(\sum_{k\in S^{(c,l)}} Z_k^{(c)(l)}, \sum_{k\in S^{(2,r)}} Y_{2k}^{(i)(r)}\Big)}_{C_2}$$
$$- \frac{1}{n_c^{(l)} m_1^{(r)}}\underbrace{\mathrm{Cov}\Big(\sum_{k\in S^{(c,l)}} Z_k^{(c)(l)}, \sum_{k\in S^{(1,r)}} Y_{1k}^{(i)(r)}\Big)}_{C_3}$$
$$+ \frac{1}{m_2^{(l)} n_c^{(r)}}\underbrace{\mathrm{Cov}\Big(\sum_{k\in S^{(2,l)}} Y_{2k}^{(i)(l)}, \sum_{k\in S^{(c,r)}} Z_k^{(c)(r)}\Big)}_{C_4}$$
$$+ \frac{1}{m_2^{(l)} m_2^{(r)}}\underbrace{\mathrm{Cov}\Big(\sum_{k\in S^{(2,l)}} Y_{2k}^{(i)(l)}, \sum_{k\in S^{(2,r)}} Y_{2k}^{(i)(r)}\Big)}_{C_5}$$

$$
\begin{aligned}
&-\frac{1}{m_2^{(l)}m_1^{(r)}}\underbrace{\mathrm{Cov}(\sum_{k\in S^{(2,l)}} Y_{2k}^{(i)(l)}, \sum_{k\in S^{(1,r)}} Y_{1k}^{(i)(r)})}_{C_6} \\
&-\frac{1}{m_1^{(l)}n_c^{(r)}}\underbrace{\mathrm{Cov}(\sum_{k\in S^{(1,l)}} Y_{1k}^{(i)(l)}, \sum_{k\in S^{(c,r)}} Z_{k}^{(c)(r)})}_{C_7} \\
&-\frac{1}{m_1^{(l)}m_2^{(r)}}\underbrace{\mathrm{Cov}(\sum_{k\in S^{(1,l)}} Y_{1k}^{(i)(l)}, \sum_{k\in S^{(2,r)}} Y_{2k}^{(i)(r)})}_{C_8} \\
&+\frac{1}{m_1^{(l)}m_1^{(r)}}\underbrace{\mathrm{Cov}(\sum_{k\in S^{(1,l)}} Y_{1k}^{(i)(l)}, \sum_{k\in S^{(1,r)}} Y_{1k}^{(i)(r)})}_{C_9}].
\end{aligned}
$$

A consistent estimator $\widehat{\boldsymbol{V}}$ of $\boldsymbol{V}$ is achieved by separately estimating terms involving C_1–C_9. Details are shown in the Appendix. Test procedures described in Sect. 4.5 can be directly applied by using the newly constructed covariance matrix estimator $\widehat{\boldsymbol{V}}$ in (4.11) and (4.12).

4.7 Simulation Study

In this section, we examine the performance of the proposed Wald-type statistic Q_n in (4.11) and that of the ANOVA-type statistic $\widehat{F}_n$ in (4.12). The evaluations focus on (a) control of the preassigned Type-I error level ($\alpha = 0.05$) under $H_0 : \boldsymbol{p} = \frac{1}{2}\mathbb{1}_d$ and (b) achieved powers to detect specific alternatives. Also, a simulation study will be conducted to investigate the accuracy of these test procedures for data sets with general missing patterns.

4.7.1 Simulation Settings

The simulation seeks to generate evidence on the performance of the tests along the two criteria in various scenarios that cover a wide spectrum of reasonable models. The study involves multivariate data with strong/weak and positive/negative correlations for small and moderate sample sizes. The observations $\boldsymbol{X}_j^{(c)}$ and $\boldsymbol{X}_{gk}^{(i)}$, $j = 1, \cdots, n_c$, $g = 1, 2$, $k = 1, \cdots, n_g$, will be generated from Discretized Multivariate Normal, Multivariate Log-Normal, and Multivariate Cauchy distributions, which represent discrete, skewed, and heavily tailed data, respectively. Covariance

Table 4.2 Complete and incomplete sample sizes combinations

Setting	n_c	n_1	n_2
1	10	30	30
2	30	10	10
3	30	30	10
4	10	10	30

or scale matrix of the data will be set to

$$\boldsymbol{\Sigma} = \begin{bmatrix} \sigma_1^2 \mathrm{I}_d + \rho_1\sigma_1^2(\mathrm{J}_d - \mathrm{I}_d) & \rho_{12}\sigma_1\sigma_2\mathrm{J}_d \\ \rho_{12}\sigma_1\sigma_2\mathrm{J}_d & \sigma_2^2\mathrm{I}_d + \rho_2\sigma_2^2(\mathrm{J}_d - \mathrm{I}_d) \end{bmatrix},$$

where J_d is the d-dimensional square matrix of all ones. The impact of between and within treatment group correlations can be investigated by varying values of ρ_1, ρ_2, and ρ_{12}. Further, homoscedastic and heteroscedastic scenarios are covered by setting $\sigma_1^2 = \sigma_2^2$ and $\sigma_1^2 \neq \sigma_2^2$, respectively. For the correlations and variances, we investigate for $(\rho_1, \rho_2, \rho_{12}) \in \{(0.1, 0.1, 0.1), (-0.1, -0.1, -0.1), (0.1, 0.9, 0.5)\}$ and $(\sigma_1^2, \sigma_2^2) \in \{(1, 1), (1, 5)\}$. With this covariance matrix $\boldsymbol{\Sigma}$, we consider three multivariate distributions:

- Discretized Multivariate Normal: Data for the complete as well as incomplete cases are generated from multivariate normal distributions, and then each component is rounded to the nearest integer. More precisely, defining $[\cdot]$ as the rounding operator, data for the complete cases are generated as $\boldsymbol{X}_j^{(c)} = (X_{1j}^{(c)(1)}, \cdots, X_{1j}^{(c)(d)}, X_{2j}^{(c)(1)}, \cdots, X_{2j}^{(c)(d)})$, where $X_{gj}^{(c)(d)} = [W_{gk}^{(c)(d)}]$ and $\boldsymbol{W}_j^{(c)} = (W_{1j}^{(c)(1)}, \cdots, W_{1j}^{(c)(d)}, W_{2j}^{(c)(1)}, \cdots, W_{2j}^{(c)(d)}) \sim N(\boldsymbol{0}, \boldsymbol{\Sigma})$. Data for incomplete cases are generated in the same manner.
- Multivariate Log Normal: Data for the complete as well as incomplete cases are generated from multivariate normal distributions, and then each component is exponentiated. Specifically, data for complete cases are generated as $\boldsymbol{X}_j^{(c)}=(X_{1j}^{(c)(1)}, \cdots, X_{1j}^{(c)(d)}, X_{2j}^{(c)(1)}, \cdots, X_{2j}^{(c)(d)})$, where $X_{gj}^{(c)(d)} = \exp(W_{gj}^{(c)(d)})$ and $\boldsymbol{W}_j^{(c)} \sim N(\boldsymbol{0}, \boldsymbol{\Sigma})$. Data for incomplete cases are generated similarly.
- Multivariate Cauchy: Both the complete and incomplete cases are generated from the multivariate Cauchy distributions $\boldsymbol{C}(\boldsymbol{0}, \boldsymbol{\Sigma})$.

Four combinations of sample sizes listed in Table 4.2 will be considered.

Dimensions of the multivariate data will be set to $d = 2, 3, 5$. For every combination of the sample size, dimension, covariance matrices, and distributions, 1000 simulations are performed. The empirical sizes or powers are calculated from these replications. All the computations are done in R (version 4.2.3) (RStudio Team, 2020).

Two different methods for handling missing values in nonparametric multivariate analysis are considered for comparison:

- The method of Brunner et al. (2002) which is designed for independent multivariate samples. We keep data from incomplete cases only for each treatment group so that the problem reduces to that of two independent samples. This method is a special case of the methods developed in this chapter by setting $n_c = 0$.
- A special case of the methods derived in this manuscript where $n_1 = n_2 = 0$. In this case, only data from complete cases will be used.

The goal of the simulation is to obtain information on whether the test procedures proposed in this manuscript, which use all available data, have superior performance over the tests that use only partial data.

For brevity of notations, the alternative methods will be referred to as Incomplete and Complete. In the simulation tables, test procedures for Incomplete and Complete are denoted by $Q_n^{(j)}$ and $F_n^{(j)}$, where $j = 1, 2$ represent Wald-type and ANOVA-type statistics, respectively.

4.7.2 Type-I Error Rate

Achieved Type-I error rates are presented in Tables 4.3, 4.4, and 4.5. From these tables, we note that dependence structures as well as distributions have minor effects on Type-I error rates. The achieved Type-I error rates for each method are close to each other no matter data are generated from discrete, skewed, or heavily tailed distributions. We can also see that the ANOVA-type statistics F_n, $F_n^{(1)}$, and $F_n^{(2)}$ are quite stable for all settings, and F_n has an advantage over $F_n^{(1)}$ and $F_n^{(2)}$ in preserving the preassigned significance level of $\alpha = 0.05$ in most of the cases. However, although the Wald-type statistics Q_n, $Q_n^{(1)}$, and $Q_n^{(2)}$ are all too liberal, Q_n performs better than $Q_n^{(1)}$ and $Q_n^{(2)}$ generally. Further, performances of Incomplete and Complete methods are slightly affected by sample size settings, i.e., $Q_n^{(1)}$ and $F_n^{(1)}$ have better performance under Setting 1 where more samples are allocated to incomplete cases, while $Q_n^{(2)}$ and $F_n^{(2)}$ perform better under Setting 4 where more samples are allocated to complete cases.

There is no obvious pattern showing that the dimension will affect the performance for the ANOVA-type statistics, but it does affect the performance for the Wald-type statistics. The achieved Type-I error rates for Q_n, $Q_n^{(1)}$, and $Q_n^{(2)}$ increase with d, and the greatest increase is observed for $Q_n^{(2)}$ at sample size Settings 1 and 4. Variances of samples also make a difference. For fixed sample sizes and correlations, data that are generated from heterogeneous distributions tend to have more liberal performance too.

Table 4.3 Achieved Type-I error rate ($\times 100$) for data generated from Discretized Multivariate Normal distribution with missing pattern as in Table 4.1 for $d = 2, 3, 5$. Here, Q_n is the Wald-type statistic proposed in (4.11); F_n is ANOVA-type statistic for small sample approximation proposed in (4.12); $Q_n^{(1)}$ and $F_n^{(1)}$ are Wald-type and ANOVA-type tests for the Incomplete method; $Q_n^{(2)}$ and $F_n^{(2)}$ are Wald-type and ANOVA-type tests for the Complete method. The nominal Type-I error rate is $\alpha = 0.05$

			$(\sigma_1^2, \sigma_2^2) = (1, 1)$						$(\sigma_1^2, \sigma_2^2) = (1, 5)$					
Sample size setting	$(\rho_1, \rho_2, \rho_{12})$	d	Q_n	F_n	$Q_n^{(1)}$	$F_n^{(1)}$	$Q_n^{(2)}$	$F_n^{(2)}$	Q_n	F_n	$Q_n^{(1)}$	$F_n^{(1)}$	$Q_n^{(2)}$	$F_n^{(2)}$
1	(0.1,0.1,0.1)	2	6.3	4.7	6.7	5.9	11.8	6.5	6.5	5.7	7.2	6.3	13	7.0
		3	7.1	5.6	8.1	5.6	20.6	5.0	7.9	5.8	6.4	4	19.4	6.1
		5	8.7	4.6	9.0	5.6	40.2	6.1	10.4	5.6	10.8	5.1	40.3	5.4
	(0.1,0.9,0.5)	2	5.8	6.3	5.6	6.3	9.6	5.2	5.7	8.4	6.5	7.5	10.1	7.2
		3	7.8	7.6	8.3	7.5	15.3	4.9	5.3	8.3	5.5	7.9	15.0	9.5
		5	7.3	5.9	8.7	8.0	36	3.8	5.5	10.6	6.6	11.1	30.7	10.8
2	(0.1,0.1,0.1)	2	6.5	4.9	10.2	5.4	7.7	4.9	6.8	5.8	11.9	7.5	7.9	5.2
		3	8.5	6.3	13.2	7.4	8.4	4.7	7.7	4.7	15.4	7.0	8.6	4.6
		5	9.2	4.4	25.3	6.9	12.6	5.2	10.7	5.7	26.9	6.2	13.9	6.3
	(0.1,0.9,0.5)	2	6.0	4.7	10.8	7.7	7.1	5.8	5.8	6.6	9.8	10.2	7.0	6.2
		3	6.8	5.2	13.7	9.0	8.0	4.5	8.1	8.5	11.3	11.0	7.9	8.6
		5	9.4	5.9	25	9.9	11.9	5.0	6.3	8.6	12.0	12.2	9.7	9.1
3	(0.1,0.1,0.1)	2	5.6	4.8	9.5	6.0	6.9	5.5	6.7	5.7	13.8	8.8	7.2	5.6
		3	6.9	5.4	13.4	5.7	9.2	5.8	7.9	6.3	16.6	5.2	9.9	6.8
		5	8.5	5.0	19.5	6.7	13.4	5.7	11.5	6.1	30.9	6.7	14.0	5.3
	(0.1,0.9,0.5)	2	5.2	6.3	9.6	9.2	5.0	4.1	7.0	7.7	9.6	11.1	7.3	6.8
		3	5.8	6.5	9.8	9.4	8.4	4.6	6.1	9.7	10.9	11.8	6.1	7.3
		5	7.9	9.0	15.1	13.8	11.3	4.6	5.7	9.6	13.4	13.9	9.7	9.4
4	(0.1,0.1,0.1)	2	9.0	6.8	9.6	6.3	14.2	8.0	7.0	5.5	7.5	5.7	11.9	7.4
		3	8.0	4.9	11.4	6.6	20.8	6.9	8.7	5.8	8.7	6.3	19.6	6.6
		5	13.5	5.1	23.9	7.2	40.5	4.7	10.1	5.5	11.4	4.9	40.2	6.3
	(0.1,0.9,0.5)	2	8.6	7.2	10.6	8.1	11.8	6.2	6.1	6.0	5.8	6.3	10.9	7.5
		3	8.7	5.5	14.3	6.0	16.0	4.2	8.7	8.3	11.0	8.4	14.8	7.4
		5	14.1	6.9	27.6	7.2	35.3	5.3	7.7	8.9	13.5	9.4	30.5	9.9

4.7.3 Power Study

To investigate power of the two tests based on Q_n and F_n, bivariate situation ($d = 2$) is considered with three multivariate distributions. In this situation, the first sample is drawn with mean $\boldsymbol{\mu} = (0, 0)$, and the second one is drawn with mean $\boldsymbol{\mu} = (\delta_1, \delta_2)$. Three types of location shift alternatives $(\delta_1, \delta_2) = \delta(1, k)$ for $k = 0, 1, 2$ are considered, where $\delta \in \{0.3, 0.6, 0.9\}$. Power simulation results are displayed in Tables 4.6, 4.7, and 4.8.

Table 4.4 Achieved Type-I error rate (×100) for data generated from Multivariate Log-Normal distribution with missing pattern as in Table 4.1 for $d = 2, 3, 5$. Here, Q_n is the Wald-type statistic proposed in (4.11); F_n is ANOVA-type statistic for small sample approximation proposed in (4.12); $Q_n^{(1)}$ and $F_n^{(1)}$ are Wald-type and ANOVA-type tests for the Incomplete method; $Q_n^{(2)}$ and $F_n^{(2)}$ are Wald-type and ANOVA-type tests for the Complete method. The nominal Type-I error rate is $\alpha = 0.05$

			$(\sigma_1^2, \sigma_2^2) = (1, 1)$						$(\sigma_1^2, \sigma_2^2) = (1, 5)$					
Sample Size Setting	$(\rho_1, \rho_2, \rho_{12})$	d	Q_n	F_n	$Q_n^{(1)}$	$F_n^{(1)}$	$Q_n^{(2)}$	$F_n^{(2)}$	Q_n	F_n	$Q_n^{(1)}$	$F_n^{(1)}$	$Q_n^{(2)}$	$F_n^{(2)}$
1	(0.1,0.1,0.1)	2	7.1	6.5	6.9	5.5	11.7	6	5.6	4.9	5.9	4.8	12.5	7.7
		3	7.2	4.7	7.1	5.8	22.2	6.5	7.1	4.7	6.3	4.1	16.9	6.2
		5	6.6	3.9	7.9	4.8	37.2	4.5	10.7	7	11.1	5.8	41.5	6.2
	(−0.1, −0.1, −0.1)	2	5.6	5	7.1	6.3	13.8	8.1	7.6	5.7	7.1	5.9	13.9	6.9
		3	6.3	4.9	6.1	4.4	20.3	6.6	7	4.6	7.2	5.3	21.5	6.1
		5	11.4	6.1	10.9	6.5	40.7	5.5	9	5.7	11.5	5.3	40.1	6.4
2	(0.1,0.1,0.1)	2	6	5.4	9.5	7	6.3	4.7	7	6.5	11.8	6.5	7.4	6.3
		3	5.6	4.6	12.5	5.5	8.4	4.8	7.9	4.7	15.9	6.2	7.8	5.6
		5	9.1	5.8	20.3	5.4	12.8	5.8	9.8	5.4	28	5.3	13.1	6.8
	(−0.1, −0.1, −0.1)	2	6.7	6	9.9	6.2	8	6.8	8	5.9	11.8	7.8	8.6	6.8
		3	7.1	5.6	15.7	6.6	9.5	4.8	8	6.4	14.8	6.4	9.7	5.6
		5	11	4.9	19.5	4.9	13.7	6.2	12.5	6.5	27.1	6	15.3	6.2
3	(0.1,0.1,0.1)	2	6.6	5.8	8.1	6.1	7.1	5.7	6.5	5.6	11.8	6.6	8.1	5.8
		3	7.2	5.5	14.9	6.9	9.1	5.6	7.1	5.1	16.5	6.9	9.8	5.2
		5	8.4	5.7	18.8	5.2	13.7	5.7	10.5	5.1	33.3	6.5	13.6	4.9
	(−0.1, −0.1, −0.1)	2	6.7	5.6	9.4	5.9	8.4	6.5	6.6	5.5	13.2	8.2	7.1	5.6
		3	7.2	4.3	10.4	5.4	9.7	5	7.3	4.9	19.1	7	8.5	5.2
		5	9.1	5.6	19.4	6.1	13.4	5.6	8.6	4.7	35.2	6.5	12.6	5.7
4	(0.1,0.1,0.1)	2	7.8	5.4	10	6.3	13.5	6.2	7	5.7	7.7	6	14.1	7.5
		3	9.4	5.9	12.3	6.1	19.5	6.6	6.1	4.4	7.9	5.8	18.4	5
		5	12.6	5.1	20.4	6.2	40.3	5.3	8.8	5	10.4	4.5	42.3	5.6
	(−0.1, −0.1, −0.1)	2	7.3	5.4	9.8	6.1	14.7	6.5	6.8	5.3	7.3	6.6	12.9	7.6
		3	9.8	6.9	13	6.4	20.3	6.9	7.4	4.8	9	5.9	20.1	5.6
		5	11.3	5.2	19.1	5.9	40.6	5.6	11.8	6.2	12.5	6.2	42.1	7

Looking at the power results in these three tables, it is clear to see that data generated from homogeneous distribution yield higher power than the heterogeneous ones for fixed sample size and location shift. Also, mean shift $\boldsymbol{\mu}_2 = (\delta, 2\delta)$ yields higher power than $\boldsymbol{\mu}_2 = (\delta, \delta)$, which in turn yields higher power than $\boldsymbol{\mu}_2 = (\delta, 0)$. This is expected because $\boldsymbol{\mu}_2 = (\delta, 2\delta)$ is a stronger departure from the null compared to $\boldsymbol{\mu}_2 = (\delta, \delta)$ and $\boldsymbol{\mu}_2 = (\delta, 0)$ in the sense that $\| (\delta, 2\delta) \|_2^2 > \| (\delta, \delta) \|_2^2 > \| (\delta, 0) \|_2^2$.

Furthermore, larger values δ produce higher power for a given location alternative. Q_n achieves the highest power among all Wald-type statistics, and similarly,

Table 4.5 Achieved Type-I error rate (×100) for data generated from Multivariate Cauchy distribution with missing pattern as in Table 4.1 for $d = 2, 3, 5$. Here, Q_n is the Wald-type statistic proposed in (4.11); F_n is ANOVA-type statistic for small sample approximation proposed in (4.12); $Q_n^{(1)}$ and $F_n^{(1)}$ are Wald-type and ANOVA-type tests for the Incomplete method; $Q_n^{(2)}$ and $F_n^{(2)}$ are Wald-type and ANOVA-type tests for the Complete method. The nominal Type-I error rate is $\alpha = 0.05$

			$(\sigma_1^2, \sigma_2^2) = (1, 1)$						$(\sigma_1^2, \sigma_2^2) = (1, 5)$					
Sample size setting	$(\rho_1, \rho_2, \rho_{12})$	d	Q_n	F_n	$Q_n^{(1)}$	$F_n^{(1)}$	$Q_n^{(2)}$	$F_n^{(2)}$	Q_n	F_n	$Q_n^{(1)}$	$F_n^{(1)}$	$Q_n^{(2)}$	$F_n^{(2)}$
1	(0.1,0.1,0.1)	2	6.9	5.8	7.6	6.5	11.9	6.3	6.2	5.2	5.8	4.9	13.8	6.1
		3	7.6	5.8	6.5	4.3	20.8	6.6	6.4	4.4	6.7	4.3	20.8	7
		5	8	4.5	8.5	4.9	47.5	6.6	9.1	5.3	10.5	5.9	43.9	5.9
	(−0.1, −0.1, −0.1)	2	7.5	6.2	8.1	6.5	13.2	7.7	6.4	5.2	6.1	5.3	15.3	8.6
		3	7.3	5.2	5.9	4.1	22.9	6.6	7	4.8	8.4	5.2	22.9	7.4
		5	10.9	6.2	9.2	5.6	48	7.3	9.6	4.3	9.5	4.9	46.7	8.3
2	(0.1,0.1,0.1)	2	6.2	4.7	12.5	6.8	6.5	4.3	7.8	6.4	10	5.5	7.4	5.7
		3	7.2	5.3	15.3	6.4	9.2	5.3	8	5.8	14.7	6.7	10.2	5.2
		5	10.2	4.4	23	4.8	16	4.6	11.2	6.3	26.2	6.4	15.8	6.1
	(−0.1, −0.1, −0.1)	2	6.4	5.4	10.9	7.5	8.3	6.3	6	4.9	9.8	5.8	7.3	4.7
		3	9.8	7.4	14.2	6	10.1	6.8	7.4	5.1	13.7	4.5	9.4	4.9
		5	11.2	4.2	23.7	5.6	15.8	5	12.1	5.3	25.4	6.2	14.8	5.9
3	(0.1,0.1,0.1)	2	8	6.1	10.2	5.9	9.1	7.3	6.6	5.8	10.8	6.9	7.3	5.9
		3	7.9	7	15.2	7.2	9.3	5.4	7.5	5.1	14	5.7	10.1	6.4
		5	10.5	5.2	19.4	5.7	17	5.5	10.7	5.9	29.4	5.3	16.3	6.3
	(−0.1, −0.1, −0.1)	2	8.9	7	9.7	5.5	10.5	7.4	5	4.5	10.8	7.3	6.9	5.7
		3	6.3	4.1	10.9	4.8	10.6	6.1	6.8	5	16.3	6.6	8.1	5.3
		5	7.4	3.3	17.1	3.8	14.6	5.1	10.6	6.3	28.5	8	13.7	4.7
4	(0.1,0.1,0.1)	2	7	5.5	10	6.6	13.6	8.2	6.7	4.8	9.2	6	12.1	6.9
		3	7.7	4.5	12.2	5.4	19.8	5.2	9.3	5.4	9.6	5.5	19.9	6.3
		5	12.2	6.1	19.6	5.9	45.5	5.9	10.3	4.6	13	4.5	43.6	6.3
	(−0.1, −0.1, −0.1)	2	7.5	5.6	9.7	6.8	16.7	8.3	6.2	5.7	7.4	5.4	14.6	8.5
		3	9.5	5.1	12.4	5.5	24.3	7.2	10.3	6.4	11.9	6.8	22.6	6.4
		5	12.1	4.6	18.8	5.6	44.3	6.6	12.5	5.1	16.3	4.4	44.6	6.2

F_n attains higher power compared to $F_n^{(1)}$ and $F_n^{(2)}$. We also note that powers for Incomplete and Complete methods are related to sample size allocations. More specifically, $Q_n^{(1)}$ and $F_n^{(1)}$ perform better in Settings 1 and 4 since incomplete data make up higher proportion in the data set. For the same reason, $Q_n^{(2)}$ and $F_n^{(2)}$ perform better in Settings 2 and 3 as complete data weight more in this case. Different from the Type-I error simulation results, the data distributions greatly affect the powers.

Table 4.6 Achieved power (×100) for data generated from Discretized Multivariate Normal distribution with missing pattern as in Table 4.1 for $d = 2$. Here, Q_n is the Wald-type statistic proposed in (4.11); F_n is ANOVA-type statistic for small sample approximation proposed in (4.12); $Q_n^{(1)}$ and $F_n^{(1)}$ are Wald-type and ANOVA-type tests in the Incomplete method; $Q_n^{(2)}$ and $F_n^{(2)}$ are Wald-type and ANOVA-type tests in the Complete method. The correlation coefficients are $(\rho_1, \rho_2, \rho_{12}) = (0.1, 0.1, 0.1)$

			$(\sigma_1^2, \sigma_2^2) = (1, 1)$						$(\sigma_1^2, \sigma_2^2) = (1, 5)$					
Sample size setting	δ_1	δ_2	Q_n	F_n	$Q_n^{(1)}$	$F_n^{(1)}$	$Q_n^{(2)}$	$F_n^{(2)}$	Q_n	F_n	$Q_n^{(1)}$	$F_n^{(1)}$	$Q_n^{(2)}$	$F_n^{(2)}$
1	0	0.3	21.6	20.2	18.7	17.3	20.5	11.3	11.3	10	10.9	9	13.4	7.3
	0.3	0.3	35.9	36.5	28.6	28.5	26.6	17.3	15.2	14	13.5	12.1	16.9	8.9
	0.6	0.6	91.8	92.4	79.3	81	49.3	38.6	44.8	44.8	37	36	25.7	18
	0.9	0.9	100	100	99.3	99.6	77.9	72.2	79.2	80.3	66.1	65.9	40.2	32.3
	0.3	0.6	77.3	76.6	61.7	62.7	37.8	26.5	32.6	30.6	25.3	23.9	21.9	15.5
	0.3	0.9	96.4	96.4	89.5	89.8	57.9	45.8	53.9	52.5	39.9	38	29.9	20.9
2	0	0.3	22.8	20.7	15.2	10.4	21	17.4	11.9	10.7	14.2	9.5	11.6	9.4
	0.3	0.3	41.9	38.8	18.7	13.5	34.9	30.4	17.4	15	13.3	8.9	16.3	14.2
	0.6	0.6	94.6	94.8	42.6	38.9	86.9	86.1	47	45.5	20	14.2	40.9	38.3
	0.9	0.9	100	100	72.5	70.4	99.6	99.5	80.5	80.5	34.7	28.3	69.2	68.4
	0.3	0.6	77.4	76.7	31.2	25.9	68.8	65.2	31.3	29.4	16.9	11.5	27.2	24.9
	0.3	0.9	97.3	97.2	51.3	44.7	93.2	92.8	56.1	54.3	25.4	19.9	46.4	43.1
3	0	0.3	26	23.2	15.9	11.3	20.8	17.9	12.5	10.5	13.8	8	12.6	9.5
	0.3	0.3	47.9	47.3	22.3	18	37.2	32.6	17.1	15.8	15.1	9.3	13.7	11.9
	0.6	0.6	96.9	97.1	58	54	87.5	87	46.4	46	23.6	17.2	37.9	35.8
	0.9	0.9	100	100	87	86.5	99.5	99.6	81.5	81.6	36.4	30.1	70.2	68.4
	0.3	0.6	83.5	83.3	36	32.5	68.7	64.9	31.6	30.9	19.9	14.2	26.1	23.8
	0.3	0.9	99	98.9	68.4	62.4	93.9	92	59.6	56.9	27.7	20.1	47.4	44.3
4	0	0.3	15.7	12.6	14.8	10.1	17	9.5	10	8.1	8.6	7.2	13.4	7.5
	0.3	0.3	29.6	27.8	22.5	18.9	22.8	13.6	13	12.5	11.6	9.4	16	9.3
	0.6	0.6	77.6	78.5	53.8	49.9	51	41.2	42.9	42.6	29.9	29.1	25	17.2
	0.9	0.9	98.4	98.4	86.4	84.5	78.7	72	71	71.4	54.3	54.3	39.3	30.9
	0.3	0.6	59.8	57.7	38.8	31.8	38	28.4	26.7	24.2	18.5	15.1	24.7	15.9
	0.3	0.9	87.6	86.1	66.9	62.5	58.1	46.2	47.9	46	35.3	32.7	27.3	18.8

While the achieved power for data from Multivariate Discretized Normal distribution is generally close to those from the Multivariate Log-Normal distribution, they both are greater than the powers for data from Multivariate Cauchy distribution.

4.7.4 Multiple Imputation

Another common method for handling missing data is Multiple Imputation introduced in (Rubin, 2004). In the context of our problem, missing or deficient values are replaced with two or more acceptable values generated from a predictive

Table 4.7 Achieved power ($\times 100$) for data generated from Multivariate Log-Normal distribution with missing pattern as in Table 4.1 for $d = 2$. Here, Q_n is the Wald-type statistic proposed in (4.11); F_n is ANOVA-type statistic for small sample approximation proposed in (4.12); $Q_n^{(1)}$ and $F_n^{(1)}$ are Wald-type and ANOVA-type tests in the Incomplete method; $Q_n^{(2)}$ and $F_n^{(2)}$ are Wald-type and ANOVA-type tests in the Complete method. The correlation coefficients are $(\rho_1, \rho_2, \rho_{12}) = (-0.1, -0.1, -0.1)$

			$(\sigma_1^2, \sigma_2^2) = (1, 1)$						$(\sigma_1^2, \sigma_2^2) = (1, 5)$					
Sample size setting	δ_1	δ_2	Q_n	F_n	$Q_n^{(1)}$	$F_n^{(1)}$	$Q_n^{(2)}$	$F_n^{(2)}$	Q_n	F_n	$Q_n^{(1)}$	$F_n^{(1)}$	$Q_n^{(2)}$	$F_n^{(2)}$
1	0	0.3	18.3	17.1	17.4	14.8	17.4	10.6	11.4	9.5	10.7	7.7	16	9.7
	0.3	0.3	41.6	37.1	32.4	27.6	27.7	17.8	16.9	14.1	15.5	13.3	16.9	8.1
	0.6	0.6	93.9	92.4	86.8	83.6	44.9	34.1	48.4	44.4	40.3	35.3	22.8	15.8
	0.9	0.9	100	100	99.6	99.3	76.9	68	82.5	79.3	72.8	68.9	34.5	24.6
	0.3	0.6	77.7	74.5	69.2	64.1	34.7	24	30.6	26.8	25.4	22.3	20.3	13.5
	0.3	0.9	96.7	95.6	92.4	90.5	54.6	44.5	55.9	52.9	45.7	41.5	28	18.6
2	0	0.3	21.4	19.4	13.7	9.9	18.4	15.9	11.6	9.5	14.1	9.6	11.4	9.3
	0.3	0.3	38.1	33.8	19.5	13.6	30.4	28.2	16	13.7	14.1	7.5	14.9	13
	0.6	0.6	92.3	92.1	49.1	39.2	82.6	80	46.6	43.5	24	16.2	38.2	34.8
	0.9	0.9	100	99.9	78.5	72.8	98.7	98.7	78.9	76.1	39.1	28.3	67.9	63.8
	0.3	0.6	71.5	69.6	33.7	25.1	59.6	55.8	31.5	27.6	17.7	11.4	26.2	22.1
	0.3	0.9	95.4	94.8	53.8	43.4	88.2	86	53.9	51.7	26.5	17.7	44.7	40.4
3	0	0.3	27.2	25.3	16.3	12.3	20.8	16.9	11.4	10.7	14.2	9.2	11	8.4
	0.3	0.3	44	41	24.5	18.7	30.9	26.7	16.2	13.1	16.6	9.9	14.4	11.8
	0.6	0.6	95.4	95	59.9	51.7	80.3	78.4	46.9	41.4	26.3	17.6	32.8	28.5
	0.9	0.9	100	100	91	87.4	98.8	98.3	82.5	79.3	41.3	33	65.9	63.3
	0.3	0.6	81.3	78.5	46.5	37.1	57.5	54.8	34.6	31.8	22	14	26.3	22.1
	0.3	0.9	98.2	98.2	68.5	58.9	89.8	88.1	57.3	52.6	29.8	21.7	45	39.9
4	0	0.3	17.9	15.4	17.2	12.9	19.2	11	9.2	8.5	11.1	8.5	11.9	7.1
	0.3	0.3	31.7	26.8	25	18	24.6	15.2	17.5	14.8	15.2	11.1	16.3	9.5
	0.6	0.6	80.5	76.3	62.1	53.2	44.2	34.5	42.9	38.9	36.2	30.2	25.1	17.2
	0.9	0.9	99.4	99	92.5	89.9	75.2	68.5	74.4	70.5	58.6	52.8	38.9	27.7
	0.3	0.6	60.1	55.1	46.2	36.5	35.7	23.6	28.3	24.4	22.1	18.5	21.3	12.3
	0.3	0.9	88.6	86.3	71.1	62.4	54	40.5	51.7	46.7	40.6	34.8	27.3	18.4

distribution. Hotelling's two sample T^2 test will be conducted on each of the completed data to test equality of mean vectors in the two groups, i.e., $H_0 : \boldsymbol{\mu}_1 = \boldsymbol{\mu}_2$ vs. $H_1 : \boldsymbol{\mu}_1 \neq \boldsymbol{\mu}_2$. We refer to this test procedure as Imputation. However, due to the computational cost of Imputation, only a small-scale simulation is conducted to compare its performance with the methods introduced in this chapter. In the covariance matrix, $(\rho_1, \rho_2, \rho_{12}) = (-0.1, -0.1, -0.1)$ or $(0.1, 0.1, 0.1)$ and $(\sigma_1, \sigma_2) = (1, 1)$ or $(1, 5)$ are used. The achieved Type-I error rates and powers from Imputation are displayed in Tables 4.9 and 4.10. In Table 4.9, for discretized multivariate normal distribution or multivariate log-normal distribution

Table 4.8 Achieved power ($\times 100$) for data generated from Multivariate Cauchy distribution with missing pattern as in Table 4.1 for $d = 2$. Here, Q_n is the Wald-type statistic proposed in (4.11); F_n is ANOVA-type statistic for small sample approximation proposed in (4.12); $Q_n^{(1)}$ and $F_n^{(1)}$ are Wald-type and ANOVA-type tests in the Incomplete method; $Q_n^{(2)}$ and $F_n^{(2)}$ are Wald-type and ANOVA-type tests in the Complete method. The correlation coefficients are $(\rho_1, \rho_2, \rho_{12}) = (0.1, 0.9, 0.5)$

			$(\sigma_1^2, \sigma_2^2) = (1, 1)$						$(\sigma_1^2, \sigma_2^2) = (1, 5)$					
Sample size setting	δ_1	δ_2	Q_n	F_n	$Q_n^{(1)}$	$F_n^{(1)}$	$Q_n^{(2)}$	$F_n^{(2)}$	Q_n	F_n	$Q_n^{(1)}$	$F_n^{(1)}$	$Q_n^{(2)}$	$F_n^{(2)}$
1	0	0.3	12.7	10.3	11	9.3	14.9	9.7	8.8	7.2	8.2	7.2	10.9	5.9
	0.3	0.3	12.8	14.9	10.1	11.6	15.3	10.1	7.5	9.8	7.8	8.7	10.8	7.2
	0.6	0.6	38.4	45.2	28.6	35.4	30.3	20.8	15.5	20.9	12.5	15.5	14	11.4
	0.9	0.9	63.8	71.2	47.4	54.7	45.7	36.8	29.2	37.1	19	28.1	21.3	17.8
	0.3	0.6	28.7	29.4	20.9	21.9	24.4	15.5	13	14.7	11.4	11.6	13.3	10.1
	0.3	0.9	49.2	48.7	35.3	34.9	34.3	24	25.7	24.4	20.2	18.8	19.8	12.4
2	0	0.3	15.2	12.2	10.5	6.7	13.7	11.2	10	8.1	9.2	8.5	8.8	6.5
	0.3	0.3	17.5	17.9	9.7	8.1	20.6	17.2	8.4	9.5	8.7	7.3	8.4	9.2
	0.6	0.6	49.5	53.9	17.9	16.4	52.2	50.7	19.9	22.8	11.9	12.1	19.8	21.6
	0.9	0.9	78.7	83.4	24.6	25.7	76.9	76.9	35.8	42.9	15.1	15.5	32.6	37.8
	0.3	0.6	38.6	40.7	16.5	13.9	40.8	37.8	14.8	17.4	9.8	9.1	15.3	14.8
	0.3	0.9	63.6	62.9	23.7	19	61.5	59	31	30.6	14.3	12.6	27.4	25.8
3	0	0.3	15.3	11.6	13	10.9	13.9	11.6	8.3	7.1	9.4	8.5	9.5	6.7
	0.3	0.3	17	21.1	11.8	12.7	19.9	17.4	7.8	9.6	10.1	10.3	9.9	9.1
	0.6	0.6	48.7	57.7	18.7	23.3	53	52.9	16.5	22	13.2	13.9	18.9	20.6
	0.9	0.9	79	87.2	30.1	34.3	75.8	77.5	34.3	42.9	15.8	17.9	33.9	39
	0.3	0.6	38.5	40	15.9	15.9	41.6	38.5	16.6	18	12.2	11.3	16.6	16.1
	0.3	0.9	62.4	63.2	28.2	23	58.4	56.6	30.5	27.4	16	12.7	28.3	26.7
4	0	0.3	11.5	8.6	11.5	7.7	14.6	8.4	9.1	7.1	9	6.6	10	6.7
	0.3	0.3	15.3	14.1	16.1	11.7	16.6	9.4	8.9	9	10.2	8.4	11.2	8.9
	0.6	0.6	34.4	36.5	25	22.5	32.3	23.6	15.7	16.4	13.1	11.7	13.8	10.2
	0.9	0.9	54.1	58.4	37.3	33.7	48.2	38.8	27.8	31.1	21.2	20.6	21.2	17.9
	0.3	0.6	26.4	24.9	20.7	16.4	23.3	15.1	13.3	13.4	11.2	10.1	14	10.3
	0.3	0.9	40.7	38.7	28.8	22.5	35.8	25.8	23.6	22.8	17.1	14.9	20.6	15.8

with homoscedasticity, F_n and Imputation achieve similar Type-I error rates. However, when data are generated from multivariate log-normal distribution with heteroscedasticity, the achieved Type-I error rates are too liberal and nearly 1. Also, for data generated from multivariate Cauchy distribution, the achieved Type-I error rates are too conservative compared to F_n. Overall, Imputation achieves smaller powers compared with Q_n and F_n. Specifically, for data that are generated from multivariate Cauchy distribution, the achieved powers are way too small.

Table 4.9 Achieved Type-I error rate ($\times 100$) for data generated from Discretized Multivariate Normal, Multivariate Log-Normal, and Multivariate Cauchy distributions with missing pattern as in Table 4.1 for $d = 2, 3, 5$. Here, Q_n is the Wald-type statistic proposed in (4.11); F_n is ANOVA-type statistic for small sample approximation proposed in (4.12); Multiple Impute is the test procedure in Imputation alternative method with five chains. The nominal Type-I error rate is $\alpha = 0.05$, and sample sizes are as in Setting 1

			Discretized multivariate normal			Multivariate log normal			Multivariate Cauchy		
$(\rho_1, \rho_2, \rho_{12})$	(σ_1^2, σ_2^2)	d	Q_n	F_n	Multiple impute	Q_n	F_n	Multiple impute	Q_n	F_n	Multiple impute
(−0.1, −0.1, −0.1)	(1,1)	2	5.2	4.2	4.6	7.2	6.3	5.6	5.4	4.4	2.4
		3	7.5	5.7	5.9	7.1	5.3	5.8	7.3	5.3	2.1
		5	12	7.1	5.3	8.0	4.8	5.0	7.9	4.0	1.1
	(1,5)	2	7.2	6.8	6.1	6.5	5.3	73.4	7.0	5.8	2.9
		3	7.1	5.7	4.8	5.4	4.3	85.7	7.8	5.8	2.7
		5	6.6	3.8	4.5	9.2	5.0	97.3	9.1	5.4	1.0
(0.1,0.1,0.1)	(1,1)	2	5.5	5.3	4.7	7.1	6.3	6.0	5.5	4.3	3.2
		3	7.2	4.9	3.6	6.4	4.3	6.0	6.6	4.5	2.1
		5	9.7	6.0	4.0	9.6	5.4	6.3	10.2	5.3	0.8
	(1,5)	2	5.1	4.7	5.6	7.2	6.3	72.2	6.4	5.4	2.8
		3	8.0	6.1	6.3	6.3	3.7	87	8.2	6.7	2.4
		5	8.8	5.9	4.8	8.9	5.0	95	8.9	4.8	1.1

4.7.5 General Missing Pattern

For multivariate data that have general missing structures, we anticipate performance to be affected by sample size allocations. We consider three allocations which are aimed to cover practical situations, and we refer to them as Designs 1–3:

Design 1: Fix the total sample size n and assign $n/15$ subjects per missing pattern.
Design 2: Fix the total sample size n and vary the proportion of complete cases a such that $n_1 = na$ (complete sample size) and $n_2 = \cdots = n_{15} = n(1 - a)/14$.
Design 3: Fix $n_2, \cdots, n_{15} = 100$ (i.e., a large number of incomplete cases) and vary the complete sample size n_1.

The achieved Type-I error rates and powers are shown in Tables 4.11, 4.12, 4.13 and 4.14, 4.15, 4.16, respectively. The performances of the methods under Discretized Multivariate Normal distribution and Multivariate Log-Normal distribution are similar.

In Table 4.11, the ANOVA-type statistic preserves preassigned significance level very well in all settings, while Wald-type statistic tends to be slightly liberal. In Tables 4.12 and 4.13, performances of Wald-type and ANOVA-type statistics are very close, and they both control preassigned significance level well. Furthermore, their performances are not affected by the distributions, covariance structures, or sample sizes allocations.

Table 4.10 Achieved power (×100) for data generated from Discretized Multivariate Normal, Multivariate Log-Normal, and Multivariate Cauchy distributions with missing pattern as in Table 4.1 for $d = 2, 3, 5$. Here, Q_n is the Wald-type statistic proposed in (4.11); F_n is ANOVA-type statistic for small sample approximation proposed in (4.12); Multiple Impute is the test procedure in Imputation alternative method with five chains. The nominal Type-I error rate is $\alpha = 0.05$, and sample sizes are as in Setting 1

				Discretized Multivariate Normal			Multivariate Log-Normal			Multivariate Cauchy		
$(\rho_1, \rho_2, \rho_{12})$	(σ_1^2, σ_2^2)	δ_1	δ_2	Q_n	F_n	Multiple impute	Q_n	F_n	Multiple impute	Q_n	F_n	Multiple impute
(−0.1, −0.1, −0.1)	(1,1)	0	0.3	20	18.1	9	19.9	17	Impute	10	8.9	2.7
		0.3	0.3	40	35	16.1	40.3	35.9	17.8	17.3	14.9	3.5
		0.6	0.6	93	91.1	58.7	94.2	93	45.5	44.8	42.5	3.9
		0.9	0.9	99.9	99.9	89.4	100	100	72.9	75.6	73.3	7.2
		0.3	0.6	77.7	75	40.2	77.3	73.8	30.8	31.9	28.6	3.2
		0.3	0.9	97.2	96.7	68.9	97.5	97.1	48.4	52.7	48.9	5.7
	(1,5)	0	0.3	10.9	9.1	6.4	13.2	12	31.1	7.5	6.1	2.2
		0.3	0.3	17.4	14	9.6	15.3	13	31.5	9.7	8.7	3
		0.6	0.6	47.3	43.2	21.9	47.6	44.8	37.4	21.4	18.4	3.2
		0.9	0.9	80.1	76.8	46.5	81.8	78.2	44.4	40.8	36.2	4.6
		0.3	0.6	32.2	28	13.3	31.2	27.9	33.5	15.8	13.2	3.1
		0.3	0.9	55.9	52.9	27.2	58.4	54.5	37.8	27.3	22.7	4.3
(0.1,0.1,0.1)	(1,1)	0	0.3	22.2	20.3	10.8	21.8	20	11.3	10	8.7	2.3
		0.3	0.3	36	35	15.7	38.1	38.1	16.1	16.3	15.5	2.2
		0.6	0.6	90	90.6	51.6	90.3	90.4	41.2	41.9	43	4
		0.9	0.9	100	100	89	99.9	99.9	72.1	70.1	72	7.4
		0.3	0.6	70	69	35.8	75.8	76	30.1	30.6	30.5	4.3
		0.3	0.9	95.3	95.2	63.6	97.1	97.1	50.8	49.8	49.2	4.6
	(1,5)	0	0.3	12.4	10.9	6.6	8.6	7.2	30.8	8.9	7.9	1.8
		0.3	0.3	16.3	16.2	9.1	15.5	14.3	31.3	10.2	9.1	2.7
		0.6	0.6	45.9	45.1	20.3	44.5	44.9	38.4	20.3	19.2	2.3
		0.9	0.9	76.9	77.3	41.5	78.5	78.9	42.7	36.6	37.7	4.3
		0.3	0.6	30.4	28.8	13.6	30.9	30.5	34.1	17.2	15.6	2.7
		0.3	0.9	53.8	52.4	23.5	51.1	50.5	37.8	25.6	24.1	3.5

The power reacts are consistent with Sect. 4.7.3. The ANOVA-type statistics tend to achieve higher powers than the Wald-type statistics and, further, homogeneous data yield more powers compared to heterogeneous data. Furthermore, we see that powers generally increase with the total sample size n, the proportion of complete cases (in Table 4.15), and the complete sample size (in Table 4.16). It is also worth mentioning that the results in Table 4.16 are quite favorable in the sense that most of them approach unity even when δ is small.

Table 4.11 Achieved Type-I error rate (×100) for data generated from Discretized Multivariate Normal, Multivariate Log-Normal, and Multivariate Cauchy distributions with general missing pattern for $d = 2$. Here, n is the total sample size in Design 1; Q_n is the Wald-type statistic proposed in (4.11); F_n is ANOVA-type statistic for small sample approximation proposed in (4.12). The nominal Type-I error rate is $\alpha = 0.05$

Design 1			Discretized multivariate normal		Multivariate log-normal		Multivariate Cauchy	
n	$(\rho_1, \rho_2, \rho_{12})$	(σ_1, σ_2)	Q_n	F_n	Q_n	F_n	Q_n	F_n
75	(−0.1, −0.1, −0.1)	(1,1)	6.2	4.9	6.4	5.6	6.1	4.6
		(1,5)	5.9	5.5	5.4	5.0	6.5	5.6
	(0.1,0.1,0.1)	(1,1)	7.7	6.1	5.5	4.4	6.7	6.0
		(1,5)	7.6	6.1	6.5	5.2	6.7	6.3
150	(−0.1, −0.1, −0.1)	(1,1)	7.1	6.5	5.4	5.0	6.2	5.6
		(1,5)	6.3	5.7	5.9	5.5	5.8	5.4
	(0.1,0.1,0.1)	(1,1)	5.4	4.7	5.5	5.3	4.9	3.4
		(1,5)	5.7	5.0	5.6	4.8	4.9	4.6
300	(−0.1, −0.1, −0.1)	(1,1)	5.5	5.5	5.9	5.4	5.1	4.8
		(1,5)	7.1	7.2	4.7	4.5	4.9	4.3
	(0.1,0.1,0.1)	(1,1)	5.6	5.4	4.9	4.5	4.7	4.5
		(1,5)	3.6	3.6	4.5	3.9	8.0	7.5

Table 4.12 Achieved Type-I error rate (×100) for data generated from Discretized Multivariate Normal, Multivariate Log-Normal, and Multivariate Cauchy distributions with general missing pattern for $d = 2$. Here, n is the total sample size in Design 2; Q_n is the Wald-type statistic proposed in (4.11); F_n is ANOVA-type statistic for small sample approximation proposed in (4.12). The nominal Type-I error rate is $\alpha = 0.05$

Design 2				Discretized multivariate normal		Multivariate log-normal		Multivariate Cauchy	
n	$(\rho_1, \rho_2, \rho_{12})$	(σ_1^2, σ_2^2)	a	Q_n	F_n	Q_n	F_n	Q_n	F_n
210	(−0.1, −0.1 − 0.1)	(1,1)	0.2	5.6	4.9	5.1	4.9	4.4	4.6
			0.4	5.1	4.9	6.2	6.2	4.8	5.0
			0.6	5.8	5.4	5.1	5.0	5.7	5.7
			0.8	5.5	5.1	4.6	4.1	5.8	5.6
		(1,5)	0.2	5.2	5.3	4.3	4.1	7.1	6.3
			0.4	5	4.5	4.6	4.0	5.3	5.2
			0.6	6.2	6.2	6.2	5.6	4.4	4.4
			0.8	6.4	6.2	5.9	6.0	5.6	5.2
	(0.1,0.1,0.1)	(1,1)	0.2	4.9	4.7	5.2	4.8	4.9	4.8
			0.4	5.4	5.0	5.9	4.9	5.9	5.5
			0.6	5.5	5.4	7.0	6.4	6.4	5.9
			0.8	5.4	4.9	4.8	4.5	5.3	4.7
		(1,5)	0.2	5.0	4.8	5.9	5.5	5.4	5.3
			0.4	6.5	5.9	6.7	5.6	4.5	4.4
			0.6	5.0	4.8	4.6	4.4	6.9	6.1
			0.8	4.8	5.1	4.5	4.7	4.9	4.4

Table 4.13 Achieved Type-I error rate (×100) for data generated from Discretized Multivariate Normal, Multivariate Log-Normal, and Multivariate Cauchy distributions with general missing pattern for $d = 2$. Here, n_1 is the complete sample size in Design 3; Q_n is the Wald-type statistic proposed in (4.11); F_n is ANOVA-type statistic for small sample approximation proposed in (4.12). The nominal Type-I error rate is $\alpha = 0.05$

Design 3			Discretized multivariate normal		Multivariate log-normal		Multivariate Cauchy	
$(\rho_1,\rho_2,\rho_{12})$	(σ_1,σ_2)	n_1	Q_n	F_n	Q_n	F_n	Q_n	F_n
(−0.1, −0.1, −0.1)	(1,1)	5	6.6	6.3	4.8	4.6	5.4	5.6
		10	6.6	6.6	6.7	6.7	4.8	4.6
		20	4.3	4.1	4.3	4.3	5.6	5.6
	(1,5)	5	5.0	5.0	4.9	5.0	4.9	4.8
		10	4.9	4.4	5.1	5.1	5.1	5.6
		20	5.8	5.6	5.8	5.6	5.6	5.9
(0.1,0.1,0.1)	(1,1)	5	5.1	4.8	6.7	6.7	4.5	4.3
		10	4.9	4.8	5.2	5.2	4.7	4.7
		20	5.9	5.8	3.8	3.9	4.1	4.0
	(1,5)	5	5.2	4.6	6.4	6.1	5.2	5.2
		10	6.4	6.6	5.8	5.5	4.2	4.4
		20	4.2	4.1	6.3	6.2	5.4	5.2

4.8 Real Data Analysis

In this section, we analyze the ARTIS data described in Sect. 4.2. The data-analytic objective is to test the existence of air-filter intervention effect on the domain variables. Our main goal is to illustrate the application of the methods developed in this chapter with a real data and compare the results with the alternative methods presented in Sect. 4.7. For the ARTIS data, the interpretation of significant intervention effect is that at least one of the domain variables has nonparametric effect size not equal to 0.5, i.e., data collected after the air-filter intervention tend to be either greater or smaller than those collected before in at least one of the domains. More generally, we want to know whether the air-filter intervention improves quality of life for children with asthma in terms of activity limitation, emotional function, or symptoms domains.

As mentioned in Sect. 4.2, one child per family and one visit per intervention period is selected randomly to make the ARTIS data fit the data scheme assumed in this chapter. In the selected random sample, $n_c = 34$ children have paired data before and after the intervention on all the three domains, $n_1 = 7$ children have data on all three domains only in the pre-intervention period, and $n_2 = 1$ child has data on all three domains only in the post-intervention period. The estimates of $\boldsymbol{p}$ are shown in Table 4.17 for the methods derived in this chapter (All) and, also, for Incomplete and Complete methods.

From Table 4.17, at $\alpha = 0.05$, the ANOVA-type statistic detects significant intervention effect for both All and Incomplete methods, while the Wald-type

Table 4.14 Achieved power (×100) for data generated from Discretized Multivariate Normal, Multivariate Log-Normal, and Multivariate Cauchy distribution with general missing pattern for $d = 2$. Here, n is the total sample size in Design 1; Q_n is the Wald-type statistic proposed in (4.11); F_n is ANOVA-type statistic for small sample approximation proposed in (4.12). The correlation coefficients are $(\rho_1, \rho_2, \rho_{12}) = (0.1, 0.1, 0.1)$. The nominal Type-I error rate is $\alpha = 0.05$

Design 1				$n = 75$		$n = 150$		$n = 300$	
Distribution	(σ_1^2, σ_2^2)	δ_1	δ_2	Q_n	F_n	Q_n	F_n	Q_n	F_n
Discretized multivariate normal	(1,1)	0	0.3	20.8	18.9	35.6	34.8	67.8	67.2
		0.3	0.3	37.0	34.6	61.6	61.7	92.4	93.0
		0.6	0.6	92.8	92.3	99.8	99.7	100	100
		0.9	0.9	99.9	99.9	100	100	100	100
		0.3	0.6	77.8	75.6	95.7	95.6	100	100
		0.3	0.9	95.7	94.9	100	100	100	100
	(1,5)	0	0.3	11.9	10.4	14.0	13.3	24.7	23.6
		0.3	0.3	15.5	14.1	23.0	22.2	44.5	44.9
		0.6	0.6	44.1	43.2	74.6	74.9	96.5	96.5
		0.9	0.9	77.9	79.2	98.3	98.7	100	100
		0.3	0.6	28.4	27.6	55.4	55.1	85.2	85.2
		0.3	0.9	55.4	52.6	84.0	83.6	99.4	99.4
Multivariate Cauchy	(1,1)	0	0.3	11.2	10.0	17.2	15.9	26.0	25.2
		0.3	0.3	16.7	14.4	25.6	24.2	46.8	45.6
		0.6	0.6	46.7	45.3	74.1	74.1	96.7	97.1
		0.9	0.9	74.5	75.0	97.1	97.4	100	100
		0.3	0.6	29.4	27.6	56.0	54.2	84.9	85.6
		0.3	0.9	53.8	52.0	82.2	82.4	98.8	98.9
	(1,5)	0	0.3	9.0	7.4	8.4	7.7	11.5	11.2
		0.3	0.3	10.4	10.0	10.4	10.4	19.9	19.8
		0.6	0.6	21.9	19.4	34.2	33.4	63.0	63.0
		0.9	0.9	38.7	36.8	68.3	67.6	93.3	93.5
		0.3	0.6	15.3	14.3	22.9	21.9	41.4	40.4
		0.3	0.9	24.9	23.6	41.8	41.4	72.8	73.9

statistic does not pick any significant affect. However, note that in the current data set, ANOVA-type statistic is more reliable compared with Wald-type statistic due to the extreme small sample sizes. Therefore, taking all available data into consideration, the air-filter intervention does have significant tendency to result in larger PAQLQ scores for the three domains. In other words, the intervention does improve the quality of life for children with asthma in homes using wood-burning stoves. And this conclusion holds if one takes only the incomplete data into consideration. However, since the total sample size for Incomplete method is $n_1 + n_2 = 8$ and there is only one sample in the post-intervention group, the results from this method are rather biased and, therefore, its effect size estimates are not reliable. It is interesting that the test by taking just the complete data into consideration is not significant, and the reason for that is the PAQLQ scores differ

Table 4.15 Achieved power ($\times 100$) for data generated from Multivariate Normal, Multivariate Log-Normal, and Multivariate Cauchy distribution with general missing pattern for $d = 2$. Here, n is the total sample size in Design 2; Q_n is the Wald-type statistic proposed in (4.11); F_n is ANOVA-type statistic for small sample approximation proposed in (4.12). The correlation coefficients are $(\rho_1, \rho_2, \rho_{12}) = (0.1, 0.1, 0.1)$. The nominal Type-I error rate is $\alpha = 0.05$

Design 2					$a = 0.2$		$a = 0.4$		$a = 0.6$		$a = 0.8$	
n	Distribution	(σ_1^2, σ_2^2)	δ_1	δ_2	Q_n	F_n	Q_n	F_n	Q_n	F_n	Q_n	F_n
210	Discretized multivariate normal	(1,1)	0	0.3	56.2	55.1	59.8	59	68.2	67.2	73.6	73
			0.3	0.3	83.6	84.1	89.6	89	92.5	92.4	95.9	95.7
			0.6	0.6	100	100	100	100	100	100	100	100
			0.9	0.9	100	100	100	100	100	100	100	100
			0.3	0.6	99.8	99.8	99.9	99.9	100	100	100	100
			0.3	0.9	100	100	100	100	100	100	100	100
		(1,5)	0	0.3	20.4	20.3	24.6	24.1	27.2	26.6	26.7	26.9
			0.3	0.3	37.2	36.6	43.5	43.5	47.5	47.8	49.2	49.3
			0.6	0.6	91.1	91.4	94.7	95.5	97.2	97.5	98.4	98.6
			0.9	0.9	100	100	100	100	100	100	100	100
			0.3	0.6	74.9	74.6	83.1	82.8	86	85.7	89.8	90.1
			0.3	0.9	96.2	95.9	98.7	98.5	99.2	99.1	99.3	99.2
	Multivariate Cauchy	(1,1)	0	0.3	21.1	20	24.9	24.1	27.9	27.3	29.8	29.7
			0.3	0.3	38.3	37.9	43.8	43.5	49.8	49.4	55.6	56.1
			0.6	0.6	91.7	91.8	94.4	94.6	96.9	97.7	98.1	98
			0.9	0.9	99.9	99.9	100	100	100	100	100	100
			0.3	0.6	74.4	74.1	83.6	84	85	86	88.4	88.7
			0.3	0.9	95.7	95.4	97.2	97.4	98.8	99.1	99.7	99.6
		(1,5)	0	0.3	9.1	9	12.5	11.2	13.3	13.1	14	13.7
			0.3	0.3	16	16.2	19.1	18.4	19.1	19.6	21	21.4
			0.6	0.6	51.2	50.6	55.9	56.6	64.7	65.9	72	72
			0.9	0.9	84.5	85.5	89.5	89.7	92.6	92.7	97.2	97.4
			0.3	0.6	35.1	34.7	38.9	38.1	47.6	46.8	48.2	48
			0.3	0.9	62.3	61.7	67.5	67.1	72.9	73.3	78.5	78.1

mainly among the subjects who do not have complete data collected. The Imputation method does not provide effect size estimates. Thus, the only conclusion that can be drawn is that there is no significant difference between mean PAQLQ scores of the domains between pre-intervention and post-intervention periods.

4.9 Discussion

In many studies, multivariate data from subjects that belong to the same or different treatment groups are collected. In this chapter, we have proposed methods that can be used to compare treatment groups for this type of data with general missing

Table 4.16 Achieved power ($\times 100$) for data generated from Multivariate Normal, Multivariate Log-Normal, and Multivariate Cauchy distribution with general missing pattern for $d = 2$. Here, n_1 is the complete sample size in Design 3; Q_n is the Wald-type statistics proposed in (4.11); F_n is ANOVA-type statistics for small sample approximation proposed in (4.12). The correlation coefficients are $(\rho_1, \rho_2, \rho_{12}) = (0.1, 0.1, 0.1)$. The nominal Type-I error rate is $\alpha = 0.05$

Design 3				$n_1 = 5$		$n_1 = 10$		$n_1 = 20$	
Distribution	(σ_1^2, σ_2^2)	δ_1	δ_2	Q_n	F_n	Q_n	F_n	Q_n	F_n
Discretized multivariate normal	(1,1)	0	0.3	99.8	99.8	100	100	100	100
		0.3	0.3	100	100	100	100	100	100
		0.6	0.6	100	100	100	100	100	100
		0.9	0.9	100	100	100	100	100	100
		0.3	0.6	100	100	100	100	100	100
		0.3	0.9	100	100	100	100	100	100
	(1,5)	0	0.3	78.8	78.8	78.2	78	81.1	80.9
		0.3	0.3	97.6	97.5	98.2	98.4	98.4	98.5
		0.6	0.6	100	100	100	100	100	100
		0.9	0.9	100	100	100	100	100	100
		0.3	0.6	100	100	100	100	100	100
		0.3	0.9	100	100	100	100	100	100
Multivariate Cauchy	(1,1)	0	0.3	82	82	82.9	82.5	84.3	83.8
		0.3	0.3	99	98.9	97.9	98	97.9	98
		0.6	0.6	100	100	100	100	100	100
		0.9	0.9	100	100	100	100	100	100
		0.3	0.6	100	100	100	100	100	100
		0.3	0.9	100	100	100	100	100	100
	(1,5)	0	0.3	37.2	37.6	37.4	37.4	38	37.9
		0.3	0.3	67	67.1	69.6	69.6	67.5	67.4
		0.6	0.6	99.9	99.9	100	100	99.9	99.9
		0.9	0.9	100	100	100	100	100	100
		0.3	0.6	97.8	97.7	96.9	97.2	97.2	97.2
		0.3	0.9	99.9	99.9	100	100	100	100

patterns. Commonly used approaches include removing incomplete samples, i.e., keep complete cases only, and imputing incomplete cases from the existing data. These strategies are not effective in the sense that they either ignore valuable information or introduce imputation errors. With simulation studies, we have shown that all of these alternatives methods are not efficient in preserving the preassigned Type-I error rate or achieving reasonable power. Therefore, they cannot be recommended for general application.

This chapter aims at inferential procedures with the fewest assumptions so that ordinal or skewed data are accommodated in a seamless way. In that sense, we derived a fully nonparametric method for estimating and testing the nonparametric effect size applicable for multivariate data. Our nonparametric effect size estimators also allow comparisons among treatment groups on each response variable. In

Table 4.17 Test statistics and p-values for Domain Variables in ARTIS data. Here, Q_n and F_n are p-values for Wald-type and ANOVA-type statistics proposed in (4.11) and (4.12); $Q_n^{(1)}$ and $F_n^{(1)}$ are p-values for Wald-type and ANOVA-type tests in the Incomplete method; $Q_n^{(2)}$ and $F_n^{(2)}$ are p-values for Wald-type and ANOVA-type tests in the Complete method. The nominal Type-I error rate is $\alpha = 0.05$

	All			Incomplete			Complete			Multiple impute
	$\widehat{\mathbf{p}}$	Q_n	F_n	$\widehat{\mathbf{p}}$	$Q_n^{(1)}$	$F_n^{(1)}$	$\widehat{\mathbf{p}}$	$Q_n^{(2)}$	$F_n^{(2)}$	p-value
Activity limitation	0.549	0.101	0.037	0.857	0.100	<0.001	0.529	0.420	0.399	0.769
Emotional function	0.596			1.000			0.548			
Symptoms	0.594			1.000			0.568			

other words, unlike global tests, the proposed procedures can provide more specific information.

With our method, the marginal distribution of each response variable is estimated independently by weighing the corresponding complete and incomplete data. This strategy leads to procedures implementable using ranking routines and reduces the code complexity for calculating effect sizes and covariance matrices. However, other estimation of marginal distributions, such as taking correlation among the variables and between the treatment groups into consideration in the weighting scheme, is likely to be more accurate. Furthermore, although multiple response variables are allowed in this chapter, only the two-group case is considered. Also, clustered data are not allowed for any of the response variables. In summary, extension to multiple groups and more elaborate estimators of nonparametric effect to accommodate complex data structures will be of interest. For instance, the ARTIS data set involves twenty-three quality of life scores measured in three groups, which can be regarded as multivariate clustered data in factorial design with complete and incomplete clusters. Harrar and Cui (2023) introduces this nonparametric model to clustered data in factorial pre-post intervention design, but an extension to multivariate case is of great interest. It should be pointed out that the missing data patterns along with dependence structures among response variables and clusters may result in a rather complex covariance matrix in the asymptotic theory. We plan to investigate these problems in future researches.

Appendix

Proof of Theorem 4.4.3

To show $\| \widehat{\boldsymbol{V}} - \boldsymbol{V} \|_2^2 \to 0$, it suffices to show the L_2-consistency for each element of $\widehat{\boldsymbol{V}} - \boldsymbol{V}$, i.e., $\| \widehat{v}^{(l,r)} - v^{(l,r)} \|_2^2 \to 0$. Here, $v^{(l,r)}$ is given in (4.6) and $\widehat{v}^{(l,r)} = \widehat{v}_c^{(l,r)} + \widehat{v}_1^{(l,r)} + \widehat{v}_2^{(l,r)}$, where $\widehat{v}_j^{(l,r)}$ is the (l, r)th entry of $\widehat{\boldsymbol{V}}_j$, $j \in \{c, 1, 2\}$ as given in (4.8) and (4.9). First, rewrite

$$\widehat{v}_g^{(l,r)} = n\frac{n_g}{m_g^2(n_g-1)}\sum_{k=1}^{n_g}(\widehat{Y}_{gk}^{(i)(l)} - \widehat{\overline{Y}}_{g\cdot}^{(i)(l)})(\widehat{Y}_{gk}^{(i)(r)} - \widehat{\overline{Y}}_{g\cdot}^{(i)(r)}), \quad g = 1,2 \quad \text{and} \tag{4.14}$$

$$\widehat{v}_c^{(l,r)} = \frac{n}{n_c(n_c-1)}\sum_{k=1}^{n_c}(\widehat{Z}_k^{(c)(l)} - \widehat{\overline{Z}}_{\cdot}^{(c)(l)})(\widehat{Z}_k^{(c)(r)} - \widehat{\overline{Z}}_{\cdot}^{(c)(r)}). \tag{4.15}$$

By triangle inequality, it follows

$$\| \widehat{v}^{(l,r)} - v^{(l,r)} \|_2^2 \leq \| \widehat{v}^{(l,r)} - \tilde{v}^{(l,r)} \|_2^2 + \| \tilde{v}^{(l,r)} - v^{(l,r)} \|_2^2 .$$

Now, the proof will be complete by showing $\| \widehat{v}^{(l,r)} - \tilde{v}^{(l,r)} \|_2^2 \to 0$ and $\| \tilde{v}^{(l,r)} - v^{(l,r)} \|_2^2 \to 0$.

To show $\| \tilde{v}^{(l,r)} - v^{(l,r)} \|_2^2 \to 0$, it suffices to show $\| \widehat{v}_j^{(l,r)} - \tilde{v}_j^{(l,r)} \|_2^2 \to 0$, $j \in \{c, 1, 2\}$, by triangle equality. Proof of the special case when $l = r \in \{1, \cdots, d\}$, $j \in \{c, 1, 2\}$ follows from Theorem 5.1 in (Konietschke et al., 2012). For other cases where $l \neq r$, we give an example proof for $j = c$.

Observe that

$$\begin{aligned}
&\| \tilde{v}_c^{(l,r)} - v_c^{(l,r)} \|_2^2 \\
&= E\Bigg(\frac{n}{n_c(n_c-1)}\sum_{k=1}^{n_c}\Big[\frac{n_c}{m_2}Y_{2k}^{(c)(l)} - \frac{n_c}{m_1}Y_{1k}^{(c)(l)} - \Big(\frac{n_c}{m_2}\overline{Y}_{2\cdot}^{(c)(l)} - \frac{n_c}{m_1}\overline{Y}_{1\cdot}^{(c)(l)}\Big)\Big]\times \\
&\qquad \Big[\frac{n_c}{m_2}Y_{2k}^{(c)(r)} - \frac{n_c}{m_1}Y_{1k}^{(c)(r)} - \Big(\frac{n_c}{m_2}\overline{Y}_{2\cdot}^{(c)(r)} - \frac{n_c}{m_1}\overline{Y}_{1\cdot}^{(c)(r)}\Big)\Big] \\
&\quad - \frac{n}{n_c}\mathrm{Cov}\Big(\frac{n_c}{m_2}Y_{2k}^{(c)(l)} - \frac{n_c}{m_1}Y_{1k}^{(c)(l)}, \frac{n_c}{m_2}Y_{2k}^{(c)(r)} - \frac{n_c}{m_1}Y_{1k}^{(c)(r)}\Big)\Bigg)^2 \\
&= E\Bigg(\sum_{g=1}^{2}\sum_{g'=1}^{2}(1 - 2\ell_{g\neq g'})\frac{n}{n_c(n_c-1)}\sum_{k=1}^{n_c}\Big(\frac{n_c}{m_g}Y_{gk}^{(c)(l)} - \frac{n_c}{m_g}\overline{Y}_{g\cdot}^{(c)(l)}\Big) \\
&\times \Big(\frac{n_c}{m_{g'}}Y_{g'k}^{(c)(r)} - \frac{n_c}{m_{g'}}\overline{Y}_{g'\cdot}^{(c)(r)}\Big) \\
&\quad - \sum_{g=1}^{2}\sum_{g'=1}^{2}(1 - 2\ell_{g\neq g'})\frac{n}{n_c}\frac{1}{n_c}\sum_{k=1}^{n_c}\mathrm{Cov}\Big(\frac{n_c}{m_g}Y_{gk}^{(c)(l)} - \frac{n_c}{m_{g'}}Y_{g'k}^{(c)(r)}\Big)\Bigg)^2 \\
&= E\Bigg(\sum_{g=1}^{2}\sum_{g'=1}^{2}(1 - 2\ell_{g\neq g'})\frac{n_c}{m_g}\frac{n_c}{m_{g'}}\Big[\frac{n}{n_c(n_c-1)}\sum_{k=1}^{n_c}(Y_{gk}^{(c)(l)} - \overline{Y}_{g\cdot}^{(c)(l)}) \\
&\quad \times (Y_{g'k}^{(c)(r)} - \overline{Y}_{g'\cdot}^{(c)(r)}) - \frac{n}{n_c^2}\sum_{k=1}^{n_c}\mathrm{Cov}(Y_{gk}^{(c)(l)}, Y_{g'k}^{(c)(r)})\Big]\Bigg)^2
\end{aligned}$$

$$\leq 4\sum_{g=1}^{2}\sum_{g'=1}^{2}(\frac{n_c}{m_g}\frac{n_c}{m_{g'}})^2 E\Bigg(\frac{n}{n_c(n_c-1)}\sum_{k=1}^{n_c}(Y_{gk}^{(c)(l)}-\overline{Y}_{g\cdot}^{(c)(l)})(Y_{g'k}^{(c)(r)}-\overline{Y}_{g'\cdot}^{(c)(r)})$$
$$-\frac{n}{n_c^2}\sum_{k=1}^{n_c}\mathrm{Cov}(Y_{gk}^{(c)(l)},Y_{g'k}^{(c)(r)})\Bigg)^2.$$

According to the proof of Theorem 3.5 in (Werner, 2006), we have

$$E\Bigg(\frac{n}{n_c(n_c-1)}\sum_{k=1}^{n_c}(Y_{gk}^{(c)(l)}-\overline{Y}_{g\cdot}^{(c)(l)})(Y_{g'k}^{(c)(r)}-\overline{Y}_{g'\cdot}^{(c)(r)})$$
$$-\frac{n}{n_c^2}\sum_{k=1}^{n_c}\mathrm{Cov}(Y_{gk}^{(c)(l)},Y_{g'k}^{(c)(r)})\Bigg)^2$$
$$=O(\frac{1}{n_c}).$$

This implies

$$\| \tilde{v}_c^{(l,r)}-v_c^{(l,r)} \|_2^2\leq 4\sum_{g=1}^{2}\sum_{g'=1}^{2}(\frac{n_c}{m_g}\frac{n_c}{m_{g'}})^2 O(\frac{1}{n_c})=O(\frac{1}{m_1}+\frac{1}{m_2}).$$

Next, we show $\| \widehat{v}_c^{(l,r)}-\tilde{v}_c^{(l,r)} \|_2^2\to 0$. Notice that

$$\| \widehat{v}_c^{(l,r)}-\tilde{v}_c^{(l,r)} \|_2^2$$
$$=E(\widehat{v}_c^{(l,r)}-\tilde{v}_c^{(l,r)})^2$$
$$=(\frac{n}{n_c-1})^2 *$$
$$E\Bigg(\frac{1}{n_c}\sum_{k=1}^{n_c}\underbrace{[(\widehat{Z}_k^{(c)(l)}-\widehat{\overline{Z}}_{\cdot}^{(c)(l)})(\widehat{Z}_k^{(c)(r)}-\widehat{\overline{Z}}_{\cdot}^{(c)(r)})-(Z_k^{(c)(l)}-\overline{Z}_{\cdot}^{(c)(l)})(Z_k^{(c)(r)}-\overline{Z}_{\cdot}^{(c)(r)})]}_{\Delta_k}\Bigg)^2$$
$$=(\frac{n}{n_c-1})^2 E(\frac{1}{n_c}\sum_{k=1}^{n_c}\Delta_k)^2.$$

Let $A=\frac{1}{n_c}\sum_{k=1}^{n_c}\Delta_k$. It follows that $\| \widehat{v}_c^{(l,r)}-\tilde{v}_c^{(l,r)} \|_2^2=(\frac{n}{n_c-1})^2E(A^2)$. By Jensen's Inequality and C_r-inequality,

$$
\begin{aligned}
E(A^2) &\le \frac{1}{n_c}\sum_{k=1}^{n_c} E(\Delta_k^2) \\
&\le 2E\left((Z_1^{(c)(l)} - \overline{Z}_{\cdot}^{(c)(l)})^2[(\widehat{Z}_1^{(c)(r)} - \widehat{\overline{Z}}_{\cdot}^{(c)(r)}) - (Z_1^{(c)(r)} - \overline{Z}_{\cdot}^{(c)(r)})]^2\right) \\
&\quad + 2E\left((\widehat{Z}_1^{(c)(r)} - \widehat{\overline{Z}}_{\cdot}^{(c)(r)})^2[(\widehat{Z}_1^{(c)(l)} - \widehat{\overline{Z}}_{\cdot}^{(c)(l)}) - (Z_1^{(c)(l)} - \overline{Z}_{\cdot}^{(c)(l)})]^2\right).
\end{aligned} \tag{4.16}
$$

Note that the random variables $Y_{gk}^{(c)(l)}$ and $\widehat{Y}_{gk}^{(c)(l)}$ are uniformly bounded by 1 so that $|Y_{gk}^{(c)(l)} - \overline{Y}_{g\cdot}^{(c)(l)}| \le 1$ and $|\widehat{Y}_{gk}^{(c)(l)} - \widehat{\overline{Y}}_{g\cdot}^{(c)(l)}| \le 1$. Then, by C_r-inequality, it follows that

$$
\begin{aligned}
E(Z_1^{(c)(l)} - \overline{Z}_{\cdot}^{(c)(l)})^2 &= E\big[\theta_2(Y_{2k}^{(c)(l)} - \overline{Y}_{2\cdot}^{(c)(l)}) - \theta_1(Y_{1k}^{(c)(l)} - \overline{Y}_{1\cdot}^{(c)(l)})\big]^2 \\
&\le 2E\big[\theta_2^2(Y_{2k}^{(c)(l)} - \overline{Y}_{2\cdot}^{(c)(l)})^2 + \theta_1^2(Y_{1k}^{(c)(l)} - \overline{Y}_{1\cdot}^{(c)(l)})^2\big] \\
&\le 2(\theta_2^2 + \theta_1^2) \\
&\le 4.
\end{aligned} \tag{4.17}
$$

Further,

$$
\begin{aligned}
&E\left((Z_1^{(c)(l)} - \overline{Z}_{\cdot}^{(c)(l)})^2[(\widehat{Z}_1^{(c)(r)} - \widehat{\overline{Z}}_{\cdot}^{(c)(r)}) - (Z_1^{(c)(r)} - \overline{Z}_{\cdot}^{(c)(r)})]^2\right) \\
&\le 16E\big[(\widehat{Z}_1^{(c)(r)} - \widehat{\overline{Z}}_{\cdot}^{(c)(r)}) - (Z_1^{(c)(r)} - \overline{Z}_{\cdot}^{(c)(r)})\big]^2 \\
&= 16E\big[(\widehat{Z}_1^{(c)(r)} - Z_1^{(c)(r)}) - (\widehat{\overline{Z}}_{\cdot}^{(c)(r)} - \overline{Z}_{\cdot}^{(c)(r)})\big]^2 \\
&\le 32E(\widehat{Z}_1^{(c)(r)} - Z_1^{(c)(r)})^2 + 32E(\widehat{\overline{Z}}_{\cdot}^{(c)(r)} - \overline{Z}_{\cdot}^{(c)(r)})^2 \\
&\le 64E(\widehat{Z}_1^{(c)(r)} - Z_1^{(c)(r)})^2,
\end{aligned}
$$

where the last step follows by Jensen's inequality. According to proof of Theorem 5.1 in (Konietschke et al., 2012), $E\big(\widehat{F}_g^{(r)}(X_{g'k}^{(c)(r)}) - F_g^{(r)}(X_{g'k}^{(c)(r)})\big)^2 = O(\frac{1}{m_g})$, $g, g' \in \{1, 2\}$, and $g \ne g'$. Then by C_r-inequality, it follows that

$$
\begin{aligned}
E(\widehat{Z}_1^{(c)(r)} - Z_1^{(c)(r)})^2 &= E\big(\theta_2(\widehat{Y}_{2k}^{(c)(r)} - Y_{2k}^{(c)(r)}) - \theta_1(\widehat{Y}_{1k}^{(c)(r)} - Y_{1k}^{(c)(r)})\big)^2 \\
&\le 2\theta_2^2 E(\widehat{Y}_{2k}^{(c)(r)} - Y_{2k}^{(c)(r)})^2 + 2\theta_1^2 E(\widehat{Y}_{1k}^{(c)(r)} - Y_{1k}^{(c)(r)})^2 \\
&= 2\theta_2^2 E\big(\widehat{F}_1^{(r)}(X_{2k}^{(c)(r)}) - F_1^{(r)}(X_{2k}^{(c)(r)})\big)^2 \\
&\quad + 2\theta_1^2 E\big(\widehat{F}_2^{(r)}(X_{1k}^{(c)(r)}) - F_2^{(r)}(X_{1k}^{(c)(r)})\big)^2 \\
&= O(\frac{1}{m_1} + \frac{1}{m_2}).
\end{aligned} \tag{4.18}
$$

Finally, applying (4.16), (4.17), and (4.18), we get $E(A^2) = O(\frac{1}{m_1} + \frac{1}{m_2})$. Together with Assumption 4.3.1, this completes the proof.

Estimator of Covariance Matrix in Sect. 4.6

We will estimate covariance matrix $\widehat{V}$ by estimating its diagonal elements and off-diagonal elements separately. Let us start with the off-diagonal elements. By independence between the subjects (clusters), it follows for $l \neq r$

$$\begin{aligned} C_1 &= \mathrm{Cov}(\sum_{k \in S^{(c,l)}} Z_k^{(c)(l)}, \sum_{k \in S^{(c,r)}} Z_k^{(c)(r)}) \\ &= \mathrm{Cov}(\sum_{k \in S^{(c,l)} \cap S^{(c,r)}} Z_k^{(c)(l)}, \sum_{k \in S^{(c,l)} \cap S^{(c,r)}} Z_k^{(c)(r)}) \\ &= \sum_{k \in S^{(c,l)} \cap S^{(c,r)}} n_k \cdot \mathrm{Cov}(Z_1^{(c)(l)}, Z_1^{(c)(r)}) \\ &:= e_1 \cdot \mathrm{Cov}(Z_1^{(c)(l)}, Z_1^{(c)(r)}). \end{aligned}$$

Similarly, we have

$$C_2 = \sum_{k \in S^{(c,l)} \cap S^{(2,r)}} n_k \cdot \mathrm{Cov}(Z_1^{(c)(l)}, Y_{21}^{(i)(r)}) := e_2 \cdot \mathrm{Cov}(Z_1^{(c)(l)}, Y_{21}^{(i)(r)}),$$

$$C_3 = \sum_{k \in S^{(c,l)} \cap S^{(1,r)}} n_k \cdot \mathrm{Cov}(Z_1^{(c)(l)}, Y_{11}^{(i)(r)}) := e_3 \cdot \mathrm{Cov}(Z_1^{(c)(l)}, Y_{11}^{(i)(r)}),$$

$$C_4 = \sum_{k \in S^{(2,l)} \cap S^{(c,r)}} n_k \cdot \mathrm{Cov}(Y_{21}^{(i)(l)}, Z_1^{(c)(r)}) := e_4 \cdot \mathrm{Cov}(Y_{21}^{(i)(l)}, Z_1^{(c)(r)}),$$

$$C_5 = \sum_{k \in S^{(2,l)} \cap S^{(2,r)}} n_k \cdot \mathrm{Cov}(Y_{21}^{(i)(l)}, Y_{21}^{(i)(r)}) := e_5 \cdot \mathrm{Cov}(Y_{21}^{(i)(l)}, Y_{21}^{(i)(r)}),$$

$$C_6 = \sum_{k \in S^{(2,l)} \cap S^{(1,r)}} n_k \cdot \mathrm{Cov}(Y_{21}^{(i)(l)}, Y_{11}^{(i)(r)}) := e_6 \cdot \mathrm{Cov}(Y_{21}^{(i)(l)}, Y_{11}^{(i)(r)}),$$

$$C_7 = \sum_{k \in S^{(1,l)} \cap S^{(c,r)}} n_k \cdot \mathrm{Cov}(Y_{11}^{(i)(l)}, Z_1^{(c)(r)}) := e_7 \cdot \mathrm{Cov}(Y_{11}^{(i)(l)}, Z_1^{(c)(r)}),$$

$$C_8 = \sum_{k \in S^{(1,l)} \cap S^{(2,r)}} n_k \cdot \mathrm{Cov}(Y_{11}^{(i)(l)}, Y_{21}^{(i)(r)}) := e_8 \cdot \mathrm{Cov}(Y_{11}^{(i)(l)}, Y_{21}^{(i)(r)}),$$

and

$$C_9 = \sum_{k \in S^{(1,l)} \cap S^{(1,r)}} n_k \cdot \mathrm{Cov}(Y_{11}^{(i)(l)}, Y_{11}^{(i)(r)}) := e_9 \cdot \mathrm{Cov}(Y_{11}^{(i)(l)}, Y_{11}^{(i)(r)}),$$

where e_j is the number of subjects that are involved in the corresponding covariance term C_j, $j = 1, \cdots, 9$. If $Y_{gk}^{(A)(l)}$, $g \in \{1, 2\}$, $A \in \{c, i\}$, $l \in \{1, \cdots, d\}$ were observable, the natural estimators $\tilde{C}_j$ of C_j, $j = 1, \cdots, 9$, would be

$$\tilde{C}_1 = \frac{e_1}{e_1 - 1} \sum_{k=1}^{e_1} (Z_k^{(c)(l)} - \overline{Z}_{\cdot}^{(c)(l)})(Z_k^{(c)(r)} - \overline{Z}_{\cdot}^{(c)(r)}),$$

$$\tilde{C}_2 = \frac{e_2}{e_2 - 1} \sum_{k=1}^{e_2} (Z_k^{(c)(l)} - \overline{Z}_{\cdot}^{(c)(l)})(Y_{2k}^{(i)(r)} - \overline{Y}_{2\cdot}^{(i)(r)}),$$

$$\tilde{C}_3 = \frac{e_3}{e_3 - 1} \sum_{k=1}^{e_3} (Z_k^{(c)(l)} - \overline{Z}_{\cdot}^{(c)(l)})(Y_{1k}^{(i)(r)} - \overline{Y}_{1\cdot}^{(i)(r)}),$$

$$\tilde{C}_4 = \frac{e_4}{e_4 - 1} \sum_{k=1}^{e_4} (Y_{2k}^{(i)(l)} - \overline{Y}_{2\cdot}^{(i)(l)})(Z_k^{(c)(r)} - \overline{Z}_{\cdot}^{(c)(r)}),$$

$$\tilde{C}_5 = \frac{e_5}{e_5 - 1} \sum_{k=1}^{e_5} (Y_{2k}^{(i)(l)} - \overline{Y}_{2\cdot}^{(i)(l)})(Y_{2k}^{(i)(r)} - \overline{Y}_{2\cdot}^{(i)(r)}),$$

$$\tilde{C}_6 = \frac{e_6}{e_6 - 1} \sum_{k=1}^{e_6} (Y_{2k}^{(i)(l)} - \overline{Y}_{2\cdot}^{(i)(l)})(Y_{1k}^{(i)(r)} - \overline{Y}_{1\cdot}^{(i)(r)}),$$

$$\tilde{C}_7 = \frac{e_7}{e_7 - 1} \sum_{k=1}^{e_7} (Y_{1k}^{(i)(l)} - \overline{Y}_{1\cdot}^{(i)(l)})(Z_k^{(c)(r)} - \overline{Z}_{\cdot}^{(c)(r)}),$$

$$\tilde{C}_8 = \frac{e_8}{e_8 - 1} \sum_{k=1}^{e_8} (Y_{1k}^{(i)(l)} - \overline{Y}_{1\cdot}^{(i)(l)})(Y_{2k}^{(i)(r)} - \overline{Y}_{2\cdot}^{(i)(r)}),$$

and

$$\tilde{C}_9 = \frac{e_9}{e_9 - 1} \sum_{k=1}^{e_9} (Y_{1k}^{(i)(l)} - \overline{Y}_{1\cdot}^{(i)(l)})(Y_{1k}^{(i)(r)} - \overline{Y}_{1\cdot}^{(i)(r)}).$$

Then we can achieve estimators $\widehat{C}_j$ of C_j by replacing the unobservable random variables $Y_{gk}^{(A)(l)}$ and $\overline{Y}_{g\cdot}^{(A)(l)}$ with their empirical counterparts $\widehat{Y}_{gk}^{(A)(l)}$ and $\widehat{\overline{Y}}_{g\cdot}^{(A)(l)}$ in $\tilde{C}_j, j = 1, \cdots, 9$. Estimators of diagonal elements ($l = r$) can be obtained analogously. In fact, in this case, due to independence among subjects, it is easy to verify that

$$\tilde{C}_2 = \tilde{C}_3 = \tilde{C}_4 = \tilde{C}_6 = \tilde{C}_7 = \tilde{C}_8 = 0,$$

and for the lth component, natural estimators of C_1, C_5 and C_9 are

$$\tilde{C}_1 = \frac{n_c^{(l)}}{n_c^{(l)} - 1} \sum_{k \in S^{(c,l)}} (Z_k^{(c)(l)} - \overline{Z}_{\cdot}^{(c)(l)})^2, \quad \tilde{C}_5 = \frac{n_2^{(l)}}{n_2^{(l)} - 1} \sum_{k \in S^{(2,l)}} (Y_{2k}^{(i)(l)} - \overline{Y}_{2\cdot}^{(i)(l)})^2$$

$$\text{and} \quad \tilde{C}_9 = \frac{n_1^{(l)}}{n_1^{(l)} - 1} \sum_{k \in S^{(1,l)}} (Y_{1k}^{(i)(l)} - \overline{Y}_{1\cdot}^{(i)(l)})^2.$$

Then we replace unobservable random variables with their empirical counterparts to get estimators of the diagonal elements.

The main difference between covariance matrices for data sets with simple and general missing pattern results from their off-diagonal elements. In Appendix "Proof of Theorem 4.4.3", we see that elements of covariance matrix for data sets with simple missing pattern can be estimated by summing up estimates of the three covariance decompositions, which are then proved to be consistent. However, for the general missing pattern, the off-diagonal elements consist of nine covariance decompositions. Since consistency of these covariance decompositions can be established in a manner similar to the proof in Appendix "Proof of Theorem 4.4.3", the consistency of the covariance matrix follows.

References

Akritas, M. G., & Arnold, S. F. (1994). Fully nonparametric hypotheses for factorial designs I: Multivariate repeated measures designs. *Journal of the American Statistical Association, 89*(425), 336–343.

Akritas, M. G., Arnold, S. F., & Brunner, E. (1997). Nonparametric hypotheses and rank statistics for unbalanced factorial designs. *Journal of the American Statistical Association, 92*(437), 258–265.

Bathke, A. C., & Harrar, S. W. (2008). Nonparametric methods in multivariate factorial designs for large number of factor levels. *Journal of Statistical Planning and Inference, 138*(3), 588–610.

Brunner, E., & Denker, M. (1994). Rank statistics under dependent observations and applications to factorial designs. *Journal of Statistical planning and Inference, 42*(3), 353–378.

Brunner, E., Dette, H., & Munk, A. (1997). Box-type approximations in nonparametric factorial designs. *Journal of the American Statistical Association, 92*(440), 1494–1502.

Brunner, E., & Munzel, U. (2000). The nonparametric Behrens-Fisher problem: asymptotic theory and a small-sample approximation. *Biometrical Journal: Journal of Mathematical Methods in Biosciences, 42*(1), 17–25.

Brunner, E., Munzel, U., & Puri, M. L. (2002). The multivariate nonparametric Behrens–Fisher problem. *Journal of Statistical Planning and Inference, 108*(1–2), 37–53.

Cui, Y., Konietschke, F., & Harrar, S. W. (2021). The nonparametric Behrens–Fisher problem in partially complete clustered data. *Biometrical Journal, 63*(1), 148–167.

Harrar, S. W., & Bathke, A. C. (2008). Nonparametric methods for unbalanced multivariate data and many factor levels. *Journal of Multivariate Analysis, 99*(8), 1635–1664.

Harrar, S. W., & Cui Y. (2023). Nonparametric methods for clustered data in pre-post intervention design. *Journal of Statistical Planning and Inference, 222*(1–21), 0378–3758. https://doi.org/10.1016/j.jspi.2022.05.009

Konietschke, F., & Brunner, E. (2009). Nonparametric analysis of clustered data in diagnostic trials: Estimation problems in small sample sizes. *Computational Statistics & Data Analysis, 53*(3), 730–741.

Konietschke, F., Harrar, S. W., Lange, K., & Brunner, E. (2012). Ranking procedures for matched pairs with missing data—asymptotic theory and a small sample approximation. *Computational Statistics & Data Analysis, 56*(5), 1090–1102.

Munzel, U., & Brunner, E. (2000a). Nonparametric methods in multivariate factorial designs. *Journal of Statistical Planning and Inference, 88*(1), 117–132.

Munzel, U., & Brunner, E. (2000b). Nonparametric tests in the unbalanced multivariate one-way design. *Biometrical Journal: Journal of Mathematical Methods in Biosciences, 42*(7), 837–854.

Noonan, C. W., Semmens, E. O., Smith, P., Harrar, S. W., Montrose, L., Weiler, E., McNamara, M., & Ward, T. J. (2017). Randomized trial of interventions to improve childhood asthma in homes with wood-burning stoves. *Environmental health perspectives, 125*(9), 097010.

RStudio Team. (2020). *RStudio: Integrated development environment for R*. RStudio, PBC.

Rubin, D. B. (2004). *Multiple imputation for nonresponse in surveys* (Vol. 81). John Wiley & Sons.

Ruymgaart, F. H. (1980). A unified approach to the asymptotic distribution theory of certain midrank statistics. In *Statistique non parametrique asymptotique* (pp. 1–18). Springer.

Sen, P. K., & Puri, M. L. (1971). *Nonparametric methods in multivariate analysis*. John Wiley & Sons.

Werner, C. (2006). *Nichtparametrische analyse von diagnostischen tests*. Ph. D. thesis, Niedersächsische Staats-und Universitätsbibliothek Göttingen.

Chapter 5
Estimating Average and Individual Treatment Effects in the Presence of Time-Dependent Covariates

Tshiamo Kgoale, Albert Whata, Justine B. Nasejje, Najmeh Nakhaei Rad, and Tshilidzi Mulaudzi

5.1 Introduction

Survival analysis is not just about predicting the duration of events, it is a powerful tool for understanding causal relationships. In survival analysis, we do not consider calculating survival probabilities only when events occur, but also look at the causes and interventions that have an effect on those events (Austin, 2014). This approach enables us to understand the causal effects of treatments or interventions on individuals or populations in fields such as epidemiology, medicine, and social sciences. A fundamental component of causal inference in survival analysis is the potential outcomes framework, sometimes known as the "counterfactual framework" (VanderWeele, 2016; Geneletti, 2005). It allows us to make a comparison between what actually occurred and what may have occurred in different conditions. This framework is useful for evaluating how interventions or treatments affect patients (Bavli, 2019). It involves careful analysis and statistical

T. Kgoale
Department of Mathematical Sciences, Sol Plaatje University, Kimberley, South Africa
e-mail: 201902605@spu.ac.za

A. Whata (✉) · N. N. Rad
Department of Statistics, University of Pretoria, Pretoria, South Africa
e-mail: albert.whata@up.ac.za; najmeh.nakhaeirad@up.ac.za

J. B. Nasejje
School of Statistics and Actuarial Science, University of the Witwatersrand, Johannesburg, South Africa
e-mail: justine.nasejje@wits.ac.za

T. Mulaudzi
University of Venda, Limpopo, South Africa
e-mail: tshilidzi.mulaudzi@univen.ac.za

D.-G. Chen, C. A. Coelho (eds.), *Biostatistics Modeling and Public Health Applications*, Emerging Topics in Statistics and Biostatistics,
https://doi.org/10.1007/978-3-031-69690-9_5

modeling to estimate both the average and individual treatment effects, providing a complete understanding of the causal relationships.

Censoring is an important aspect in survival analysis, as some participants may not encounter the event of interest throughout the research period (Leung et al., 1997; Clark et al., 2003). To properly predict survival probabilities while accounting for censoring, advanced statistical methods must be employed. Survival probabilities are estimated using the survival function, denoted as $S(t)$ which represents the probability of a patient surviving beyond time t, i.e., $Pr(T > t)$, which can be estimated using both parametric and nonparametric methods. For example, the Kaplan–Meier estimator is a nonparametric method used when subjects are continuously observed. Other sophisticated models such as the Cox proportional hazards (PH) model help in identifying factors that influence survival outcomes (Cox, 1972). These models do not assume specific distributions, making them versatile for causal inference in survival analysis. Recently, machine learning (ML) and deep learning models, such as random survival forest, DeepSurv, and DeepHit, have been applied in survival analysis (Ishwaran et al., 2008; Katzman et al., 2018; Lee et al., 2018). It is important to note that these models have a good predictive performance, especially on datasets with complex covariate relationships. However, these models diverge from classical survival approaches by not prioritizing causal analysis and the assessment of treatment effects.

The aim of this chapter therefore is to employ ML techniques to assess causality, estimate and predict survival functions, evaluate heterogeneous treatment effects, and bridge the gap between predictive modeling and causal understanding in complex healthcare contexts, with a focus on time-dependent outcomes within electronic health records (EHR) data. In fact, we use advanced deep learning techniques for causal analysis, focusing on predicting survival functions and evaluating heterogeneous treatment effects. The causal inference in survival analysis and the potential outcomes framework explored in this chapter provide a powerful and comprehensive evaluation of survival probabilities in the presence of time-dependent covariates. By using the potential outcomes framework, this method establishes a robust approach for estimating treatment effects in the presence of time-dependent covariates that impact survival outcomes. Many ML methods concentrate on predicting outcomes without exploring the complex causal relationships. In survival analysis, relying on machine learning primarily for predictions restricts its effectiveness in uncovering causal relationships. Additionally, there is a gap in the literature concerning the use of longitudinal EHR data to identify causal effects on survival. We adapted models, such as DeepSurv, DeepHit, and MTL-DNN, to now predict survival probabilities under both treatment and control conditions. This adaptation is very important because these models lack a built-in explanatory mechanism for causal inference. Through this adaptation, this chapter offers a more comprehensive evaluation of treatment effects, especially considering the influence of time-dependent covariates.

This chapter is outlined as follows: Sect. 5.2 describes the ML methods that will be employed for causal inference in survival analysis. Section 5.3 details the simulation and experimental procedures. Section 5.4 presents and discusses the results. Finally, Sect. 5.5 concludes this chapter.

5.2 Methodology

In this section, we present an overview of ML within the context of survival analysis. The discussion includes the challenge of causal inference, the survival analysis challenge, and the estimation of treatment effects within these models. Furthermore, we present the methodologies used to evaluate the performance differences among the machine learning models considered in this chapter for survival analysis.

5.2.1 Machine Learning Methods for Causal Inference in Survival Analysis

The Cox model (Cox, 1972; Xiao et al., 2010) is frequently used to estimate treatment effects using time-dependent confounders. The Cox model models the hazard function represented as: $h(t \mid X) = h_0 \exp(\beta' X)$, where β is a constant vector and h_0 represents the baseline hazard of experiencing an event at time t_0. It quantifies the absolute likelihood of an event occurring at time t given the covariates X. The Cox model calculates the likelihood of an event occurring at time t in both treatment and control settings, regardless of the prior history of X or treatment conditions. To incorporate time-dependent effects and covariates, β can be extended to $\beta(t)$ using a piece-wise constant Cox model (Yang & Prentice, 2015) and X to $X(t)$, respectively.

On the other hand, ML covers various scientific methods for predicting and classifying data (Hastie et al., 2009). Recently, it has gained attention for building prediction models from data (Zupan et al., 2000). While ML provides advantages over the Cox model, such as describing nonlinear connections and developing interpretable models, its application in survival analysis was initially constrained by challenges in handling censored data (Zupan et al., 2000). Despite these limitations, various ML-based methods have been devised for analyzing continuous survival data (Nemati et al., 2020). For instance, in survival analysis the random survival forest (RSF), an extension of the random forest methodology, has been employed (Ishwaran et al., 2008; Jiang, 2019; Nasejje et al., 2022). The RSF has recently been expanded to incorporate time-varying variables (Zhang et al., 2018).

This chapter explores using ML such as DeepSurv, DeepHit, and MTL-DNN for causal survival analysis in the presence of time-dependent covariates. DeepSurv (Katzman et al., 2018) originally designed for continuous time and time-independent covariates has proven to be highly effective in modeling time-to-event datasets due to its adaptable and robust architecture. This flexibility allows it to handle the dynamic nature of covariates over time, integrating the history window of events and evolving risk factors, making it particularly powerful for survival analysis in medical and clinical research where patient history windows significantly influence outcomes. On the other hand, techniques like DeepHit (Lee et al., 2018) can effectively model time-dependent covariates because it treats survival time as discrete and the time horizon as finite. Importantly, this chapter explores the usage of the DeepSurv, DeepHit, and MTL-DNN in estimating the average treatment effect (ATE) with time-dependent covariates. Previous work, described by Katzman et al. (2018), extended DeepSurv for a personalized treatment recommender system.

In healthcare, ML holds significant promise for improving diagnostic accuracy, particularly in domains like radiography (Obermeyer & Emanuel, 2016). The landscape of ML applications in healthcare has witnessed substantial evolution over the past decade. Earlier models, such as support vector machines, random forests, and Lasso, were employed to predict outcomes like hospitalization (Hong et al., 2018). However, these models often offered only incremental improvements over traditional regression methods. In recent years, the surge of deep learning models, driven by enhanced hardware capabilities and the availability of extensive healthcare data, has been noteworthy (Shickel et al., 2017). Unlike traditional ML approaches that rely on feature engineering, deep learning models directly extract features from the data, unveiling previously unnoticed correlations (Radovanović et al., 2018). Causal inference, historically a fundamental element of statistics and epidemiology, has gained increased attention and has been integrated with machine learning techniques in recent research endeavors (Crown, 2019). For example, in the presence of continuous survival data, a range of ML-based methods have been developed to estimate treatment effects (Nemati et al., 2020).

5.2.2 The Causal Inference Problem

Rubin Causal Model

In this chapter, we use the Rubin Causal Model (RCM) by Holland (1986) to evaluate casual inference. We consider a population of units U in the RCM. These are the subjects that may be affected by causes or treatments (Holland, 1986). For a given unit and time interval of t_1 to t_2, we define the causal effect of one treatment, E, over another, C, as the difference between what would have happened at time t_2 if the unit had been exposed to E initiated at time t_1 and what would have happened at time t_2 if the unit had been exposed to C initiated at t_1. This definition brings about an important aspect which is the notion of potential. It is important to note that each unit be potentially exposable to any one of the causes (Holland, 1986).

Causal inference is primarily concerned with the effects of causes on specific units, that is, with ascertaining the value of the casual effect $Y_t(u)$ - $Y_c(u)$. Since each unit, C in U, has a value for both Y_t and Y_c, the causal effect can therefore be defined at the level of individual units. However, $Y_t(u)$ and $Y_c(u)$ can never be observed on the same unit, and therefore, it is impossible to observe the effect of t on u, and this presents a problem which is referred to by Holland (1986) as the *Fundamental Problem of Causal Inference*. In other words one cannot return to time t_1 given the other treatment (Rubin, 1974).

Counterfactuals Theory and Potential Outcomes Theory

In causal inference, the counterfactual theorem tells us that certain information necessary for making causal inferences may not be observable. Therefore, it is crucial to make specific assumptions. Therefore, the causal effect of an action or treatment is determined by comparing two potential outcomes. The potential outcomes include the one that is realized and observed, as well as the one that is not realized and, therefore, not observed. A classic example of potential outcomes widely used in the literature is related to taking aspirin (Holland, 1986). When taking an aspirin, one potential outcome would be the result of taking the aspirin, while the alternative potential outcome corresponds to not taking an aspirin, resulting in a different observed outcome. The causal effect depends on potential outcomes and is independent of the observed outcome. The potential outcomes framework allows us to define the causal effect as the comparison of outcomes at the same time. It is important to note that the causal effect is not determined by comparing outcomes at different times, as is the case in before-and-after studies.

Estimation of Treatment Effects

We consider a random sample of size N from a large population. For each unit i in the sample ($i = 1, \ldots, N$), A_i denotes whether the treatment of interest was administered, where $A_i = 1$ signifies that the unit received the active treatment, and $A_i = 0$ indicates that the unit received the control treatment. Adopting the potential outcome notation established by Rubin (1974), $S_0(t)$ represents the outcome for each unit i under control, while $S_1(t)$ signifies the outcome under treatment. The observed variables include A_i and $S_i(t)$, where $S_i(t) = A_i \cdot S_1(t) + (1 - A_i) \cdot S_0(t)$. Additionally, a vector of covariates is observed and denoted by X_i. We estimate the population ATE using

$$\mathrm{E}[S_1(t) - S_0(t)],$$

and the weighted average treatment effects as expressed by

$$\tau_{\text{wate}} = \frac{\int_{\mathcal{X}} [E[S_1(t) - S_0(t) \mid X = x] \cdot g(x)] \, dF(x)}{\int_{\mathcal{X}} g(x) dF(x)}, \tag{5.1}$$

where $g(\cdot)$ represents a known function of the covariates. However, in this chapter, we estimate the function $g(x)$ using the propensity score $p(x) = \Pr(A_i = 1 \mid X = x)$. Under the assumption of unconfoundedness, this results in the average effect for those who received the treatment

$$ATE_{\text{treated}} = E[S_1(t) - S_0(t) \mid A_i = 1].$$

A fundamental challenge arises as we observe either $S_0(t)$ or $S_1(t)$ for each unit i, but never both. To address this identification problem, we consistently uphold the unconfoundedness assumption throughout our study, as proposed by Rubin (1978) and Rosenbaum and Rubin (1983). This assumption is closely related to the selection-on-observables assumption by Barnow et al. (1980). It posits that, given the observed covariates, the treatment indicator is independent of the potential outcomes. Formally, we express this as follows:

Assumption 5.2.1 (Unconfounded Treatment Assignment) $A_i \perp (S_0(t), S_1(t)) \mid X$.

Under the assumption of unconfoundedness, we can estimate the average treatment effect (ATE) conditional on the covariates: ATE is given by $E[S_1(t) - S_0(t) \mid X = x]$. Therefore

$$
\begin{aligned}
ATE &= E[S_1(t) - S_0(t) \mid X = x] \\
&= E[S_1(t) \mid A_i = 1, X = x] - E[S_0(t) \mid A_i = 0, X = x].
\end{aligned}
$$

To bypass the need for matching units based on all covariates, we adopt a procedure by Rosenbaum and Rubin (1983, 1984) that is centered on the propensity score:

$$
p(x) = \Pr(A_i = 1 \mid X = x) = E[A_i \mid X = x], \tag{5.2}
$$

where $p(x)$ is assumed to be bounded away from zero and one. The key understanding here is that the treatment and potential outcomes are independent when considering all covariates. This independence also holds when conditioned on the propensity score. In simple terms, as shown by Rosenbaum and Rubin (1983), the idea of unconfoundedness implies:

$$
A_i \perp (S_0(t), S_1(t) \mid p(X),
$$

indicating that adjusting for the propensity score is sufficient to eliminate biases associated with covariate differences.

In this chapter, for the estimation of treatment effects in survival analysis, we begin by assuming that we have N units, of which N_0 are in the control group and N_1 are treated; this means that $N = N_1 + N_0$. Each unit is associated with covariates X, which can be heterogeneous and comprise both continuous and categorical variables such as process codes and laboratory vital signs. In addition, we have a treatment indicator A, with $A = 0$ for control subjects and $A = 1$ for the treated. Using the potential-outcomes framework given in Sect. 5.2.2, we define $S_0(t)$ and $S_1(t)$ as the potential outcomes for a certain subject under treatment and control, respectively. We only observe one of the possible outcomes in practice, namely the factual outcome $S_1(t)$, whereas the counterfactual outcome $S_0(t)$ is not observed. The expected difference between $S_1(t)$ and $S_0(t)$ for an individual unit (person), conditioned on X, is commonly referred to as the *individualized treatment effect* (ITE) or the *heterogeneous treatment effect*. In addition, the ATE is evaluated using 5.1.

Model Evaluation

In this chapter, the evaluation of DeepSurv, DeepHit, and MTLR-DNN models is conducted using metrics such as the absolute percent bias, outlined in 5.3. The absolute percent bias serves as an important metric that provides a quantitative measure to assess the accuracy and reliability of the DeepSurv, DeepHit, and MTLR-DNN models in capturing treatment effects. This metric quantifies the bias present in the models' estimated treatment effects. Specifically, it measures the absolute percentage bias in the estimated ATE or ITE when compared to true ATE or ITE. We use the following formula to calculate the absolute percent bias

$$Bias(t) = \frac{1}{nk} \sum_{ik} \left| \frac{\hat{\phi}_{ik}(t) - \phi_{ik}(t)}{\phi_{ik}(t)} \right|. \tag{5.3}$$

Here, n represents the sample size, k denotes the number of simulations, and $\hat{\phi}_{ik}(t)$ and $\phi_{ik}(t)$ are the estimated and true values, respectively, for the treatment effect at time t in the i-th simulation and k-th iteration.

Log-Rank Test

A statistical comparison of two survival curves is a fundamental aspect in the evaluation of treatments concerning survival outcomes. The null hypothesis, which states that there is no difference in survival between the two treatments, is tested using the log-rank test (Kleinbaum & Klein, 2012). In this test, the expected number of events in each group, denoted as E_1 and E_2, is calculated, while O_1 and O_2 represent the observed events in each respective group. The log-rank test statistic is calculated using the formula

$$\frac{(O_1 - E_1)^2}{E_1} + \frac{(O_2 - E_2)^2}{E_2}.$$

Here, E_2 represents the total expected occurrences for group 2, and E_1 is derived by subtracting E_2 from the sum of observed events in both groups ($O_1 + O_2$). By comparing the computed test statistic with the critical value from a chi-square table for one degree of freedom, one can determine the statistical significance, providing a rigorous and objective assessment of potential differences in survival outcomes between the treatments under consideration.

The Concordance

The concordance statistic (C-statistic), introduced by Harrell Jr. et al. (1996) for Cox models, is a widely adopted measure of goodness-of-fit in survival models. The C-statistic is calculated using the following formula:

$$\text{C-statistic} = \frac{\text{Number of concordant pairs}}{\text{Total number of pairs}}.$$

In this chapter, we employ the C-statistic to assess the predictive accuracy of the DeepSurv, DeepHit, and MTLR-DNN models, quantifying the agreement between observed and predicted survival probabilities. The C-statistic is computed as the percentage of concordant pairs among subjects receiving different treatments. A higher C-statistic signifies improved discrimination between treatment and control subjects. Acceptable discrimination typically falls within C-statistic values ranging from 0.7 to 0.8, while excellent discrimination lies between 0.8 to 0.9. Values ≥ 0.9 indicate outstanding discrimination (Hosmer Jr. et al., 2013).

5.3 Simulations and Experiments

5.3.1 Data

In this chapter, we used both simulated and real datasets to explain how treatment effects are estimated in the context of deep learning methods in survival analysis.

Simulated Data

We used simulated data generated according to the techniques proposed by Crowther and Lambert (2013) to simulate complex distributions of survival times. The data simulation procedure is outlined below:

1. D continuous confounding variables $X(t_1), X(t_2), \ldots, X(t_D) \sim N(\sqrt{t}, V)$ starting at $t = t" - u$ ending at $t = t' + q$, and the normal distribution's variance is represented by V and the feature dimension is represented by D;
2. The exposure binary: $B(t) \sim Binom(\nu.I(\sum_{d=1}^{3})X(t_D)) > (\sum_{d=1}^{3})X(t_i)) + 0.5.(1-\nu))$, and I is an indicator function and ν controls the level of overlap. When $\nu = 0$, there is 50% likelihood of taking the treatment in spite of $X(t)$; when $\nu = 1$, the indicator function is followed by allocation, causing the first three confounders of $X(t)$ to influence the outcome; when $\nu = \frac{1}{2}$, the likelihood of getting the treatment depends on the indicator function (partially) and is $(\frac{1}{2}.I + \frac{1}{4})100\%$.
3. HR: $h(t) = \frac{log(t)}{\lambda}(\frac{1}{10})B(t) + \beta \sum_{i=1}^{D} X(t))$, and $\beta = 1$.

4. The survival likelihood $S(t) = exp(-h(t))$.
5. The censorship likelihood $SC(t) = exp(-\frac{log(t)}{\lambda})$, and $\lambda = 30$.
6. An event indication produced utilizing *root-finding* Crowther and Lambert (2013) each at t: $E(t) = I(S(t) < U \sim Uni(0, 1))$, and the outcome t is denoted by τ_s if $E_i(\tau_s) =$, if not $\tau_s = q + 1$.
7. A censoring indication produced utilizing *root-finding* method: $C(t) = I(S(t) < U \sim Uniform(0, 1))$, during censorship t is denoted by τ_c if $C(\tau_c) = 1$, if not $\tau_c = q$.
8. The survival result given by the indicator function: $Y = I(\tau_s \leq \tau_c)$.

This chapter employs the parameter settings that were recommended by Crowther and Lambert (2013) to simulate biologically plausible data. These parameters are set with $V = \frac{5}{10}$, $D = \frac{12}{2}$, $\nu = \frac{9}{10}$, and $N = 1500$. Additionally, the simulation data is designed to have an estimation period with a length of 10 time steps.

Real Data

In addition to the simulation study, we applied DeepSurv, DeepHit, and MTL-DNN to the primary biliary cirrhosis (PBC) study. The PBC dataset used in this analysis originates from a clinical investigation involving 312 individuals diagnosed with primary biliary cirrhosis (PBC). The study was done as part of a clinical trial at the Mayo Clinic from January 1974 to May 1984. The study aimed to assess the effectiveness of D-penicillamine as a treatment for PBC. The primary outcome was the patients' survival time (time to death) (Murtaugh et al., 1994). Throughout the trial, different patient data and medical measurements were recorded as covariates. These records were obtained when the patients were enrolled and then annually thereafter. The dataset includes twelve covariates selected for their clinical importance and simplicity of assessment in the study (Murtaugh et al., 1994).

5.3.2 *Experiments*

We used three advanced survival analysis models DeepSurv, DeepHit, and MTLR-DNN to estimate treatment effects within simulated time-to-event and the real-life data. To determine the best learning rate for each model, a systematic grid search was conducted. For DeepSurv, an optimal learning rate of 0.01, with a batch size of 32, and 50 training epochs, was identified. DeepHit performed best with a learning rate of 0.001, a batch size of 64, and 100 training epochs. Similarly, MTLR-DNN utilized a learning rate of 0.001, a batch size of 128, and 30 training epochs. These specific hyperparameter configurations contributed to the models' high predictive power. Besides hyperparameter tuning, the study enhanced the models by adapting them to estimate survival probabilities for both control and treatment groups. This modification enabled a comprehensive evaluation of the models' performance under treatment and control groups at different time points.

In addition to hyperparameter tuning, the models were adapted to estimate survival probabilities for both the treatment and control groups, allowing a comprehensive evaluation of their performance across various time points. The dataset was split into the treatment and control groups. Subsequently, DeepSurv, DeepHit, and MTL-DNN models were customized to estimate survival probabilities separately for each of these groups. Following this, the estimated survival probabilities were used to calculate the ATEs and ITEs. To avoid matching units based on all covariates, we employ the propensity score ($p(x)$), as defined in 5.2. This approach acknowledges that, when considering all covariates, the treatment and control (potential) outcomes become independent. The integration of propensity scores, reflecting the probability of receiving treatment given observed covariates, enhances the precision of average treatment effect calculations. This method provides a valuable alternative to exhaustive covariate matching.

To assess bias in ATE estimation, the Kaplan–Meier estimator was employed as a reliable benchmark for the true population ATE. Moreover, we computed C-statistic and the log-rank statistic to offer a comprehensive evaluation of the models' performance in both treatment and control groups. These statistical measures contribute to our understanding of the models' effectiveness in capturing survival dynamics and estimating treatment effects using simulated and real-life data.

5.4 Results and Discussion

5.4.1 Simulated Data

Kaplan–Meier Survival Functions for the Treatment and Control

Using simulated data, we determined survival probabilities under treatment and control conditions based on treatment status, event occurrence, and follow-up time. Subsequently, we applied the Kaplan–Meier method to estimate survival probabilities and generate corresponding survival curves for both control and treatment groups. These curves were plotted to illustrate survival probabilities over specified follow-up time intervals for both groups. The follow-up times begin either at the start of the study or when a participant is deemed at risk, and it continues until the event occurs, the study concludes, or the participant is lost. Figure 5.1 illustrates how survival curves behave for the control and treatment groups, where the control group is depicted in orange, and the treatment group is represented in blue.

The vertical axis displays the chance of survival or the proportion of survivors, while the horizontal axis depicts time points, or the follow-up time points. The participants have a 1.0 or 100% survival chance at time zero. At time point 2, the probability of survival under treatment is approximately 0.60 or 60%, and the probability of survival under control is approximately 0.75 or 75%. At the follow-

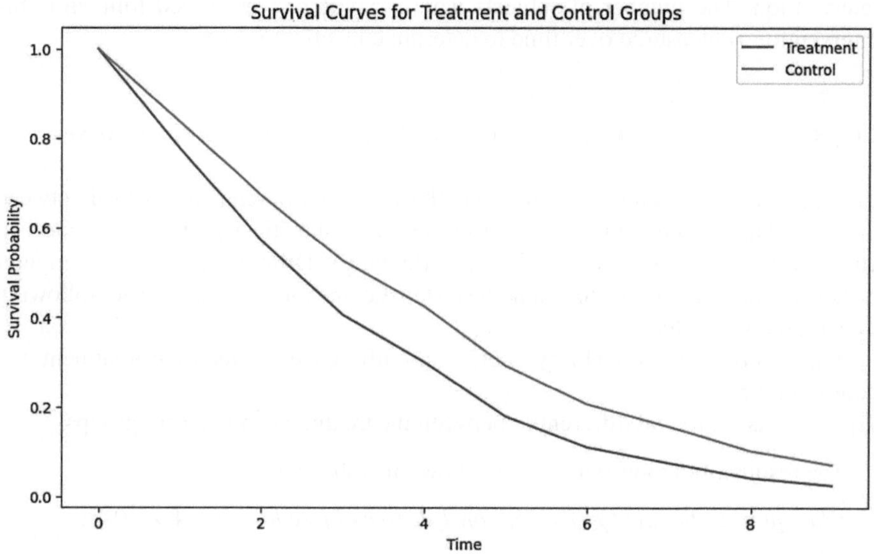

Fig. 5.1 Estimated survival functions for the treatment and control

up time point 8, the probability of survival is approximately 0.10 or 10% and 0.20 or 20% for the treatment and control status, respectively. In addition, the median survival is approximately at time point 3 and time point 4 for the treatment and control, respectively. This means that a subject has a 50% probability of surviving for at least time point 3 for the treatment, given that they have survived up to time point 2. Similarly, a subject has a survival time (i.e., 50% probability of surviving) of at least 4 time units for the control, given that they have survived up to three time units. As Fig. 5.1 illustrates, the survival curve of the treatment (blue) lies below the survival curve of the control (orange), which means survival under the treatment is lower compared to survival under the control. This indicates that the survival rate under the control is better than that under treatment because the treatment was simulated to have detrimental impact compared to the control group.

In this chapter, we consider the treatment group to be subjects who could be under a newer therapy (treatment 1) and the control group to be subjects who could be under a standard therapy (Treatment 2). Figure 5.1 shows that there is a gap in the vertical direction between the two survival curves. This vertical gap indicates that, at a given time point, there was a higher chance of survival for participants under treatment 2 compared to subjects under treatment 1. At each time point, we can therefore estimate the ITE as well as the ATE. The results obtained in this section are very important because the survival curves can be used in real life to measure the proportion of subjects that are still living for a certain amount of time after treatment. Also, we can compare the proportion of subjects receiving the standard treatment to those receiving the newer treatment to quantify the effect of the treatment or intervention. Moreover, the therapy could be a community trial or a clinical study intervention. The number of subjects who survived or were saved following this intervention is measured over time to determine its effectiveness.

Log Rank Test for the Comparison of the Kaplan–Meier Survival Curves

The log-rank test examines the null hypothesis of no difference in survival between the control and treatment groups. This test analyzes statistically whether the survival curves for each group are identical (overlapping). Different statistical computer packages implement the log-rank test statistic in various ways. The following hypothesis was tested:

H_0: In terms of survivability, there is no difference between the treatment and control groups.

H_1: There is a survival differential between the treatment and control groups.

The results of the log-rank test are shown in Table 5.1.

Chi-squared statistic (χ^2) = *25.9 on 1 degree of freedom,* $p = 4 \times 10^{-7}$.

The results of the log-rank test yield a chi-squared test statistic of 25.9 on 1 degree of freedom, and the corresponding *p-value* is *4e-07*. Since this *p-value* is less than 0.05, we reject the null hypothesis and infer that there is enough evidence to claim there is a significant difference in survival between the two groups.

Estimating True Population Individual Treatment Effects with the Kaplan–Meier Method

In clinical studies for causal inference, it is crucial to estimate the ITE on the survival period. This information holds significant importance for tailored medical decision-making and patient care. Figure 5.2 illustrates the results of the effect on survival for each individual who has received treatment 1 ($A_i = 1$) and treatment 2 ($A_i = 0$).

In addition, Fig. 5.2 represents the estimated ITE for each individual in the study at each follow-up time point. Thus, it illustrates the difference in the individual treatment effect under treatment ($A_i = 1$) and control ($A_i = 0$) for each individual at each follow-up time point. Also, ITE is defined by $ITE_i = \Delta S_i(t) = S_1(t)(x_i) - S_0(t)(x_i)$, where $S_1(t)(x_i)$ and $S_0(t)(x_i)$ represent the potential outcomes of a pair of treatments $A_i = 1$ and $A_i = 0$, and x_i consists of some covariates. ITE_i is counterfactual because one of $Y_i^{T_1}(x_i) - Y_i^{T_0}(x_i)$ is counterfactual. The inclusion

Table 5.1 The log-rank test for survival curve comparison

	N	Observed (O_i)	Expected (O_i)	$\frac{(O_i-E_i)^2}{E_i}$	$\frac{(O_i-E_i)^2}{V_i}$
Treatment 1 = 0	5050	4445	4631	7.46	25.9
Treatment 2 = 1	4950	4725	4539	7.61	25.9

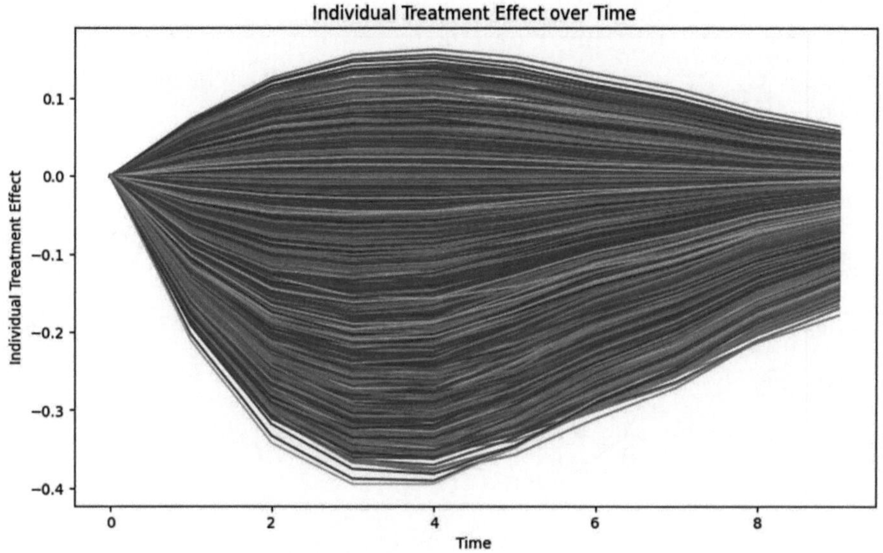

Fig. 5.2 Individual treatment effects for survival

of x_i in $S_i(t)(x_i)$ indicates that the survival function is conditional on the covariate values x_i. In other words, it represents the probability that individual i survives beyond time t given the specific values of covariates x_i. This notation is commonly used in survival analysis to denote a conditional survival function, which takes into account the influence of covariates on the survival probability.

Figure 5.2 shows that, for most individuals, ITE_i becomes increasingly negative up to follow-up time 3, reaching approximately −0.390, and remains constant from time points 3–4. After follow-up time point 4, ITE_i becomes less negative. However, there are some individuals who experienced a positive treatment effect, reaching a maximum of approximately 0.200. Overall, these results indicate that, for most individuals, treatment 1 $A_i = 1$ had a negative impact on the survival probability.

The estimation of ITE is a significant area of study in causal inference. Estimating ITE on survival time offers insights into how an individual may benefit from a pair of therapies with the potential to extend survival time. This has become a focal point in personalized healthcare. A patient or a doctor can choose a treatment based on the findings shown in Fig. 5.2. This means that the doctor or patient can access quantitative data and helpful therapeutic advice that cannot be gained through randomized control trials (RCTs). For example, if we consider a study that examines whether patients with underlying health conditions could benefit from a new drug, Coviphen, to treat COVID-19, we can compare the survival probabilities of patients with underlying medical conditions who were administered Coviphen to those given a standard drug. If the study shows that the new drug, Coviphen, did

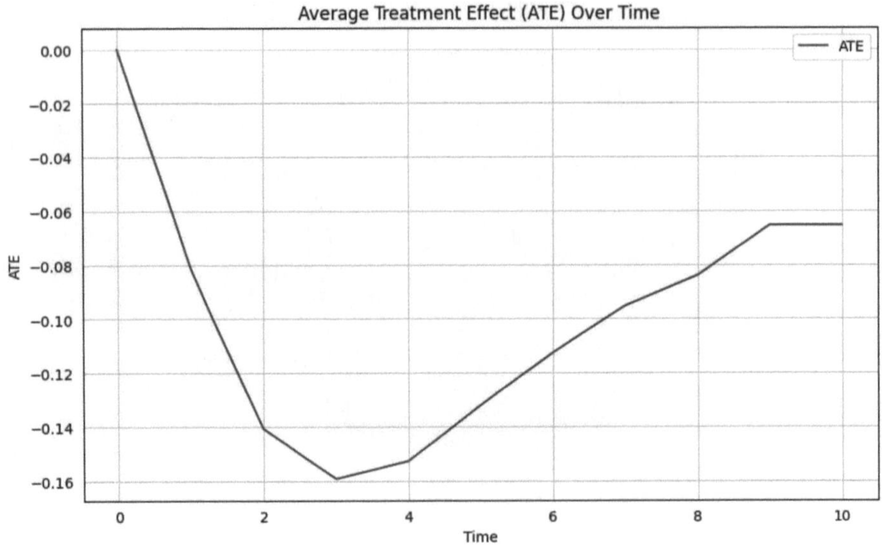

Fig. 5.3 Average treatment effects for survival

not significantly improve patients' survival times, individuals would obtain valuable information about the effectiveness of Coviphen before opting for the treatment.

Estimating True Population Average Treatment Effects with the Kaplan–Meier Method

Examining whether the treatment's impact changes across patient subgroups is crucial in a number of clinical research. Figure 5.3 displays the estimation of ATE as a function of variations in survival probability using the Kaplan–Meier Method.

ATE is an average of ITEs for study participants, and it is formulated by $ATE_i = E[Y_i(1) - Y_i(0)]$. The green curve estimates the ATE at each follow-up time. It shows that it is increasingly negative up to follow-up time $\approx$2.9 and remains constant from time points 2.9–4. Afterward the curve is decreasingly negative up to the follow-up time 9. Since the results are largely negative, it shows that treatment 1 had a negative impact on the survival probability compared to treatment 2. The KM average treatment effect is **−0.0989**. The data was simulated in such a way that treatment 1 would have a negative treatment compared to treatment 2. The KM ATE will be used as the true population treatment effect in evaluating bias for the deep learning algorithms that will be employed in this chapter.

5.4.2 *Comparison of the Predictive Performances of DeepSurv, DeepHit, and MTL-DNN*

We present a comparative analysis of DeepSurv, DeepHit, and MTL-DNN using simulated data. In Fig. 5.4a, we observe the *C*-statistic generated by the three models, which have been adapted to sequentially estimate survival probabilities under both treatment and control groups. These estimated survival probabilities are then used to estimate the average treatment effects.

Figure 5.4b assesses the predictive performances of the three models using combined data that includes both the control and treatment groups. The *C*-statistic values obtained from this combined data are as follows: DeepHit (0.9997), MTL-DNN (0.9996), and DeepSurv (0.8928). The higher *C*-statistic values for DeepHit and MTL-DNN, in comparison to DeepSurv, indicate that these two models perform better than DeepSurv.

Estimating of ATE and Bias of DeepSurv, DeepHit, and MTL-DNN

The ATE graphs show a similar pattern to that of the ATE of the Kaplan–Meier observed in Sect. 5.4.1 (Fig. 5.5).

Table 5.2 shows the bias, standard deviation (SD), and 95% confidence intervals (CI) for the ATE produced by DeepSurv, DeepHit, and MTL-DNN.

Table 5.2 shows that the ATE values which represent the impact of a treatment regime on survival are negative for all models, indicating a negative effect. DeepHit and MTL-DNN have slightly lower ATE values than DeepSurv. DeepSurv has the lowest standard deviation indicating that its ATE estimates are more stable. In addition, DeepSurv has the highest bias, while DeepHit and MTL-DNN show lower bias which indicates that these two models align more closely with the true population treatment effects.

5.4.3 *Real Clinical Data*

In addition to the simulated data, we applied DeepSurv, DeepHit, and MTL-DNN to the PBC data. The results of the treatment effect estimation using the clinical PBC data are shown in Table 5.3 including the ATE, SD, and average *C*-statistic obtained from the DeepSurv, DeepHit, and MTL-DNN models.

Table 5.3 displays that DeepHit emerged as the top performer, surpassing other models with the highest average *C*-statistic, indicating superior overall predictive accuracy. The *C*-statistic results for DeepHit remain higher than those of DeepSurv and MTL-DNN, consistent with the observations from the simulated data analysis. The SD values for all the models indicate prediction stability, with DeepHit and MTL-DNN demonstrating lower variability than DeepSurv. Moreover, the ATE

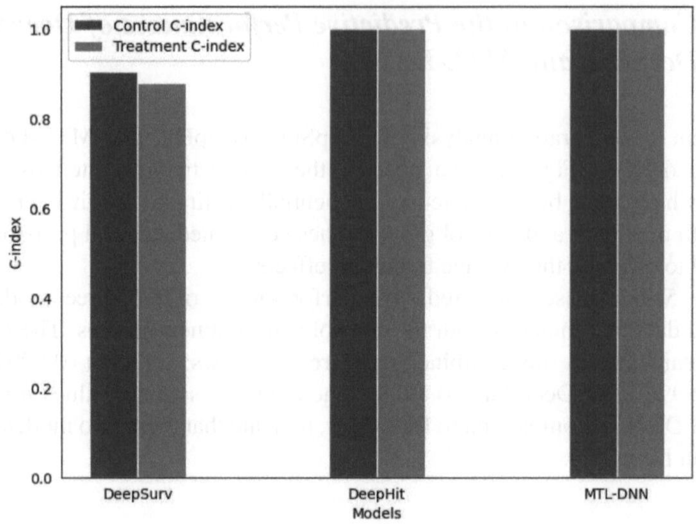

(a)

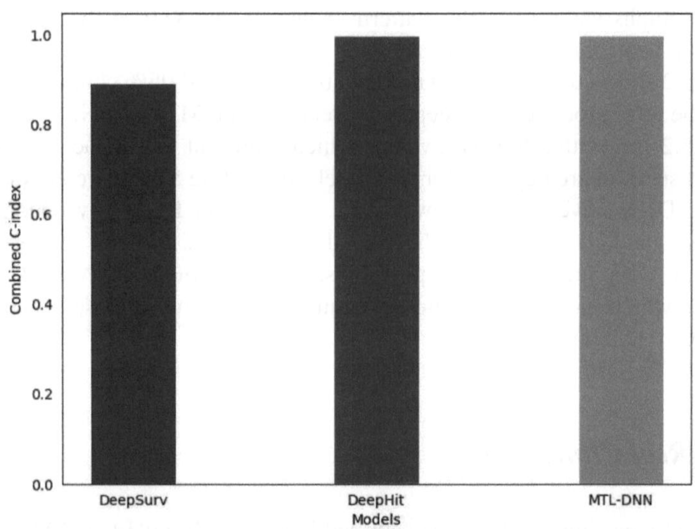

(b)

Fig. 5.4 *C*-statistic comparisons. (**a**) Comparison of the *C*-statistic for the control and treatment groups of DeepSurv, DeepHit, and MTL-DNN. (**b**) Comparison of the predictive performance of DeepSurv, DeepHit, and MTL-DNN with the control and treatment conditions combined

for DeepSurv is 0.1047, with a 95% CI ranging from 0.0867 to 0.1227. This suggests that patients receiving D-penicillamine treatment exhibit, on average, a positive 10.47% increased risk on their survival time (time-to-death) compared to

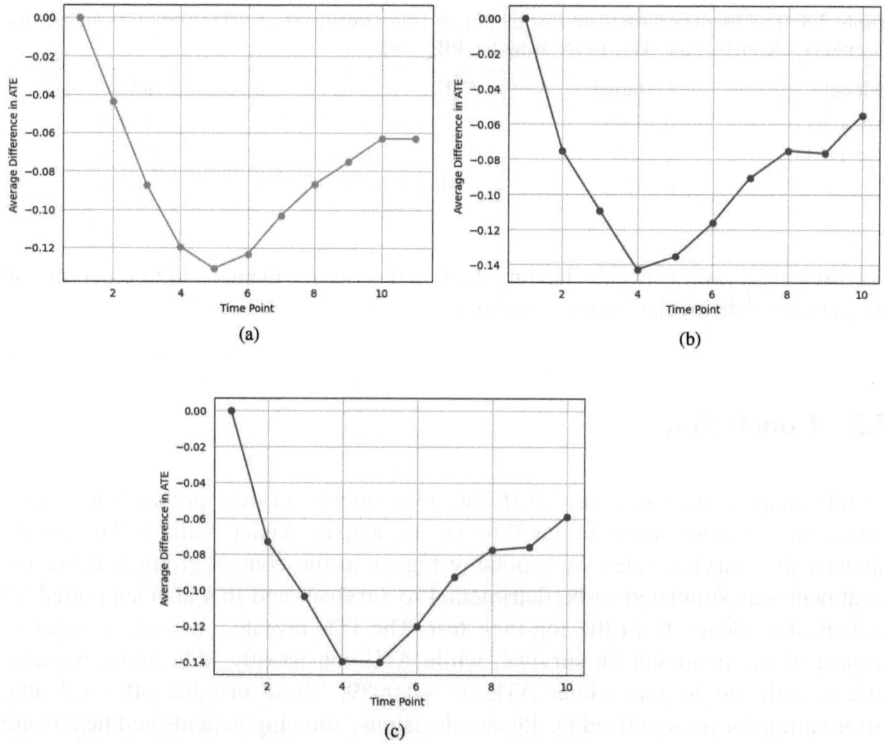

Fig. 5.5 Comparison of ATE for DeepSurv, DeepHit, and MTL-DNN. (**a**) DeepSurv ATE. (**b**) DeepHit ATE. (**c**) MTL-DNN ATE

Table 5.2 The bias, SD, and 95% CI for the ATE produced by DeepSurv, DeepHit, and MTL-DNN

	ATE	SD	Bias
DeepSurv	−0.0815 (−0.1043, −0.0586)	0.0387	0.0174
DeepHit	−0.0875 (−0.1135, −0.0615)	0.0419	0.0114
MTL-DNN	−0.0881 (−0.1140, −0.0622)	0.0418	0.0108

the untreated group. This means that D-penicillamine medication may be linked to an elevated risk of time to death, which could affect survival rates, according to the positive ATE. In contrast, the ATE values of DeepHit and MTL-DNN are lower, at 0.0726 and 0.0481, respectively. These disparate ATE values demonstrate how the estimated treatment effects varied between the models. These findings align with the results by Gong et al. (2004). The authors found that D-penicillamine significantly elevated the risk of adverse events with relative risk (RR) values of 3.11 (95% CI 2.33 to 4.16) in a fixed model and 4.18 (with 95% CI from 1.38 to 12.69) in a random model. Gong et al. (2004) concluded that D-penicillamine did not demonstrate a reduction in the risk of mortality but substantially increased the

Table 5.3 The average *C*-statistic (for treatment 1 and treatment 2), ATE, 95% CI, and SD for DeepSurv, DeepHit, and MTL-DNN using the PBC data

Model	*C*-statistic	ATE	SD
DeepSurv	0.95315	0.1047 (0.0867, 0.1227)	0.0964
DeepHit	0.9889	0.0726 (0.0384, 0.1069)	0.0553
MTL-DNN	0.9577	0.0481 (0.0124, 0.0838)	0.0576

occurrence of adverse events, leading them to discourage the use of D-penicillamine for patients with primary biliary cirrhosis.

5.5 Conclusion

In this chapter, we used simulated data to examine survival probabilities under treatment and control conditions through the Kaplan–Meier method. The results showed that survival rates were notably higher in the control group beacuse the treatment was simulated to be detrimental to survival, and this also supported by statistical evidence from the log-rank test. The ITE revealed an overall negative impact of the treatment on survival, while ATE consistently indicated a negative effect, with the Kaplan–Meier ATE at -0.0989. These insights offer valuable information for personalized healthcare decisions, allowing patients and healthcare providers to make informed choices based on survival probabilities associated with different treatments.

Moving beyond traditional survival analysis, we compared the predictive performances of DeepSurv, DeepHit, and MTL-DNN models. The *C*-statistic demonstrated that DeepHit and MTL-DNN outperformed DeepSurv, particularly when considering the combined data of treatment and control groups. Additionally, ATE estimation and bias analysis for the ML models indicated that DeepHit and MTL-DNN closely aligned with the true population treatment effects. Despite the limitations, including the use of simulated data, this study provides valuable insights into survival analysis and the comparative performance of ML models.

The results of the treatment effect estimation using the PBC dataset underscore the inherent trade-offs between prediction accuracy and treatment impact estimation in survival analysis methods. This clinical study highlights the importance of carefully balancing predictive accuracy and treatment impact estimation when selecting a survival analysis model for real-world applications.

Future research will explore additional deep learning models for survival data, including Cox-time (Kvamme et al., 2019), Dynamic-DeepHit (Lee et al., 2019), and joint modeling approaches. The objective is to improve the ability to accurately model time-dependent covariates and their interactions with other covariates in predicting survival outcomes.

Acknowledgments The research is supported in part by the RDP grant at the University of Pretoria and the National Research Foundation (NRF) of South Africa, Ref.: RA210106581084, grant No. 150170. The opinions expressed and conclusions arrived at are those of the authors and are not necessarily to be attributed the NRF.

References

Austin, P. C. (2014). The use of propensity score methods with survival or time-to-event outcomes: reporting measures of effect similar to those used in randomized experiments. *Statistics in Medicine, 33*(7), 1242–1258.

Barnow, B. S., Cain, G. G., Goldberger, A. S., et al. (1980). *Issues in the analysis of selectivity bias* (Vol. 4). University of Wisconsin, Inst. for Research on Poverty.

Bavli, H. J. (2019). Counterfactual causation. *Arizona State Law Journal, 51*, 879.

Clark, T. G., Bradburn, M. J., Love, S. B., & Altman, D. G. (2003). Survival analysis part i: basic concepts and first analyses. *British Journal of Cancer, 89*(2), 232–238.

Cox, D. R. (1972). Regression models and life-tables. *Journal of the Royal Statistical Society: Series B (Methodological), 34*(2), 187–202.

Crown, W. H. (2019). Real-world evidence, causal inference, and machine learning. *Value in Health, 22*(5), 587–592.

Crowther, M. J., & Lambert, P. C. (2013). Simulating biologically plausible complex survival data. *Statistics in Medicine, 32*(23), 4118–4134.

Geneletti, S. G. (2005). *Aspects of casual inference in a non-counterfactual framework*. University of London, University College London (United Kingdom).

Gong, Y., Klingenberg, S. L., & Gluud, C. (2004). D-penicillamine for primary biliary cirrhosis. *Cochrane Database of Systematic Reviews*, (4).

Harrell Jr., F. E., Lee, K. L., & Mark, D. B. (1996). Multivariable prognostic models: issues in developing models, evaluating assumptions and adequacy, and measuring and reducing errors. *Statistics in Medicine, 15*(4), 361–387.

Hastie, T., Tibshirani, R., Friedman, J. H., & Friedman, J. H. (2009). *The elements of statistical learning: Data mining, inference, and prediction* (Vol. 2). Springer.

Holland, P. W. (1986). Statistics and causal inference. *Journal of the American Statistical Association, 81*(396), 945–960.

Hong, W. S., Haimovich, A. D., & Taylor, R. A. (2018). Predicting hospital admission at emergency department triage using machine learning. *PloS One, 13*(7), e0201016.

Hosmer Jr., D. W., Lemeshow, S., & Sturdivant, R. X. (2013). *Applied logistic regression* (Vol. 398). John Wiley & Sons.

Ishwaran, H., Kogalur, U. B., Blackstone, E. H., & Lauer, M. S. (2008). Random survival forests. *The Annals of Applied Statistics, 2*(3), 841–860.

Jiang, S. (2019). Prediction based on random survival forest. *American Journal of Biomedical Science & Research, 6*(2), 109–11.

Katzman, J. L., Shaham, U., Cloninger, A., Bates, J., Jiang, T., & Kluger, Y. (2018). DeepSurv: Personalized treatment recommender system using a Cox proportional hazards deep neural network. *BMC Medical Research Methodology, 18*(1), 1–12.

Kleinbaum, D. G., & Klein, M. (2012). Kaplan-Meier survival curves and the log-rank test. In *Survival analysis* (pp. 55–96). Springer.

Kvamme, H., Borgan, Ø., & Scheel, I. (2019). Time-to-event prediction with neural networks and Cox regression. *Journal of Machine Learning Research, 20*(129), 1–30.

Lee, C., Yoon, J., & Van Der Schaar, M. (2019). Dynamic-DeepHit: A deep learning approach for dynamic survival analysis with competing risks based on longitudinal data. *IEEE Transactions on Biomedical Engineering, 67*(1), 122–133.

Lee, C., Zame, W., Yoon, J., & Van Der Schaar, M. (2018). DeepHit: A deep learning approach to survival analysis with competing risks. In *Proceedings of the AAAI conference on artificial intelligence* (Vol. 32).

Leung, K.-M., Elashoff, R. M., & Afifi, A. A. (1997). Censoring issues in survival analysis. *Annual Review of Public Health, 18*(1), 83–104.

Murtaugh, P. A., Dickson, R. E., Van Dam, G. M., Malinchoc, M., Grambsch, P. M., Langworthy, A. L., & Gips, C. H. (1994). Primary biliary cirrhosis: Prediction of short–term survival based on repeated patient visits. *Hepatology, 20*(1), 126–134.

Nasejje, J. B., Mbuvha, R., & Mwambi, H. (2022). Use of a deep learning and random forest approach to track changes in the predictive nature of socioeconomic drivers of under-5 mortality rates in Sub-Saharan Africa. *BMJ Open, 12*(2), e049786.

Nemati, M., Ansary, J., & Nemati, N. (2020). Machine-learning approaches in covid-19 survival analysis and discharge-time likelihood prediction using clinical data. *Patterns, 1*(5), 100074.

Obermeyer, Z., & Emanuel, E. J. (2016). Predicting the future big data, machine learning, and clinical medicine. *The New England Journal of Medicine, 375*(13), 1216.

Radovanović, S., Delibašić, B., Jovanović, M., Vukićević, M., & Suknović, M. (2018). Framework for integration of domain knowledge into logistic regression. In *Proceedings of the 8th International Conference on Web Intelligence, Mining and Semantics* (pp. 1–8).

Rosenbaum, P. R., & Rubin, D. B. (1983). The central role of the propensity score in observational studies for causal effects. *Biometrika, 70*(1), 41–55.

Rosenbaum, P. R., & Rubin, D. B. (1984). Reducing bias in observational studies using subclassification on the propensity score. *Journal of the American statistical Association, 79*(387), 516–524.

Rubin, D. B. (1974). Estimating causal effects of treatments in randomized and nonrandomized studies. *Journal of Educational Psychology, 66*(5), 688.

Rubin, D. B. (1978). Bayesian inference for causal effects: The role of randomization. *The Annals of Statistics, 6*(1), 34–58.

Shickel, B., Tighe, P. J., Bihorac, A., & Rashidi, P. (2017). Deep EHR: A survey of recent advances in deep learning techniques for electronic health record (EHR) analysis. *IEEE Journal of Biomedical and Health Informatics, 22*(5), 1589–1604.

VanderWeele, T. J. (2016). Commentary: On causes, causal inference, and potential outcomes. *International Journal of Epidemiology, 45*(6), 1809–1816.

Xiao, Y., Abrahamowicz, M., & Moodie, E. E. (2010). Accuracy of conventional and marginal structural Cox model estimators: A simulation study. *The International Journal of Biostatistics, 6*(2), 1–30.

Yang, S., & Prentice, R. L. (2015). Assessing potentially time-dependent treatment effect from clinical trials and observational studies for survival data, with applications to the women's health initiative combined hormone therapy trial. *Statistics in Medicine, 34*(11), 1801–1817.

Zhang, Z., Reinikainen, J., Adeleke, K. A., Pieterse, M. E., & Groothuis-Oudshoorn, C. G. (2018). Time-varying covariates and coefficients in Cox regression models. *Annals of Translational Medicine, 6*(7), 121.

Zupan, B., Demšar, J., Kattan, M. W., Beck, J. R., & Bratko, I. (2000). Machine learning for survival analysis: A case study on recurrence of prostate cancer. *Artificial intelligence in Medicine, 20*(1), 59–75.

Part II
Imaging Data Analysis

Chapter 6
Detection of Quadratic Interactions in Brain Functional Connectivity

Xuze Zhang, Yuichi Goto, Benjamin Kedem, and Shuo Chen

6.1 Introduction

The human brain consists of functionally interconnected regions. This is referred to as brain functional connectivity (FC), which is measured during the resting state of functional magnetic resonance imaging (fMRI) and represents a manifestation of spontaneous low-frequency fluctuations in blood oxygen level-dependent (BOLD) signals. Pairwise FC is typically measured in terms of correlation, coherence, and other suitable measures. The complete map of the human brain functional connectivity, or neural pathways, is referred to as the *connectome*.

Mohanty et al. (2020) conducted an exploratory study on several FC measures including Pearson's correlation, cross-correlation, coherence, wavelet coherence, mutual information, Euclidean distance, cityblock distance, dynamic time warping, and Wasserstein metric. The authors highlighted the fact that "brain regions may appear connected functionally under one definition but disconnected under another." The same authors found that (i) Pearson's correlation may provide an incomplete characterization of FC, (ii) there exist several alternative measures that

X. Zhang (✉) · B. Kedem
Department of Mathematics and Institute for Systems Research, University of Maryland, College Park, MD, USA
e-mail: xzhang51@umd.edu; bnk@umd.edu

Y. Goto
Faculty of Mathematics, Kyushu University, Fukuoka, Japan
e-mail: yuichi.goto@math.kyushu-u.ac.jp

S. Chen
Maryland Psychiatric Research Center, School of Medicine, University of Maryland, College Park, MD, USA
e-mail: shuochen@umd.edu

D.-G. Chen, C. A. Coelho (eds.), *Biostatistics Modeling and Public Health Applications*, Emerging Topics in Statistics and Biostatistics,
https://doi.org/10.1007/978-3-031-69690-9_6

can capture interactions between brain signals in different ways, and (iii) no single measure of FC stands out in the context of classification or prediction. This echoes the sentiment in Horwitz (2003), who addresses of the "elusive concept of brain connectivity."

Despite these shortcomings, coherence has been a widely used FC measure. It is a time series method, akin to the statistical correlation, used to determine if two or more brain regions are spectrally connected, that is, loosely speaking, if two or more brain regions have "similar neuronal oscillatory activity" (Bowyer, 2016). However, coherence measures the strength of linear relationships only but fails to measure nonlinear relations expressed, for example, as nonlinear impulse response models (Zhao et al., 2019; Cao et al., 2022). In particular, coherence fails to measure spectral relationships due to *quadratic interaction terms*. This can be rectified by the so-called *lagged coherence* (Kedem-Kimelfeld, 1975) and/or its offshoot *maximum residual coherence* which provide the contribution of specific quadratic interaction terms to covariation of brain regions, over and beyond the coherence by itself (Khan et al., 2014; Kedem, 2016). It will be clear from the definition of lagged coherence below that there are cases where the coherence is rather low but that the lagged coherence points to an increased covariation activity due to quadratic interactions.

This chapter explores the use of lagged coherence in measuring the contribution of interactions to functional connectivity, exemplified by case-control schizophrenia data, following the recent development in Goto et al. (2023).

6.2 Linearization and Orthogonalization of a Quadratic System

Kimelfeld (1974) considered a quadratic system

$$Y(t) = K_0 + \sum_{s=-\infty}^{\infty} \ell_s X(t-s) + \sum_{r_1=-\infty}^{\infty} \sum_{r_2=-\infty}^{\infty} c_{r_1,r_2} X(t-r_1) X(t-r_2), \quad (6.1)$$

where K_0 is a constant and $EX(t) = EY(t) = 0$. Assume that $\{X(t)\}$ is a real-valued fourth-order stationary process with absolutely summable fourth-order cumulants, and $\{\ell_s\}$ and $\{c_{r_1,r_2}\}$ are absolutely summable real-valued series. The quadratic terms can be expressed as *lag processes*

$$\widetilde{X}_u(t) = X(t)X(t+u) - R_{XX}(u)$$

for $u \in \mathbb{N}$, where $R_{XX}(u)$ is the covariance function of $X(t)$. Equation (6.1) can be rewritten in terms of $\{\widetilde{X}_u(t)\}$, that is,

$$Y(t) = \sum_{s=-\infty}^{\infty} \ell_s X(t-s) + \sum_{u=0}^{\infty} \sum_{r=-\infty}^{\infty} b_{u,r} \widetilde{X}_u(t-r), \tag{6.2}$$

where $\{b_{u,r}\}$ is a set of absolutely summable real-valued series.

Thus, the quadratic filter of $\{X(t)\}$ in (6.1) can be considered as linear filters of lag processes in (6.2). According to Kimelfeld (1974), for sufficiently large n, $Y(t)$ can be approximated by $X(t)$ and $\widetilde{X}_u(t)$ for a finite set of u, $u_1, \ldots, u_n$ in mean square, and then we may express $Y(t)$ as

$$Y(t) = \sum_{s=-\infty}^{\infty} \ell_s X(t-s) + \sum_{k=1}^{n} \sum_{r=-\infty}^{\infty} b_{u_k,r} \widetilde{X}_{u_k}(t-r), \tag{6.3}$$

and $Y(t)$ admits the spectral representation

$$Y(t) = \int_{-\pi}^{\pi} e^{it\lambda} L(\lambda) dZ_X(\lambda) + \sum_{k=1}^{n} \int_{-\pi}^{\pi} e^{it\lambda} B_k(\lambda) dZ_{\widetilde{X}_{u_k}}(\lambda), \tag{6.4}$$

where $L(\lambda) = \sum_{s=-\infty}^{\infty} e^{-is\lambda} \ell_s$ and $B_k(\lambda) = \sum_{r=-\infty}^{\infty} e^{-ir\lambda} b_{u_k,r}$ for $k = 1, \ldots, n$.

Now, suppose that the fourth-order cumulants of $\{X(t)\}$ satisfy

$$\sum_{t_1,t_2,t_3=-\infty}^{\infty} \left(1 + \sum_{i=1}^{3} t_i^2\right) |\mathrm{cum}\,(X(0), X(t_1), X(t_2), X(t_3))| < \infty,$$

and

$$\sum_{s=-\infty}^{\infty} s^2 |\ell_s| < \infty, \quad \sum_{r=-\infty}^{\infty} r^2 |b_{u_k,r}| < \infty, \; k = 1, \ldots, n.$$

Let $Z_X(\lambda)$ and $Z_{\widetilde{X}_{u_k}}$ be the spectral measures corresponding to $X(t)$ and $\widetilde{X}_{u_k}(t)$ for $k = 1, \ldots, n$. Then $\{Y(t)\}$ can be decomposed into two orthogonal processes $\{G_1(t)\}$ and $\{G_2(t)\}$ such that

$$G_1(t) = \int_{-\pi}^{\pi} e^{it\lambda} H(\lambda) dZ_X(\lambda),$$

and

$$\begin{aligned} G_2(t) &= \sum_{k=1}^{n} G_{2,k}(t) \\ &= \sum_{k=1}^{n} \left(\int_{-\pi}^{\pi} e^{it\lambda} A_k(\lambda) dZ_X(\lambda) + \int_{-\pi}^{\pi} e^{it\lambda} B_k(\lambda) dZ_{\widetilde{X}_{u_k}}(\lambda) \right), \end{aligned}$$

where

$$L(\lambda) = H(\lambda) + \sum_{k=1}^{n} A_k(\lambda), \quad H(\lambda) = \frac{f_{XY}(\lambda)}{f_{XX}(\lambda)}, \quad \boldsymbol{A}(\lambda) = -\frac{\mathrm{diag}(\boldsymbol{f}_{XU}(\lambda))}{f_{XX}(\lambda)} \boldsymbol{B}(\lambda),$$

$$\boldsymbol{B}(\lambda) = \left(\boldsymbol{f}_{UU}(\lambda) - \frac{\boldsymbol{f}_{UX}(\lambda)\boldsymbol{f}_{XU}(\lambda)}{f_{XX}(\lambda)}\right)^{-1} \left(\boldsymbol{f}_{UY} - \frac{f_{XY}(\lambda)}{f_{XX}(\lambda)} \boldsymbol{f}_{UX}(\lambda)\right),$$

$\boldsymbol{A}(\lambda) = (A_1(\lambda), \ldots, A_n(\lambda))^\top$, $\boldsymbol{B}(\lambda) = (B_1(\lambda), \ldots, B_n(\lambda))^\top$, $\boldsymbol{f}_{UU}(\lambda) = (f_{\widetilde{X}_{u_i} \widetilde{X}_{u_j}}(\lambda))$, $\boldsymbol{f}_{UY}(\lambda) = (f_{\widetilde{X}_{u_1} Y}(\lambda), \ldots, f_{\widetilde{X}_{u_n} Y}(\lambda))^\top$, and $\boldsymbol{f}_{XU}^H(\lambda) = \boldsymbol{f}_{UX}(\lambda) = (f_{\widetilde{X}_{u_1} X}(\lambda), \ldots, f_{\widetilde{X}_{u_n} X}(\lambda))^\top$. Note that

$$Y(t) \in \overline{sp}(\{X(t)\}) + \sum_{k=1}^{n} \overline{sp}(\{\widetilde{X}_{u_k}(t)\}),$$

and $G_1(t)$ is indeed the projection of $\{Y(t)\}$ onto $\overline{sp}(\{X(t)\})$, while $G_2(t)$ is the projection of $Y(t)$ onto $(\overline{sp}(\{X(t)\}))^\perp$. Similar orthogonalization ideas can be found in Wiener (1958) and Hannan (1970).

6.3 Lagged Coherence and Maximum Residual Coherence

When the quadratic terms are expressed as lag processes, it is of interest to measure the intensity of each lag process. Kedem-Kimelfeld (1975) considered a quadratic system with a single lag process

$$Y(t) = \sum_{s=-\infty}^{\infty} \ell_s X(t-s) + \sum_{r=-\infty}^{\infty} b_r \widetilde{X}_u(t-r) + \epsilon(t), \tag{6.5}$$

where $\{\epsilon(t)\}$ is a zero-mean stationary noise independent of $\{X(t)\}$. Then the orthogonal decomposition of $Y(t)$ is

$$Y(t) = G_1(t) + G_2(t; u) + \epsilon(t),$$

where

$$G_1(t) = \int_{-\pi}^{\pi} e^{it\lambda} H(\lambda) dZ_X(\lambda),$$

$$G_2(t; u) = \int_{-\pi}^{\pi} e^{it\lambda} A(\lambda; u) dZ_X(\lambda) + \int_{-\pi}^{\pi} e^{it\lambda} B(\lambda; u) dZ_{\widetilde{X}_u}(\lambda),$$

with

$$H(\lambda) = \frac{f_{XY}(\lambda)}{f_{XX}(\lambda)}, \quad A(\lambda; u) = -\frac{f_{X\widetilde{X}_u}(\lambda)}{f_{XX}(\lambda)} B(\lambda; u),$$

$$\text{and} \quad B(\lambda; u) = \frac{f_{XX}(\lambda) f_{\widetilde{X}_u Y}(\lambda) - f_{\widetilde{X}_u X}(\lambda) f_{XY}(\lambda)}{f_{XX}(\lambda) f_{\widetilde{X}_u \widetilde{X}_u}(\lambda) - \left|f_{X\widetilde{X}_u}(\lambda)\right|^2}.$$

The squared coherence between $\{X(t)\}$ and $\{Y(t)\}$ can be obtained by standardizing the spectral density of $\{G_1(t)\}$ using $f_{YY}(\lambda)$, that is,

$$S_1(\lambda) = \frac{f_{G_1 G_1}(\lambda)}{f_{YY}(\lambda)} = \frac{|H(\lambda)|^2 f_{XX}(\lambda)}{f_{YY}(\lambda)} = \frac{|f_{XY}(\lambda)|^2}{f_{XX}(\lambda) f_{YY}(\lambda)},$$

which measures the linear dependence between $\{X(t)\}$ and $\{Y(t)\}$. In the same fashion, the lagged coherence is defined by standardizing $f_{G_1 G_1}(\lambda) + f_{G_2 G_2}(\lambda; u)$ using $f_{YY}(\lambda)$, that is,

$$\begin{aligned} S_2(\lambda; u) &= S_1(\lambda) + \frac{f_{G_2 G_2}(\lambda; u)}{f_{YY}(\lambda)} \\ &= S_1(\lambda) + \frac{|B(\lambda; u)|^2}{f_{YY}(\lambda)} \left(f_{\widetilde{X}_u \widetilde{X}_u}(\lambda) - \frac{\left|f_{X\widetilde{X}_u}(\lambda)\right|^2}{f_{XX}(\lambda)} \right) \qquad (6.6) \\ &= S_1(\lambda) + \frac{\left|f_{XX}(\lambda) f_{\widetilde{X}_u Y}(\lambda) - f_{\widetilde{X}_u X}(\lambda) f_{XY}(\lambda)\right|^2}{\left(f_{XX}(\lambda) f_{\widetilde{X}_u \widetilde{X}_u}(\lambda) - \left|f_{X\widetilde{X}_u}(\lambda)\right|^2\right) f_{XX}(\lambda) f_{YY}(\lambda)}. \end{aligned}$$

Then the lag process $\{\widetilde{X}_{u_0}(t)\}$ with

$$u_0 = \underset{u}{\operatorname{argmax}}\, S_2(\lambda; u), \quad -\pi \le \lambda \le \pi,$$

is considered as the most influential lag process. However, as noted by Kedem-Kimelfeld (1975), such u_0 may not exist, that is, $S_2(\lambda; u)$ may be maximized by distinct u's over different frequency bands.

Thus, it is imperative to have a criterion that is independent of λ to measure the effect of the lag process. Before we introduce the available criteria, it should be noted that $S_2(\lambda; u) - S_1(\lambda)$ is closely related to the squared partial coherency spectrum (Jenkins and Watts, 1968, p. 489). The squared partial coherency spectrum of $\{\widetilde{X}_u(t)\}$ and $\{Y(t)\}$ allowing for $\{X(t)\}$ is defined by

$$\kappa^2_{\widetilde{X}_u Y|X}(\lambda)$$

$$=\frac{\left|f_{\widetilde{X}_u Y}(\lambda)-\frac{f_{\widetilde{X}_u X}(\lambda)f_{XY}(\lambda)}{f_{XX}(\lambda)}\right|^2}{f_{\widetilde{X}_u\widetilde{X}_u}(\lambda)\left(1-\frac{\left|f_{X\widetilde{X}_u}(\lambda)\right|^2}{f_{XX}(\lambda)f_{\widetilde{X}_u\widetilde{X}_u}(\lambda)}\right)f_{YY}(\lambda)\left(1-\frac{|f_{XY}(\lambda)|^2}{f_{XX}(\lambda)f_{YY}(\lambda)}\right)}$$

$$=\frac{\left|f_{XX}(\lambda)f_{\widetilde{X}_u Y}(\lambda)-f_{\widetilde{X}_u X}(\lambda)f_{XY}(\lambda)\right|^2}{\left(f_{XX}(\lambda)f_{\widetilde{X}_u\widetilde{X}_u}(\lambda)-\left|f_{X\widetilde{X}_u}(\lambda)\right|^2\right)\left(f_{XX}(\lambda)f_{YY}(\lambda)-|f_{XY}(\lambda)|^2\right)},$$

and hence

$$\kappa^2_{\widetilde{X}_u Y|X}(\lambda)=\frac{f_{XX}(\lambda)f_{YY}(\lambda)}{f_{XX}(\lambda)f_{YY}(\lambda)-|f_{XY}(\lambda)|^2}\left(S_2(\lambda;u)-S_1(\lambda)\right).$$

Both $\kappa^2_{\widetilde{X}_u Y|X}(\lambda)$ and $S_2(\lambda; u) - S_1(\lambda)$ are measurements of the linear dependence between $\{\widetilde{X}_u(t)\}$ and $\{Y(t)\}$ with the effect of $\{X(t)\}$ removed.

Based on $S_2(\lambda; u) - S_1(\lambda)$, the maximum residual coherence is defined by

$$RS(u)=\max_{\lambda}\{S_2(\lambda;u)-S_1(\lambda)\},\tag{6.7}$$

which is independent of λ. As mentioned by both Khan et al. (2014) and Kedem (2016), the effects of lag processes can be graphically compared by the estimated values of $RS(u)$ for different u's.

We use the following example to show the problem may arise in using $S_2(\lambda; u)$ and $RS(u)$. Let $\{X(t)\}$ be an AR(1) process such that

$$X(t)=0.2X(t-1)+e(t),$$

where $e(t) \overset{i.i.d.}{\sim} N(0, 1)$. Define $\{Y(t)\}$ as

$$Y(t)=X(t)+0.7\widetilde{X}_0(t)+\widetilde{X}_{10}(t)+\epsilon(t),$$

where $\epsilon(t) \overset{i.i.d.}{\sim} N(0, 1)$. All processes have length $n = 1000$. The estimates of the cross spectral densities are obtained using the Parzen window with bandwidth $M_n = \lfloor n^{1/3.5}\rfloor$, following Assumption 3.1 in Goto et al. (2023). As shown in Fig. 6.1, neither estimated $S_2(\lambda; 0)$ nor $S_2(\lambda; 10)$ dominates the other so that it is difficult to discern which one is more prominent based on lagged coherence. Nevertheless, such decision can be readily made based on the bar plot of estimated $RS(u)$ in Fig. 6.2, which indicates that the lag process with $u = 10$ is more prominent.

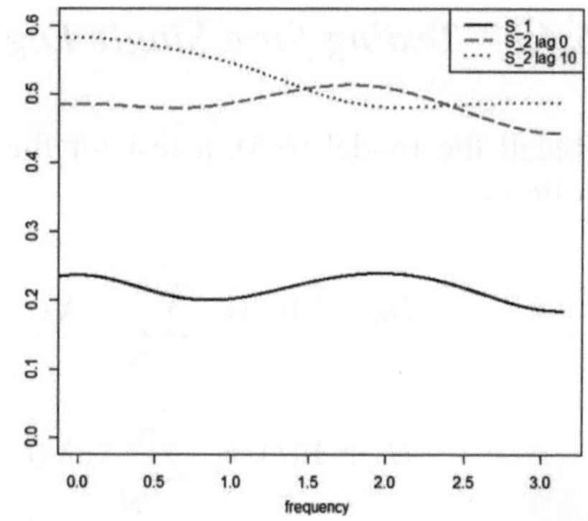

Fig. 6.1 Estimated $S_1(\lambda)$ and $S_2(\lambda; u)$ for $u = 0, 10$

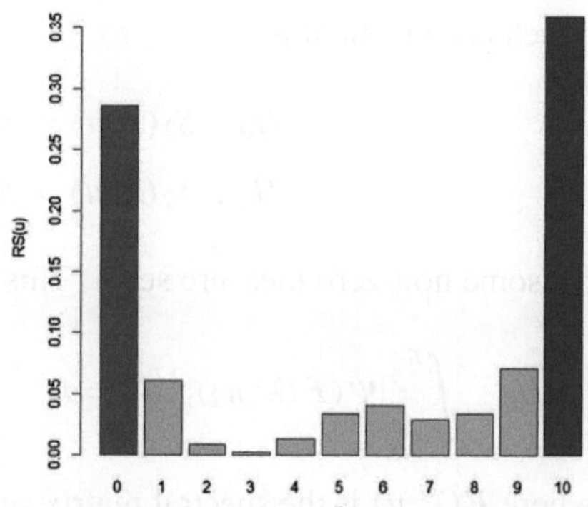

Fig. 6.2 Estimated $RS(u)$ for $u = 0, \ldots, 10$

The residual coherence $RS(u)$ maximizes $S_2(\lambda; u) - S_1(\lambda)$ over λ, and hence it does not depend on λ. Alternatively, one may construct a criterion by integrating out λ such as $\int_{-\pi}^{\pi}(S_2(\lambda; u) - S_1(\lambda))d\lambda$. Further discussions can be found in Goto et al. (2023).

6.4 Testing for the Presence of Lag Processes

The maximum residual coherence can be used to compare the effects of a set of lag processes, but it cannot guarantee that the most prominent one is statistically significant. It could be the case that none of the lag processes in this set has a significant effect. A regression method is proposed by Kedem (2016) to detect significant interaction terms within the prominent lag processes selected by the maximum residual coherence. The significance of integration terms in a lag process suggests the presence of this lag process to some extent, but it is still of interest to test for the presence of lag processes directly. In this section, we introduce a test for the presence of lag processes based on Goto et al. (2023).

6.4.1 Testing for a Single Lag Process

Recall the model (6.5), a test for the existence of $\{\widetilde{X}_u(t)\}$ can be formulated as follows:

$$H_0 : Y(t) = \sum_{s=-\infty}^{\infty} \ell_s X(t-s) + \epsilon(t),$$

$$H_a : Y(t) = \sum_{s=-\infty}^{\infty} \ell_s X(t-s) + \sum_{r=-\infty}^{\infty} b_r \widetilde{X}_u(t-r) + \epsilon(t),$$

which is equivalent to

$$H_0 : S_2(\lambda; u) = S_1(\lambda), \ \lambda \in [-\pi, \pi] \ a.e.$$
$$H_a : S_2(\lambda; u) > S_1(\lambda), \ \lambda \in A \subset [-\pi, \pi]$$

for some non-zero measure set A. This can be rephrased by

$$H_0 : \int_{-\pi}^{\pi} |\Psi(\boldsymbol{F}(\lambda; u))|^2 \, d\lambda = 0, \quad H_a : \int_{-\pi}^{\pi} |\Psi(\boldsymbol{F}(\lambda; u))|^2 \, d\lambda > 0, \tag{6.8}$$

where $\boldsymbol{F}(\lambda; u)$ is the spectral matrix such that

$$\boldsymbol{F}(\lambda; u) = \begin{bmatrix} f_{XX}(\lambda) & f_{X\widetilde{X}_u}(\lambda) & f_{XY}(\lambda) \\ f_{\widetilde{X}_u X}(\lambda) & f_{\widetilde{X}_u \widetilde{X}_u}(\lambda) & f_{\widetilde{X}_u Y}(\lambda) \\ f_{YX}(\lambda) & f_{Y\widetilde{X}_u}(\lambda) & f_{YY}(\lambda) \end{bmatrix}$$

and

$$\Psi(\boldsymbol{F}(\lambda; u)) = f_{XX}(\lambda) f_{\widetilde{X}_u Y}(\lambda) - f_{\widetilde{X}_u X}(\lambda) f_{XY}(\lambda).$$

The following assumptions are made to ensure the asymptotic properties of the test statistic to be formulated, following Goto et al. (2023).

Assumption 6.4.1

(1) The process {X(t)} is a strictly stationary process of which all moments are finite. Moreover, for any $j \in \mathbb{Z}^+$,

$$\sum_{t_1,\ldots,t_j=-\infty}^{\infty} \left(1 + \sum_{i=1}^{j} t_i^2\right) \left|\mathrm{cum}\left(X(0), X(t_1), \ldots, X(t_j)\right)\right| < \infty.$$

(2) The linear filters of $\{X(t)\}$ *and* $\widetilde{X}_u(t)$ *satisfy that*

$$\sum_{s=-\infty}^{\infty} s^2|\ell_s| < \infty \quad \text{and} \quad \sum_{r=-\infty}^{\infty} r^2|b_r| < \infty.$$

(3) The disturbance $\{\epsilon(t)\}$ *is a sequence of zero-mean i.i.d. noise independent of* $\{X(t)\}$.

The cross spectral densities in $\boldsymbol{F}(\lambda; u)$ are estimated by the kernel method based on the Parzen window

$$w(x) = \begin{cases} 1 - 6|x|^2 + 6|x|^3, & |x| < \frac{1}{2}, \\ 2(1 - |x|)^3, & \frac{1}{2} \leq |x| \leq 1, \\ 0, & otherwise \end{cases}$$

with bandwidth $M_n = \lfloor n^{1/3.5} \rfloor$. Following Goto et al. (2023), the test statistic is given by

$$Z_n(u) = \frac{\frac{n}{M_n}\int_{-\pi}^{\pi} \left|\Psi(\widehat{\boldsymbol{F}}(\lambda; u))\right|^2 d\lambda - \sqrt{M_n}\eta_{w,2}\int_{-\pi}^{\pi} \psi(\widehat{\boldsymbol{F}}(\lambda; u))d\lambda}{\sqrt{4\pi\eta_{w,4}\int_{-\pi}^{\pi} \left|\psi(\widehat{\boldsymbol{F}}(\lambda; u))\right|^2 d\lambda}}, \tag{6.9}$$

where

$$\begin{aligned} &\psi(\boldsymbol{F}(\lambda; u)) \\ &= \left(f_{XX}(\lambda) f_{\widetilde{X}_u\widetilde{X}_u}(\lambda) - |f_{X\widetilde{X}_u}(\lambda)|^2\right)\left(f_{XX}(\lambda) f_{YY}(\lambda) - |f_{XY}(\lambda)|^2\right), \end{aligned}$$

$$\eta_{w,2} = \int_{-\infty}^{\infty} w^2(x)dx, \quad \text{and} \quad \eta_{w,4} = \int_{-\infty}^{\infty} w^4(x)dx.$$

By Theorems 3.1 and 3.2 in Goto et al. (2023), under Assumption 6.4.1 and H_0, $Z_n(u)$ converges weakly to a standard normal distribution as $n \to \infty$.

6.4.2 Testing for Multiple Lag Processes

When the goal is to test whether $\{Y(t)\}$ is a quadratic system of $\{X(t)\}$, it is more persuasive to test the presence of multiple lag processes instead of a single one. But if the test (6.8) is directly applied to multiple lag processes, there will be a multiplicity issue. Nonetheless, with a slight modification of (6.8) and (6.9), a test for multiple lag processes can be formulated based on Goto et al. (2023). The hypotheses for testing lag processes corresponding to a set of lags $\boldsymbol{u} = (u_1, \ldots, u_k)^\top$ are given by

$$H_0: \int_{-\pi}^{\pi} \|\boldsymbol{\Phi}(\boldsymbol{F}_{-}(\lambda; \boldsymbol{u}))\|_2^2 \, d\lambda = 0, \quad H_a: \int_{-\pi}^{\pi} \|\boldsymbol{\Phi}(\boldsymbol{F}_{-}(\lambda; \boldsymbol{u}))\|_2^2 \, d\lambda > 0, \tag{6.10}$$

where

$$\begin{aligned} \boldsymbol{\Phi}(\boldsymbol{F}_{-}(\lambda; \boldsymbol{u})) =& (\Phi_1(\boldsymbol{F}_{-}(\lambda; \boldsymbol{u})), \ldots, \Phi_k(\boldsymbol{F}_{-}(\lambda; \boldsymbol{u})))^\top, \\ \Phi_j(\boldsymbol{F}_{-}(\lambda; \boldsymbol{u})) =& \Psi(\boldsymbol{F}(\lambda; u_j)), \ j = 1, \ldots, k, \end{aligned}$$

and $\boldsymbol{F}_{-}(\lambda; \boldsymbol{u})$ is the spectral matrix of all processes such that

$$\boldsymbol{F}_{-}(\lambda; \boldsymbol{u}) = \begin{bmatrix} f_{XX}(\lambda) & f_{X\widetilde{X}_{u_1}}(\lambda) & \cdots & f_{X\widetilde{X}_{u_k}}(\lambda) & f_{XY}(\lambda) \\ f_{\widetilde{X}_{u_1}X}(\lambda) & f_{\widetilde{X}_{u_1}\widetilde{X}_{u_1}}(\lambda) & \cdots & f_{\widetilde{X}_{u_1}\widetilde{X}_{u_k}}(\lambda) & f_{\widetilde{X}_{u_1}Y}(\lambda) \\ \vdots & \vdots & \ddots & \vdots & \vdots \\ f_{\widetilde{X}_{u_k}X}(\lambda) & f_{\widetilde{X}_{u_k}\widetilde{X}_{u_1}}(\lambda) & \cdots & f_{\widetilde{X}_{u_k}\widetilde{X}_{u_k}}(\lambda) & f_{\widetilde{X}_{u_k}Y}(\lambda) \\ f_{YX}(\lambda) & f_{Y\widetilde{X}_{u_1}}(\lambda) & \cdots & f_{Y\widetilde{X}_{u_k}}(\lambda) & f_{YY}(\lambda) \end{bmatrix}.$$

Then the test statistic $\widetilde{Z}_n(\boldsymbol{u})$ is given by

$$\widetilde{Z}_n(\boldsymbol{u}) = \frac{\int_{-\pi}^{\pi} \left\|\boldsymbol{\Phi}(\widehat{\boldsymbol{F}}_{-}(\lambda; \boldsymbol{u}))\right\|_2^2 d\lambda - \mu_n(\widehat{\boldsymbol{F}}_{-}(\lambda; \boldsymbol{u}))}{\sigma_n(\widehat{\boldsymbol{F}}_{-}(\lambda; \boldsymbol{u}))}, \tag{6.11}$$

where

$$\begin{aligned} &\mu_n(\boldsymbol{F}_{-}(\lambda; \boldsymbol{u})) \\ =& \sqrt{M_n}\eta_{w,2} \int_{-\pi}^{\pi} \operatorname{tr}\left\{\Gamma(\boldsymbol{F}_{-}(\lambda; \boldsymbol{u})) \left(\boldsymbol{F}_{-}^\top(\lambda; \boldsymbol{u}) \otimes \boldsymbol{F}_{-}(\lambda; \boldsymbol{u})\right)\right\} d\lambda, \\ &\sigma_n^2(\boldsymbol{F}_{-}(\lambda; \boldsymbol{u})) \\ =& 4\pi \eta_{w,4} \int_{-\pi}^{\pi} \operatorname{tr}\left\{\Gamma(\boldsymbol{F}_{-}(\lambda; \boldsymbol{u})) \left(\boldsymbol{F}_{-}^\top(\lambda; \boldsymbol{u}) \otimes \boldsymbol{F}_{-}(\lambda; \boldsymbol{u})\right) (\Gamma(\boldsymbol{F}_{-}(\lambda; \boldsymbol{u})) \right. \\ &+ \left. \Gamma^H(\boldsymbol{F}_{-}(\lambda; \boldsymbol{u}))\right) \left(\boldsymbol{F}_{-}^\top(\lambda; \boldsymbol{u}) \otimes \boldsymbol{F}_{-}(\lambda; \boldsymbol{u})\right)\Big\} d\lambda, \end{aligned}$$

and

$$\Gamma(\boldsymbol{F}_{-}(\lambda; \boldsymbol{u})) = \sum_{j=1}^{k} \operatorname{vec}\left(\overline{\frac{\partial \Phi_j(\boldsymbol{Z})}{\partial \boldsymbol{Z}}}\right) \operatorname{vec}\left(\frac{\partial \Phi_j(\boldsymbol{Z})}{\partial \boldsymbol{Z}}\right)^\top \Bigg|_{\boldsymbol{Z}=\boldsymbol{F}_{-}(\lambda; \boldsymbol{u})}.$$

Again, under Assumption 6.4.1 and H_0, $\widetilde{Z}_n(\boldsymbol{u})$ converges weakly to a standard normal distribution as $n \to \infty$.

Remark 6.4.1 In (6.10), we have many lags $u_1, \ldots, u_k$, almost global u for large k. But the size k is limited by the length of the time series used for the test.

6.5 Testing for Quadratic Interactions in Brain Functional Connectivity

In this section, we compare the brain FC in parietal lobes between healthy individuals and schizophrenia patients. The data consist of BOLD time series extracted from 246 subregions based on Brainnetome Atlas (Fan et al., 2016) for 61 healthy individuals and 49 schizophrenia patients. A more detailed description can be found in Culbreth et al. (2021). Our test is applied to the 38 subregions of parietal lobes to detect possible quadratic associations between BOLD series in these subregions. Possible connections between abnormalities in parietal lobes and schizophrenia have been proposed by many research works of which a review can be referred to Chieffi et al. (2018).

The 38 subregions of parietal lobes are subregions 125–162 in Fan et al. (2016). Subregions with odd numbers are in the left hemisphere, while that with even numbers are in the right hemisphere. For each subregion, we take an average over all healthy individuals such that

$$X_{H,i}(t) = \frac{1}{61}\sum_{l=1}^{61} X_{H,i,l}(t),$$

where $X_{H,i,l}(t)$ is the observation of i-th subregion of l-th healthy individual at time t, and $X_{H,i}(t)$ is the averaged sequence at time t. Then, we take the first-order difference and remove the first two observations to obtain a sequence that is sufficiently stationary. Then center the process at 0, and denote the processed sequence as $\{D_{H,i}(t)\}$. Thus, we obtain 38 processed sequences representing the corresponding subregions for healthy control group. Similarly, we obtain the processed sequences $\{D_{P,i}(t)\}$, $i = 1, \ldots, 38$, for patient group.

Then, for $i \neq j$, perform the test (6.8) or (6.10) to detect whether the quadratic association is significant between $\{D_{H,i}(t)\}$ and $\{D_{H,j}(t)\}$. For example, one may determine whether $\{D_{H,i}(t)\}$ is a quadratic system of $\{D_{H,j}(t)\}$ by testing

$$H_0 : D_{H,i}(t) = \sum_{s=-\infty}^{\infty} \ell_s^{(H,i,j)} D_{H,j}(t-s) + \epsilon(t),$$

$$H_a : D_{H,i}(t) = \sum_{s=-\infty}^{\infty} \ell_s^{(H,i,j)} D_{H,j}(t-s) + \sum_{r=-\infty}^{\infty} b_r^{(H,i,j)} \widetilde{D}_{H,j,u}(t-r) + \epsilon(t),$$

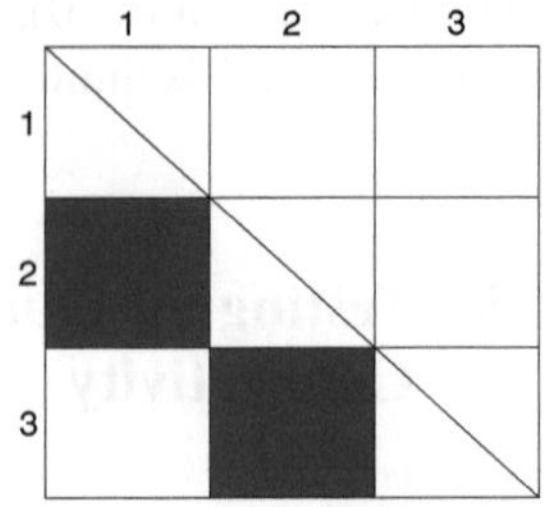

Fig. 6.3 Colored blocks obtained by the test result of the healthy control group

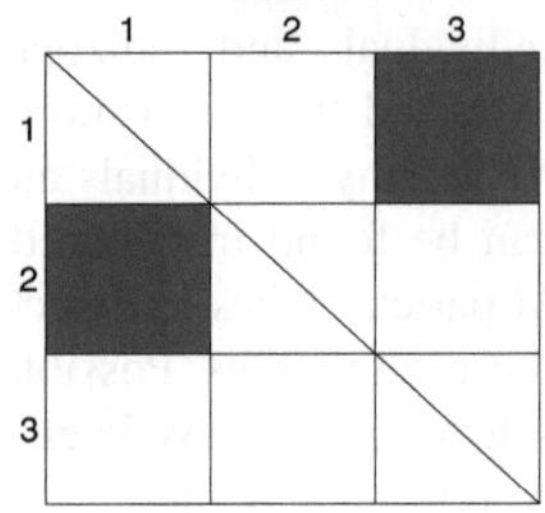

Fig. 6.4 Colored blocks obtained by the test result of the patient group

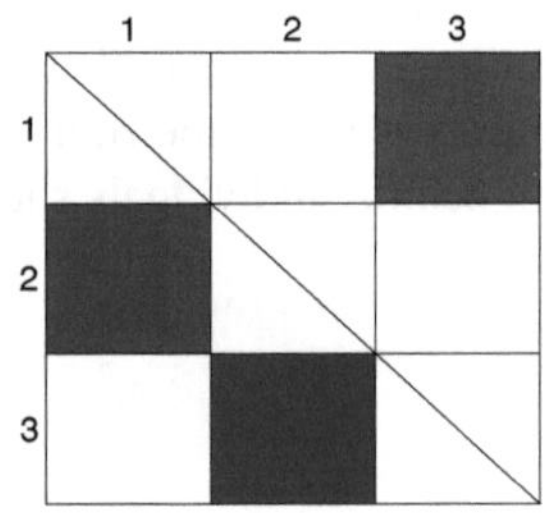

Fig. 6.5 Colored blocks obtained by adding up the result of Figs. 6.3 and 6.4

where $\{\widetilde{D}_{H,j,u}(t)\}$ is the lag process of $\{D_{H,j}(t)\}$ such that

$$\widetilde{D}_{H,j,u}(t) = D_{H,j}(t)D_{H,j}(t+u) - R_{D_{H,j}D_{H,j}}(u).$$

One may refer to (6.8) when testing for a single u and (6.10) when testing for multiple u's. Similarly, the tests are also applied to $\{D_{P,i}(t)\}$ and $\{D_{P,j}(t)\}$. Then we can use the colored blocks to show the testing result. The colored blocks represent the rejection of corresponding tests in which the row represents the output and the column represents the input. An illustrative example is given by Figs. 6.3, 6.4, and 6.5. Suppose that three time series TS_1, TS_2, and TS_3 are of interest. The two blue blocks in Fig. 6.3 indicate that TS_2 is a quadratic system of TS_1, and TS_3 is a quadratic system of TS_2 in the healthy control group. The two red blocks in Fig. 6.4 indicate that TS_2 is a quadratic system of TS_1, and TS_1 is a quadratic system of TS_3 in the patient group. Figure 6.5 is obtained by merging Figs. 6.3 and 6.4 together so that the four colors indicate the following:

1. White: There is no quadratic association between two sequences in either healthy control group or patient group.

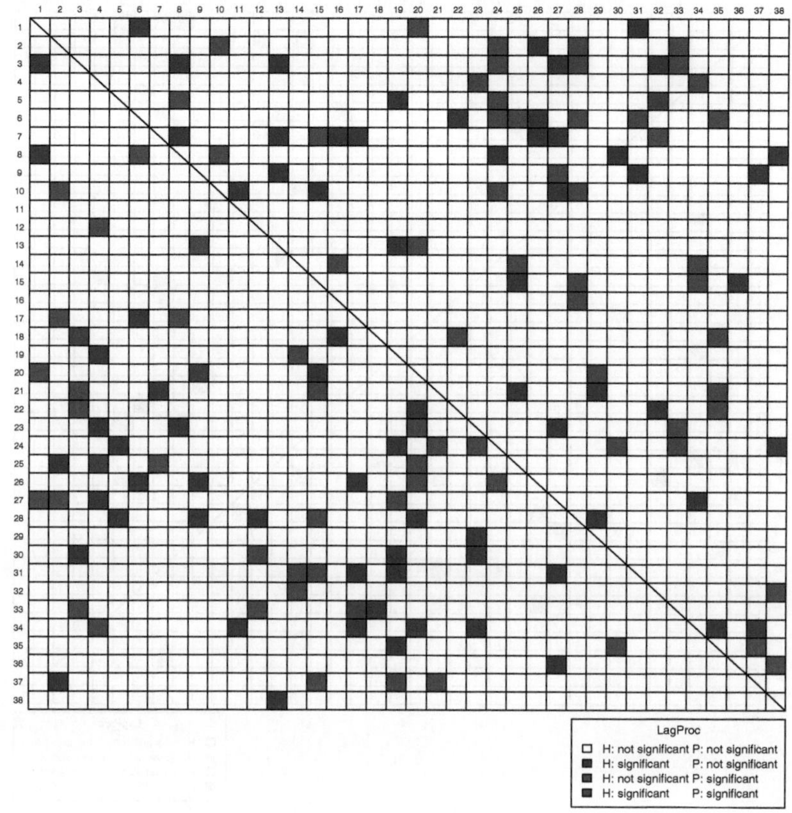

Fig. 6.6 Colored blocks based on testing for a single lag process with $u = 0$

2. Blue: The quadratic association only exists in healthy control group.
3. Red: The quadratic association only exists in patient group.
4. Purple: The quadratic association exists in both healthy control group and patient group.

Then we apply the test for (6.8) with $u = 0$ and the test for (6.10) with $\boldsymbol{u} = (0, 1, 2)^\top$ to the 38 subregions. The significance level is $\alpha = 0.05$. Figure 6.6 contains the colored blocks obtained based on the test for (6.8) with $u = 0$, while Fig. 6.7 contains that obtained based on the test (6.10) with $\boldsymbol{u} = (0, 1, 2)^\top$. The blue and red blocks depict the structural differences between healthy control group and patient group. For these pairs of subregions, the quadratic association is only detected in one of the two groups.

From Fig. 6.6, the pairs of subregions that have structural difference in linear association are marked by red and blue blocks, while the difference in quadratic association is shown by Fig. 6.7. This method serves as an exploratory tool to identify the differences of the associations of the subregions between healthy

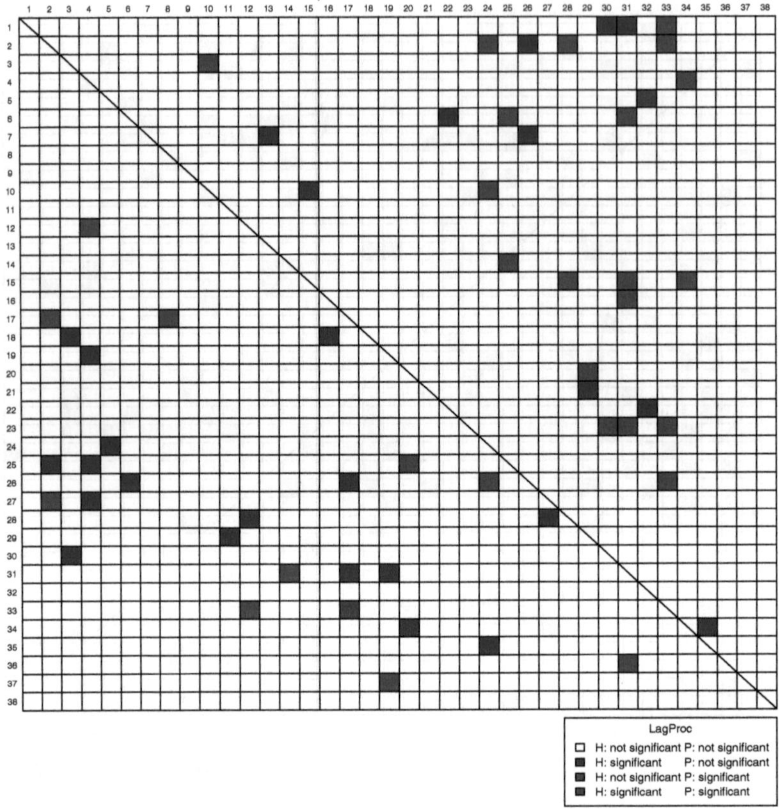

Fig. 6.7 Colored blocks based on testing for multiple lag processes with $\boldsymbol{u} = (0, 1, 2)^\top$

control group and patient group. The tests for linear and quadratic associations are demonstrated here. The quadratic association is tested based on lag processes. If the input time series have alternative forms, for example, higher order polynomials, the corresponding association can also be tested based on Goto et al. (2023). The restriction of this method is that the lag u needs to be predetermined so that we can only test for a set of lag processes. Also, further analysis is required to deal with multiplicity issue.

References

Bowyer, S. M. (2016). Coherence a measure of the brain networks: past and present. *Neuropsychiatric Electrophysiology, 2*, 1–12.

Cao, J., Zhao, Y., Shan, X., Wei, H.-l., Guo, Y., Chen, L., & Sarrigiannis, P. G. (2022). Brain functional and effective connectivity based on electroencephalography recordings: A review. *Human Brain Mapping, 43*(2), 860–879.

Chieffi, S., Ilardi, C. R., & Iavarone, A. (2018). Parietal lobe dysfunction in schizophrenia: A review. *Current Psychiatry Reviews, 14*(2), 71–83.

Culbreth, A. J., Wu, Q., Chen, S., Adhikari, B. M., Hong, L. E., Gold, J. M., & Waltz, J. A. (2021). Temporal-thalamic and cingulo-opercular connectivity in people with schizophrenia. *NeuroImage: Clinical, 29*, 102531.

Fan, L., Li, H., Zhuo, J., Zhang, Y., Wang, J., Chen, L., et al. (2016). The human Brainnetome Atlas: A new brain atlas based on connectional architecture. *Cerebral Cortex, 26* (8), 3508–3526.

Goto, Y., Zhang, X., Kedem, B., & Chen, S. (2023). Residual spectrum applied in brain functional connectivity. arXiv preprint arXiv:2305.19461.

Hannan, E. J. (1970). *Multiple time series*. John Wiley & Sons.

Horwitz, B. (2003). The elusive concept of brain connectivity. *Neuroimage, 19*(2), 466–470.

Jenkins, G. M., & Watts, D. G. (1968). *Spectral analysis and its applications*. Holden-Day.

Kedem, B. (2016). Coherence consideration in binary time series analysis. In1 *Handbook of discrete-valued time series* (p. 311).

Kedem-Kimelfeld, B. (1975). Estimating the lags of lag processes. *Journal of the American Statistical Association, 70*(351a), 603–605.

Khan, D., Katzoff, M., & Kedem, B. (2014). Coherence structure and its application in mortality forecasting. *Journal of Statistical Theory and Practice, 8*, 578–590.

Kimelfeld, B. (1974). Estimating the kernels of nonlinear orthogonal polynomial functionals. *The Annals of Statistics, 2*(2), 353–358.

Mohanty, R., Sethares, W. A., Nair, V. A., & Prabhakaran, V. (2020). Rethinking measures of functional connectivity via feature extraction. *Scientific Reports, 10*(1), 1298.

Wiener, N. (1958). *Nonlinear problems in random theory*. MIT Press.

Zhao, Y., Zhao, Y., Durongbhan, P., Chen, L., Liu, J., Billings, S., & Sarrigiannis, P. G. (2019). Imaging of nonlinear and dynamic functional brain connectivity based on EEG recordings with the application on the diagnosis of Alzheimer's disease. *IEEE Transactions on Medical Imaging, 39*(5), 1571–1581.

Chapter 7
Robust Principal Component Analysis for Retinal Image Enhancement

Habte Tadesse Likassa and Ding-Geng Chen

7.1 Introduction

Nowadays, the rapid advancement of multimedia technology and the development of methods for enhancing medical images have become crucial auxiliary tools in medical diagnosis. The enhancement of images has garnered significant attention in modern mathematical statistics, particularly in the field of biomedical image processing, laying the groundwork for medical diagnosis. Image enhancement has found applications in a variety of areas such as medical imaging (Kasten et al., 2013), batch image denoising (De Cheveigné & Simon, 2007), and computational imaging (Zhao et al., 2006). Its versatility in various image processing domains, including cataract detection (Fu et al., 2019) and image decomposition (Candès et al., 2011; Likassa & Fang, 2018), has fueled extensive research interest over the past few decades (Hu et al., 2018; Zhang & Lerman, 2014). While efforts to improve the quality of medical images for diagnostic purposes have been documented as in Candès et al. (2011), concerns persist regarding the robustness of these enhancement methods. However, this problem faces some severe challenges such as illumination variation, occlusion, outliers, and heavy sparse noise. Consequently, there is a pressing need to develop effective image enhancement techniques that not only improve image quality but also demonstrate resilience against perturbing effects.

H. T. Likassa (✉)
College of Health Solutions, Arizona State University, Phoenix, AZ, USA
e-mail: hlikassa@asu.edu

D.-G. Chen
College of Health Solutions, Arizona State University, Phoenix, AZ, USA

Department of Statistics, University of Pretoria, Pretoria, South Africa
e-mail: ding-geng.chen@asu.edu

D.-G. Chen, C. A. Coelho (eds.), *Biostatistics Modeling and Public Health Applications*, Emerging Topics in Statistics and Biostatistics,
https://doi.org/10.1007/978-3-031-69690-9_7

Principal component analysis (PCA), developed by Wall et al. (2003), is a technique that leverages sophisticated mathematical principles to transform a set of potentially correlated variables into a smaller set of variables known as principal components, commonly used for image classification purposes. However, its application in retinal image analysis is hindered by its susceptibility to nonlinear manifold embeddings, leading to incorrect results and heightened sensitivity to outliers and noise, as discussed in Vidal et al. (2005). To address these drawbacks, RPCA was developed by Candès et al. (2011) to enhance the performance of existing PCA developed by Wall et al. (2003). Since the inception of the pioneering RPCA by Candès et al. (2011), a myriad of attempts have been made to develop methods to tackle the impact of outliers and noises in high-dimensional medical image processing particularly for image enhancement (Peng et al., 2012). However, these methods often fail to perform well in the presence of significant errors within the data.

To improve the quality of retinal images, Fu et al. (2019) proposed a new robust method to reduce the influence of outliers in high-dimensional images; however, the computational load associated with the proposed method is substantial. To improve the performance, several algorithms were developed in retinal image processing. For instance, Singh et al. (2019) introduced histogram equalization techniques (HETs) for enhancing high-dimensional retinal images, Shen et al. (2020) developed a new method for enhancing the quality of retinal images in spatial domain filtering, Rosas-Romero et al. (2015) proposed a method using grayscale transformations, and Jiang et al. (2023) proposed an event-based low-illumination image enhancement. Nonetheless, these methods have limitations in generalization and occasionally produce nonexistent artifacts, which can adversely affect the accuracy of medical diagnostics. Alimanov and Islam (2023) suggested a machine learning method, from which the performance is becoming in enhancing retinal images; however, its computational complexity is expensive. To address these drawbacks, Zhu et al. (2023) proposed a simple but effective end-to-end framework for enhancing poor-quality retinal fundus images. However, it is not scalable and robust when the number of tensors and blood vessels in retinal images becomes large. Singh et al. (2022) introduced a Low-Light Image Enhancement via Deep Neural Networks (2LIM + DNN) to improve image quality. Additionally, a novel hybrid method (NHM) developed by Xian et al. (2023) is not robust when there are variations in lighting and retinal image content.

Several approaches have also been proposed to decompose and represent retinal images (Candès et al., 2011; Likassa et al., 2019; Santosh & Barpanda, 2022; Gao et al., 2021), yet these methods still struggle with achieving high-quality enhancement. Tensor RPCA by Cao et al. (2016) applied for video surveillance separation, Li et al. (2017) suggested a method for batch image denoising, while Solomon et al. (2019) proposed an extended RPCA approach for the purpose of computational image processing. Moreover, Lu et al. (2016, 2019); Wen et al. (2017); Jain et al. (2017); Liang et al. (2022) considered the tensor RPCA for high-dimensional tensor image decomposition.

Addressing the challenges in high-dimensional medical image processing involves effectively handling occlusion, illumination variations, noise, errors, and heavy non-sparse or sparse noise. This requires employing convex optimization techniques to extract the intrinsic clean part of medical images from highly corrupted ones for accurate medical diagnosis. Developing robust methods resilient to various adverse effects is crucial for solving image recovery problems. The rapid advancements in statistical methods have drawn considerable attention from researchers worldwide, particularly in addressing these challenges in image recovery and retinal image enhancement. Consequently, AT, RPI, and $L_{2,1}$ norms have been introduced in the development of RPCA to tackle these issues effectively to obtain the intrinsic clean part of the medical images from highly corrupted one for further medical diagnosis. It is thus of importance to develop robust methods to solve image recovery problems, which are resilient to different annoying effects.

This chapter is organized as follows: Sect. 7.2 focuses on enhancing medical image quality through the integration of RPCA (Candès et al., 2011) with AT + RPI, addressing limitations in existing methods and emphasizing the need for detecting noise and outlier as demonstrated by Lerman and Maunu (2018). Section 7.3 introduces an alternative approach using the $L_{2,1}$ norm to overcome RPCA with AT + RPI limitations, presenting the development of RPCA with AT and $L_{2,1}$ norms. Section 7.4 discusses the development of Tensor RPCA with AT + $L_{2,1}$ norms for multi-array image decomposition. Section 7.5 explores the application of these methods in retinal medical image analysis, supported by experimental results validating their effectiveness. Finally, Sect. 7.26 concludes the chapter with discussions and concluding remarks.

The contribution of this work to emerging topics in statistics and mathematics is summarized as follows: First, we integrate affine transformations with the low-rank plus sparse convex optimization problem, where the low-rank component is distributed across a union of subspaces rather than a single subspace. The affine transformations effectively address distortion or misalignment in batches of corrupted retinal images, resulting in more accurate image decomposition and boosted robustness against heavy sparse errors and outliers. To better enhance the quality of retinal images, second, we propose RPCA with $L_{2,1}$ norms to accurately estimate the parameters involved in the convex optimization problem by reducing the influence of handling large errors and outliers in images that can impact recovery accuracy. This norm, in conjunction with affine transformations, further enhances performance. Third, a tensor RPCA model is proposed to mitigate the influence of noise and outliers in multi-array retinal images by combining AT with $L_{2,1}$ norms. Fourth, the ADMM method is utilized to solve the new convex optimization problem, and a new set of updating equations is derived to iteratively update optimization variables, and the proposed methods outperform existing state-of-the-art techniques in retinal image analysis.

7.2 Robust PCA with AT + RPI

One of the major drawbacks of the existing methods, such as Candès et al. (2011), Zhang and Yang (2011), Lerman and Maunu (2018), Zhao et al. (2019), Liang et al. (2021), Rahmani and Atia (2015), Likassa (2020), Likassa et al. (2018), Zhang and Lerman (2014), is their inefficiency in adequately eliminating outliers and noise during image enhancement. To overcome this limitation, the subsequent section introduces a pioneering approach for enhancing images.

7.2.1 *The AT + RPI Method*

In this subsection, we introduce the concept of AT on the development of RPCA with AT. Given a set of unaligned retinal images $\boldsymbol{I_1, I_2, ..., I_n}$ of the same object, we assume that they can be transformed to similar images which are not only well aligned by a set of domain transformations $\boldsymbol{\tau_1, \tau_2, ..., \tau_n}$ but also detect the outliers in the images. Stacking the transformed images as vectors, we can construct the matrix: $\boldsymbol{Mo_\tau = [vec(I_1^0) \mid ... \mid vec(I_n^0)] \in \Re^{m\times n}}$, where $\boldsymbol{I_i^n = I_i o \tau_i}$ for $i = 1, ..., n$ is a well-aligned version of image i and operator o denotes the transformations applied to produce it. After linearizing $\boldsymbol{M_{o\tau}}$ by using the first-order Taylor expansion, we can get $\boldsymbol{M_{o\tau} + \sum_{i=1}^{n} J_i \Delta\tau u_i u_i^T \in \Re^{m\times n}}$ that satisfies $\boldsymbol{M_{o\tau} + \sum_{i=1}^{n} J_i \Delta\tau u_i u_i^T = A + E}$, where $\boldsymbol{E}$ is the sparse matrix error and $\boldsymbol{A}$ is a low-rank matrix with rank r and singular value decomposition $\boldsymbol{A = U\Sigma V^T}$.

To further improve the robustness of the proposed method, we introduce the concept of rank prior information here. Let us know $\boldsymbol{m \times r_Q}$ basis matrix $\boldsymbol{Q}$ so that $\boldsymbol{A_{new}}$ has rank smaller than $\boldsymbol{r}$. Our research work is to recover $\boldsymbol{A}$ and $\boldsymbol{E}$ from $\boldsymbol{A_{o\tau} + \sum_{i=1}^{n} J_i \Delta\tau u_i u_i^T}$ using the given prior information $\boldsymbol{Q}$ (He et al., 2014; Wei et al., 2017; Wu et al., 20001; Li et al., 2015). Moreover, let $\boldsymbol{V_{new}}$ be the right singular vectors of the reduced singular value decomposition's of $\boldsymbol{A_{new} = U_{new}\Sigma_{new}V_{new}^T}$. Furthermore, let $\boldsymbol{\gamma}$ denote the linear space of matrices with column span equal to that of the columns of $\boldsymbol{Q}$ which can be written as $\boldsymbol{\gamma := \left\{ Q \times X^T, X \in \Re^{n\times r_Q} \right\}}$, and by orthogonal compliment finally we can get

$$\boldsymbol{M_{o\tau} + \sum_{i=1}^{n} J_i \Delta\tau * u_i u_i^T = A_{new} + Q \times X^T + E} \tag{7.1}$$

Each transformation $\boldsymbol{\tau_i}$ can be represented by a vector of $\boldsymbol{p}$ parameters, yielding $\boldsymbol{\tau = [\tau_1 \mid ... \mid \tau_n] \in \Re^{p\times n}}$. Specifically, if the initial transformations $\boldsymbol{\tau}$ are known, we can change $\boldsymbol{M_{o\tau} + \sum_{i=1}^{n} J_i \Delta\tau u_i u_i^T = A_{new} + Q \times X^T + E}$, where the mathematical expression $\boldsymbol{J_i = \frac{\partial}{\partial \tau_i} vec(I_i o \tau_i) \in \Re^{m*p}}$ denotes the Jacobian transformation of the $\boldsymbol{i}$th image with regard to the transformations $\boldsymbol{\tau_i}$, and $\boldsymbol{u_i}$ denotes the standard basis for $\Re^n$. Based on the prior knowledge about partial column low rank, we propose a new method relaxing problem of convexity and inspired by Bertsekas (2015), Dhara and Dutta (2011) which is given by

$$\min_{A_{new}, E, Q, X, \Delta\tau} \|A_{new}\|_* + \lambda \|E\|_1 \text{ s.t} : M_{o\tau} + \sum_{i=1}^{n} J_i \Delta\tau u_i u_i^T = A_{new}$$

$$+Q \times X^T + E \tag{7.2}$$

7.2.2 Parameter Estimation

The above proposed method includes A_{new}, E, Q, X, and $\Delta\tau$ which can be estimated and updated. To do this, first let us denote the constraint term in convex optimization problem (7.2) $M_{o_\tau} + \sum_{i=1}^{n} J_i \Delta\tau u_i u_i^T - A_{new} - Q \times X^T - E$ by $h(A_{new}, E, X, \Delta\tau)$. We need to show how augmented Lagrangian multiplier in Peng et al. (2012), Chen et al. (2016), Lin et al. (2010) can be applied to efficiently solve our newly proposed algorithm in (7.2). As in Boyd and Vandenberghe (2004), the Lagrangian multiplier of our proposed method is given by

$$\mathcal{L}(A_{new}, E, Z, X, \Delta\tau) = \underset{A_{new}, E, X, \Delta\tau}{\operatorname{argmin}} \mathcal{L} \|A_{new}\|_* + \lambda \|E\|_1$$

$$+ \langle Z, h(A_{new}, E, X, \Delta\tau)\rangle + \frac{\tau}{2} \|h(A_{new}, E, X, \Delta\tau)\|_F^2 , \tag{7.3}$$

where Z is a Lagrangian multiplier matrix, τ is a positive penalty parameter, $\langle ., .\rangle$ denotes the matrix inner product, and $\|.\|_F$ denotes the Frobenius norm. It is difficult to solve the above Lagrangian function directly. So, we choose to minimize the augmented Lagrangian function approximately by adopting an alternating strategy. We iteratively minimize the optimization techniques using an augmented Lagrangian function as in Abidi et al. (2023) iteratively. First, when updating one parameter, we keep all the other parameters as a constant and solve for each parameter involved in the convex optimization problem.

$$A_{new}^{k+1} = \underset{A_{new}}{\operatorname{argmin}} \mathcal{L} \quad (A_{new}, E^k, X^k, \Delta\tau^k, Z^k) \tag{7.4}$$

$$E^{k+1} = \underset{E}{\operatorname{argmin}} \mathcal{L} \quad (E, A_{new}^k, X^k, \Delta\tau^k, Z^k) \tag{7.5}$$

$$X^{k+1} = \underset{X}{\operatorname{argmin}} \mathcal{L} \quad (A_{new}^{k+1}, E^{k+1}, X^k, \Delta\tau^k, Z^k)() \tag{7.6}$$

$$\Delta\tau = \underset{\Delta\tau}{\operatorname{argmin}} \mathcal{L} \quad (A_{new}^{k+1}, E^{k+1}, X^{k+1}, \Delta\tau, Z^k) \tag{7.7}$$

$$Z^{k+1} = Z^k + \tau_k h(A_{new}^{k+1}, E^{k+1}, \Delta\tau^{k+1}) \tag{7.8}$$

First, to update A_{new} in (7.4), all other variables, including E, are regarded as independent of A_{new}^{k+1}. Subsequently, the parameter corresponding to the updated A_{new}^{k+1} is determined by

$$\begin{aligned} A_{new}^{k+1} &= \underset{A_{new}}{\operatorname{argmin}} \mathcal{L} \, \|A_{new}\|_* + \langle Z, h(A_{new}, E, X, \Delta\tau)\rangle \\ &+ \frac{\tau}{2} \, \|h(A_{new}, E, X, \Delta\tau)\|_F^2 \end{aligned} \tag{7.9}$$

Again, using the concept of inner product and Frobenius norm relationship, the new updated parameter A_{new}^{k+1} can be expressed in the form of

$$\underset{A_{new}}{\operatorname{argmin}} \mathcal{L} \, \|A_{new}\|_* + \frac{1}{2\tau_k^{-1}} \left\| A_{new} - h(A_{new}, E, X, \Delta\tau) + \tau_k^{-1} \times Z_k \right\|_F^2 \tag{7.10}$$

Lastly, the solution of A_{new}^{k+1} using singular value threshold operator is given by

$$M_{\tau_k^{-1}}(h(A_{new}, E, \Delta\tau) + \tau_k^{-1} Z_k) = U_{new} E_{\frac{1}{\tau_k}}[\Sigma] V_{new}^T \tag{7.11}$$

where $E_{\frac{1}{\tau_k}}[\Sigma]$ denotes the soft-thresholding operator.

$$M_{\tau_k^{-1}}(M_{o_\tau} + \sum_{i=1}^{n} J_i \Delta\tau u_i u_i^T - Q * X^T - E + \tau_k^{-1} Z_k) = U_{new} E_{\frac{1}{\tau_k}}[\Sigma] V_{new}^T \tag{7.12}$$

Finally, we can get

$$A_{new}^{k+1} = U_{new} E_{\frac{1}{\tau_k}}[\Sigma] V_{new}^T \tag{7.13}$$

Moreover, from (7.5) we can update E^{k+1} and the augmented Lagrangian function can be expressed as

$$\begin{aligned} E^{k+1} &= \underset{E}{\operatorname{argmin}} \mathcal{L} \, \|A_{new}\|_* + \lambda \, \|E\|_1 + \langle Z, h(L_{new}, E, X, \Delta\tau)\rangle \\ &+ \frac{\tau}{2} \, \|h(A_{new}, E, X, \Delta\tau)\|_F^2 \end{aligned} \tag{7.14}$$

Using the relationship between inner product and Frobenius norm,

$$E^{k+1} = \underset{E}{\operatorname{argmin}} \mathcal{L}\lambda \, \|E\|_1 + \frac{1}{2\tau_k^{-1}} \left\| E - h(A_{new}, E, X, \Delta\tau) + \tau_k^{-1} Z_k \right\|_F^2 \tag{7.15}$$

By employing the idea of matrix value threshold on E^{k+1}, we can get

$$\boldsymbol{E}_{\frac{\lambda}{\tau_k}}[\boldsymbol{h}(\boldsymbol{A}_{new}, \boldsymbol{E}, \boldsymbol{X}, \boldsymbol{\Delta\tau}) + \boldsymbol{\tau}_k^{-1}\boldsymbol{Z}_k] \tag{7.16}$$

and lastly it is converged to

$$\boldsymbol{E}_{\frac{\lambda}{\tau_k}}[\boldsymbol{M}_{o_\tau} + \sum_{i=1}^{n} \boldsymbol{J}_i \boldsymbol{\Delta\tau} \boldsymbol{u}_i \boldsymbol{u}_i^T - \boldsymbol{A}_{new} - \boldsymbol{Q} * \boldsymbol{X}^T + \boldsymbol{\tau}_k^{-1}\boldsymbol{Z}_k] \tag{7.17}$$

Consider (7.6) to update $\boldsymbol{X}^{k+1}$, and the augmented Lagrangian function is given by

$$\begin{aligned} \boldsymbol{X}^{k+1} &= \underset{\boldsymbol{X}}{\operatorname{argmin}} \mathcal{L} \left\| \boldsymbol{A}_{new} \right\|_* + \lambda \left\| \boldsymbol{E} \right\|_1 + \langle \boldsymbol{Z}, h(\boldsymbol{A}_{new}, \boldsymbol{E}, \boldsymbol{X}, \boldsymbol{\Delta\tau}) \rangle \\ &+ \frac{\tau}{2} \left\| h(\boldsymbol{A}_{new}, \boldsymbol{E}, \boldsymbol{X}, \boldsymbol{\Delta\tau}) \right\|_F^2 \end{aligned} \tag{7.18}$$

Since $\boldsymbol{X}^{k+1}$ is independent of $\boldsymbol{A}_{new}$ and $\boldsymbol{E}$, we ignore them again applying the soft-threshold operator, and finally it is converged to

$$\boldsymbol{X}^{k+1} = \boldsymbol{Q}^*[\boldsymbol{M}_{o\tau} + \sum_{i=1}^{n} \boldsymbol{J}_i \boldsymbol{\Delta\tau}_k \boldsymbol{u}_i \boldsymbol{u}_i^T - \boldsymbol{E}^{k+1} + \boldsymbol{\tau}_k^{-1}\boldsymbol{Z}_k] \tag{7.19}$$

Consider (7.7) to update the parameter $\boldsymbol{\Delta\tau}$, and each step involves solving a convex program which has a closest optimal solution, and the corresponding augmented Lagrangian function of $\boldsymbol{\Delta\tau}^{k+1}$ is given as

$$\begin{aligned} \boldsymbol{\Delta\tau}^{k+1} &= \underset{\boldsymbol{\Delta\tau}}{\operatorname{argmin}} \mathcal{L} \left\| \boldsymbol{A}_{new} \right\|_* + \lambda \left\| \boldsymbol{E} \right\|_1 + \langle \boldsymbol{Z}, h(\boldsymbol{A}_{new}, \boldsymbol{E}, \boldsymbol{X}, \boldsymbol{\Delta\tau}) \rangle \\ &+ \frac{\tau}{2} \left\| h(\boldsymbol{A}_{new}, \boldsymbol{E}, \boldsymbol{X}, \boldsymbol{\Delta\tau}) \right\|_F^2 \end{aligned} \tag{7.20}$$

Ignoring $\boldsymbol{A}_{new}$ and $\boldsymbol{E}$ and applying threshold operator, finally

$$\boldsymbol{\Delta\tau}^{k+1} = \sum_{i=1}^{n} \boldsymbol{J}_i^+ * [(\boldsymbol{A}_{new}^{k+1} + \boldsymbol{Q} * \boldsymbol{X}^T + \boldsymbol{E}^{k+1} - \boldsymbol{M}o_\tau - \frac{\boldsymbol{1}}{\boldsymbol{\tau}_k}\boldsymbol{Z}_k)]\boldsymbol{u}_i \boldsymbol{u}_i^T \tag{7.21}$$

Using an augmented Lagrangian function given by

$$\begin{aligned} \mathcal{L}(\boldsymbol{A}_{new}, \boldsymbol{E}, \boldsymbol{Z}, \boldsymbol{X}, \boldsymbol{\Delta\tau}) &= \underset{\boldsymbol{A}_{new}}{\operatorname{argmin}} \mathcal{L} \left\| \boldsymbol{A}_{new} \right\|_* + \lambda \left\| \boldsymbol{E} \right\|_1 \\ + \langle \boldsymbol{Z}, h(\boldsymbol{A}_{new}, \boldsymbol{E}, \boldsymbol{X}, \boldsymbol{\Delta\tau}) \rangle &+ \frac{\tau}{2} \left\| h(\boldsymbol{L}_{new}, \boldsymbol{E}, \boldsymbol{X}, \boldsymbol{\Delta\tau}) \right\|_F^2 \end{aligned} \tag{7.22}$$

and from this equation, we can get

$$Z^{k+1} = Z^k + \tau_k h(A_{new}^{k+1}, E^{k+1}, \Delta\tau^{k+1}) \tag{7.23}$$

Lastly (7.23) is converged to the following expression:

$$Z^{k+1} = Z^k + \tau_k[M_{O\tau} + \sum_{i=1}^{n} J_i \Delta\tau_k u_i u_i^T - A_{new}^{k+1} - Q * X^T - E^{k+1}] \tag{7.24}$$

where $svd(.)$ denotes a singular value decomposition operator and J_i^+ denotes Moore-Penrose pseudoinverse of J_i (Prasad & Bapat, 1992). Moreover, the soft-threshold operator for scalars is given by

$$E_{\frac{\lambda}{\tau_k}}(x) = sign(x).max(|x| - \frac{\lambda}{\tau_k}, 0) \tag{7.25}$$

The effectiveness of RPCA with AT + RPI is validated through retinal image enhancement, as illustrated in Fig. 7.2, and confirmed via numerical simulations provided in Table 7.2. However, one major drawback of RPCA with AT + RPI is that the low-rank component lies in a single subspace and lacks the ability to detect outliers when gross outliers and errors occur due to the L_1 norm. To address these drawbacks, we additionally consider using the $L_{2,1}$ norm across multiple subspaces.

To make the proposed method easy to understand, the pseudo-code is summarized in Algorithm 7.1.

Algorithm 7.1: Robust PCA with AT + RPI

Input:
Data Matrix: $M \in \Re^{m\times n}$, $A^0 \in \Re^{m\times n}$, $X^0 \in \Re^{n\times r_Q}$, $E^0 \in \Re^{m\times n}$, $\Delta\tau^0 \in \Re^{p\times n}$, λ, ρ
While not converged **Do**
Update: $A_{new}^{(k+1)}$ by (13)
Update: $E^{(k+1)}$ by (17)
Update: $X^{(k+1)}$ by (19)
Update: $\Delta\tau^{(k+1)}$ by (21)
Update: $Z^{(k+1)}$ by (24)
End while
Outputs: $A, X, E, \Delta\tau, Z_1$

7.3 Robust PCA with AT + $L_{2,1}$ Norm

The drawback of RPCA with AT + RPI is its reliance on a single subspace for the low-rank component, which hampers its ability to detect outliers in the presence of gross errors, typically resulting from the L_1 norm. To address this issue, Sect. 7.3.1

introduces the $L_{2,1}$ norms into the problem formulation, aiming to mitigate this drawback.

7.3.1 The AT + $L_{2,1}$ Norm Method

Consider n images, $\{\boldsymbol{I}_i^0\} \in \Re^{w\times h}$, $i = 1, \cdots, n$, where w and h denote the weight and height of the images, respectively. All of these images contain the same objects and are highly correlated with one another. In many scenarios, these images are corrupted by occlusions and outliers. We can stack these images into a matrix: $\boldsymbol{M} = [vec(\mathbf{I}_1^0) \mid vec(\mathbf{I}_2^0) \mid \ldots \mid vec(\mathbf{I}_n^0)] \in \Re^{m\times n}$, where $vec(\cdot)$ denotes the vector stacking operator. We can decompose $\boldsymbol{M}$ into a summation of a low-rank component and a sparse error matrix (Lin et al., 2010): $\boldsymbol{M} = \boldsymbol{AC} + \boldsymbol{E}$, where we assumed that the subspaces may not be independent from each other or the data are contaminated by large noise, so the low-rank component lies in a union of subspaces, in which $\boldsymbol{A} \in \Re^{m\times n}$ is a clean low-rank dictionary, $\boldsymbol{C} \in \Re^{n\times n}$ is a coefficient matrix as the low-rank representation by $\boldsymbol{A}$, and $\boldsymbol{E} \in \Re^{m\times n}$ denotes a sparse error matrix incurred by outliers or corruptions. In practice, $\boldsymbol{I}_i^0$ are generally not well aligned, entailing the above low-rank plus sparse decomposition to be imprecise. To take account of this, inspired by Peng et al. (2012), Likassa et al. (2022), Likassa et al. (2018), Likassa and Fang (2018), Likassa et al. (2019), we apply affine transformations $\boldsymbol{\tau}_i$ to the potentially misaligned input images $\boldsymbol{I}_i^0$ to get a collection of transformed images $\boldsymbol{I}_i = \boldsymbol{I}_i^0 o \boldsymbol{\tau}_i$, where the operator o indicates the transformation. We can then stack these aligned images into a matrix and obtain $\boldsymbol{M}_{o\boldsymbol{\tau}} = [vec(\mathbf{I}_1) \mid vec(\mathbf{I}_2) \mid \ldots \mid vec(\mathbf{I}_n)] \in \Re^{m\times n}$. The aligned images can be treated as samples taken from a union of low-dimensional subspaces (Vaswani et al., 2018), which, if well aligned, should exhibit a low-rank subspace structure as the rank of the transformed images is as small as possible, up to some outliers and heavy sparse errors. Solving for the variables corresponding to the constraints $\boldsymbol{M}_{o\boldsymbol{\tau}} = \boldsymbol{AC} + \boldsymbol{E}$ is intractable due to its nonlinearity. To resolve this dilemma, we assume that the change produced by these affine transformations $\boldsymbol{\tau}_i$ is small, and an initial of $\boldsymbol{\tau}_i$ is known. We can then linearize $\boldsymbol{M}_{o\boldsymbol{\tau}}$ by using the first-order Taylor approximation as $\boldsymbol{M}_{o(\boldsymbol{\tau}+\boldsymbol{\Delta\tau})} \approx \boldsymbol{M}_{o\boldsymbol{\tau}} + \sum_{i=1}^{n} \boldsymbol{J}_i \boldsymbol{\Delta\tau} \boldsymbol{v}_i \boldsymbol{v}_i^T$, where $\boldsymbol{M}_{o\boldsymbol{\tau}} \in \Re^{m\times n}$ is the transformed image, $\boldsymbol{\Delta\tau} \in \Re^{p\times n}$ with p being the number of variables, $\boldsymbol{J}_i = \frac{\partial vec(\boldsymbol{I}_i o \boldsymbol{\tau}_i)}{\partial \boldsymbol{\tau}_i} \in \Re^{m\times p}$ denotes the Jacobian of the ith image with respect to $\boldsymbol{\tau}_i$, and $\boldsymbol{v}_i$ is the standard basis for $\Re^n$. In this way, we obtain approximate transformations to recover the low-rank component from the underlying subspaces.

To make the new approach more resilient to outliers and heavy sparse noise, the $L_{2,1}$ norm, which combines the advantages of the L_1 and L_2 norms, is used here. The $L_{2,1}$ regularizer is considered as the rotational invariant of the L_1 norm and can effectively handle outliers (Ding et al., 2006). Also, as observed in Li et al. (2018), the $L_{2,1}$ regularizer can also achieve better sparsity promotion than the L_1 norm. The L_1 norm (Peng et al., 2012) may yield a biased estimation as it ignores the extreme values and cannot handle the collinearity of features. In contrast, the $L_{2,1}$

norm is more stable and has the ability to better preserve the spatial information than the L_1 regularizer, as demonstrated in Ding et al. (2006), Li et al. (2018). Additionally, the $L_{2,1}$ norm is superior to the nonconvex norms when the signals are not sparse or when the matrix is not strictly low rank (Wen et al., 2018). The overall problem can thus be posted as an optimization problem given by

$$\begin{aligned} &\min_{\boldsymbol{A},\boldsymbol{E},\boldsymbol{C},\boldsymbol{Q},\boldsymbol{\Delta\tau}} \|\boldsymbol{A}\|_* + \|\boldsymbol{C}\|_* + \lambda_1 \|\boldsymbol{Q}\|_{2,1} + \lambda_2 \|\boldsymbol{E}\|_{2,1} \\ &\text{s.t } \boldsymbol{M_{o\tau}} + \sum_{i=1}^{n} \boldsymbol{J}_i \boldsymbol{\Delta\tau} \boldsymbol{v}_i \boldsymbol{v}_i^T = \boldsymbol{AC} + \boldsymbol{E}, \boldsymbol{C} = \boldsymbol{Q}, \boldsymbol{Q} \succeq \boldsymbol{0} \end{aligned} \tag{7.26}$$

where $\|\boldsymbol{A}\|_* = \sum_{i=1}^{min(m,n)} \sigma_i(\boldsymbol{A})$ denotes the nuclear norm of $\boldsymbol{A}$ (Rublee & Cohen, 2018), in which $\sigma_i(\boldsymbol{A})$ indicates the singular values of $\boldsymbol{A}$, λ_1, and λ_2 are the regularization parameters, and $\|\boldsymbol{E}\|_{2,1} = \sum_{i=1}^{m}(\sum_{j=1}^{n} \boldsymbol{E}_{ji}^2)^{1/2}$ denotes the $L_{2,1}$ norm of $\boldsymbol{E}$ (Kong et al., 2011). The first nuclear norm term in (7.26) enforces the dictionary $\boldsymbol{A}$ to lie in low-dimensional subspaces. The second and the third terms constrain the representation to be low rank plus sparse. The fourth term regularizes the error $\boldsymbol{E}$ to be sparse.

7.3.2 *Parameter Estimation*

To solve the optimization problem in (7.26), we use the augmented Lagrangian multiplier technique and rewrite (7.26) as

$$\begin{aligned} \mathcal{L}(\boldsymbol{A}, \boldsymbol{C}, \boldsymbol{E}, \boldsymbol{Q}, \boldsymbol{\Delta\tau}) &= \|\boldsymbol{A}\|_* + \|\boldsymbol{C}\|_* + \lambda_1 \|\boldsymbol{Q}\|_{2,1} + \lambda_2 \|\boldsymbol{E}\|_{2,1} \\ &+ \langle \boldsymbol{Z}_1, \boldsymbol{B} - \boldsymbol{AC} - \boldsymbol{E} \rangle + \frac{\mu_1}{2} \|\boldsymbol{B} - \boldsymbol{AC} - \boldsymbol{E}\|_F^2 \\ &+ \langle \boldsymbol{Z}_2, \boldsymbol{C} - \boldsymbol{Q} \rangle + \frac{\mu_2}{2} \|\boldsymbol{C} - \boldsymbol{Q}\|_F^2 \end{aligned} \tag{7.27}$$

where $\boldsymbol{Z}_1 \in \Re^{m\times n}$ and $\boldsymbol{Z}_2 \in \Re^{n\times n}$ are the Lagrangian multipliers, μ_1 and μ_2 are the penalty parameters, $\langle \boldsymbol{X}, \boldsymbol{Y} \rangle = Trace(\boldsymbol{X}^T\boldsymbol{Y})$, $||\cdot||_F$ denotes the Frobenius norm, and $\boldsymbol{B} = \boldsymbol{M_{o\tau}} + \sum_{i=1}^{n} \boldsymbol{J}_i \boldsymbol{\Delta\tau} \boldsymbol{v}_i \boldsymbol{v}_i^T$. By using augmented Lagrange multiplier with adaptive penalty (Boyd & Vandenberghe, 2004), (7.27) can be rewritten as

$$\begin{aligned} \mathcal{L}(\boldsymbol{A}, \boldsymbol{C}, \boldsymbol{E}, \boldsymbol{Q}, \boldsymbol{\Delta\tau}) &= \|\boldsymbol{A}\|_* + \|\boldsymbol{C}\|_* + \lambda_2 \|\boldsymbol{E}\|_{2,1} \\ &+ \lambda_1 \|\boldsymbol{Q}\|_{2,1} + \frac{\mu_1}{2} \left\|\boldsymbol{B} - \boldsymbol{AC} - \boldsymbol{E} + \frac{\boldsymbol{Z}_1}{\mu_1}\right\|_F^2 + \frac{\mu_2}{2} \left\|\boldsymbol{C} - \boldsymbol{Q} + \frac{\boldsymbol{Z}_2}{\mu_2}\right\|_F^2 \end{aligned} \tag{7.28}$$

Solving (7.28) directly is computationally prohibitive; thereby we consider to iteratively update the variables alternatively via ADMM (Boyd & Vandenberghe, 2004), which decomposes the original problem into a set of subproblems. In each step, we update just one variable while keeping the other variables unchanged. So the above terms like $\|\boldsymbol{B} - \boldsymbol{AC} - \boldsymbol{E}\|_F$ are convex even if it involves the matrix factorization term $\boldsymbol{AC}$ (Zhang et al., 2017).

Firstly, to update $\boldsymbol{A}$, we fix $\boldsymbol{E}$, $\boldsymbol{Q}$, $\boldsymbol{C}$, and $\boldsymbol{\Delta\tau}$, so $\boldsymbol{A}^{(k+1)}$ can be determined by

$$\boldsymbol{A}^{(k+1)} = \underset{\boldsymbol{A}}{\operatorname{argmin}} \mathcal{L}\left\{\boldsymbol{A}, \boldsymbol{E}^{(k)}, \boldsymbol{C}^{(k)}, \boldsymbol{Q}^{(k)}, \boldsymbol{\Delta\tau}^{(k)}\right\} \tag{7.29}$$

where k is the iteration index. By ignoring all irrelevant terms of $\boldsymbol{A}$, Eq. (7.29) can be simplified as

$$\boldsymbol{A}^{(k+1)} = \underset{\boldsymbol{A}}{\operatorname{argmin}} \mathcal{L}\left\{ \|\boldsymbol{A}\|_* + \frac{\mu_1^{(k)}}{2}\left\|\boldsymbol{B}^{(k)} - \boldsymbol{AC}^{(k)} - \boldsymbol{E}^{(k)} + \frac{\boldsymbol{Z}_1^{(k)}}{\mu_1^{(k)}}\right\|_F^2\right\} \tag{7.30}$$

We can then use the linear augmented direction method with the soft shrinkage operator as in Cai et al. (2010) and update $\boldsymbol{A}^{(k+1)}$ by

$$\boldsymbol{A}^{(k+1)} = \Omega_{\frac{1}{\kappa_{\boldsymbol{A}}^{(k)}}}\left\{\boldsymbol{A}^{(k)} - \frac{\boldsymbol{P}_{\boldsymbol{A}}^{(k)}}{\kappa_{\boldsymbol{A}}^{(k)}}\right\} \tag{7.31}$$

where Ω is the singular value threshold, $\boldsymbol{P}_{\boldsymbol{A}}^{(k)} = (\mu_1^{(k)})(\boldsymbol{A}^{(k)})^T\boldsymbol{C}^{(k)} - \mu_1^{(k)}(\boldsymbol{B}^{(k)} - \boldsymbol{E}^{(k)}) - (\boldsymbol{Z}_1^{(k)} + \boldsymbol{Z}_2^{(k)})(\boldsymbol{C}^{(k)})^T$, $\kappa_{\boldsymbol{A}}^{(k)} = (\mu_1^{(k)})\frac{\tau_{\boldsymbol{A}}}{2}$, $\tau_{\boldsymbol{A}} > \sigma(\boldsymbol{C}^T\boldsymbol{C})$ is the proximal parameter, in which $\sigma(\boldsymbol{C}^T\boldsymbol{C})$ denotes the spectral radius of $\boldsymbol{C}^T\boldsymbol{C}$.

Secondly, to update $\boldsymbol{E}$, we keep $\boldsymbol{A}$, $\boldsymbol{Q}$, $\boldsymbol{C}$, and $\boldsymbol{\Delta\tau}$ as constants, so $\boldsymbol{E}^{(k+1)}$ can be determined by

$$\boldsymbol{E}^{(k+1)} = \underset{\boldsymbol{E}}{\operatorname{argmin}} \mathcal{L}\left\{\boldsymbol{A}^{(k+1)}, \boldsymbol{E}, \boldsymbol{C}^{(k)}, \boldsymbol{Q}^{(k)}, \boldsymbol{\Delta\tau}^{(k)}\right\} \tag{7.32}$$

Again, by ignoring all irrelevant terms of $\boldsymbol{E}$, Eq. (7.32) can be simplified as

$$\boldsymbol{E}^{(k+1)} = \underset{\boldsymbol{E}}{\operatorname{argmin}}\left\{\lambda_2\|\boldsymbol{E}\|_{2,1} + \frac{\mu_1^{(k)}}{2}\left\|\boldsymbol{B}^{(k)} - \boldsymbol{A}^{(k)}\boldsymbol{C}^{(k)} - \boldsymbol{E} + \frac{\boldsymbol{Z}_1^{(k)}}{\mu_1^{(k)}}\right\|_F^2\right\} \tag{7.33}$$

Considering lemma by Yang et al. (2009), the update of the ith column of $\boldsymbol{E}^{(k+1)}$, $\boldsymbol{E}_i^{(k+1)}$, is given by

$$\boldsymbol{E}_i^{(k+1)} = \begin{cases} \dfrac{\left\|\boldsymbol{V}_i^{(k)}\right\|_2 - \frac{\lambda_2}{\mu_1^{(k)}}}{\left\|\boldsymbol{V}_i^{(k)}\right\|_2}\boldsymbol{V}_i^{(k)}, & \text{if } \left\|\boldsymbol{V}_i^{(k)}\right\|_2 \geq \frac{\lambda_2}{\mu_1^{(k)}} \\ 0, & \text{otherwise} \end{cases} \tag{7.34}$$

where $\|.\|_2$ denotes the Euclidean norm as in Celebi et al. (2011) and $V^{(k)} = (\boldsymbol{B}^{(k)} - \boldsymbol{A}^{(k)}\boldsymbol{C}^{(k)} + \frac{\boldsymbol{Z}_1^{(k)}}{\mu_1^{(k)}})$.

Thirdly, to find an update of $\boldsymbol{C}$, we keep $\boldsymbol{A}$, $\boldsymbol{E}$, $\boldsymbol{Q}$, and $\boldsymbol{\Delta\tau}$ as constants, and thus $\boldsymbol{C}^{(k+1)}$ can be determined by

$$\boldsymbol{C}^{(k+1)} = \underset{\boldsymbol{C}}{\operatorname{argmin}} \mathcal{L}\left\{\boldsymbol{A}^{(k+1)}, \boldsymbol{E}^{(k+1)}, \boldsymbol{C}, \boldsymbol{Q}^{(k)}, \boldsymbol{\Delta\tau}^{(k)}\right\} \tag{7.35}$$

By ignoring all irrelevant terms of $\boldsymbol{C}$, Eq. (7.35) can be simplified as

$$\boldsymbol{C}^{(k+1)} = \underset{\boldsymbol{C}}{\operatorname{argmin}} \mathcal{L}\left\{ \|\boldsymbol{C}\|_* + \frac{\mu_1^{(k)}}{2}\left\|\boldsymbol{B}^{(k)} - \boldsymbol{A}^{(k)}\boldsymbol{C} - \boldsymbol{E}^{(k)} + \frac{\boldsymbol{Z}_1^{(k)}}{\mu_1^{(k)}}\right\|_F^2 \right.$$
$$\left. + \frac{\mu_2}{2}\left\|\boldsymbol{C} - \boldsymbol{Q}^{(k)} + \frac{\boldsymbol{Z}_2^{(k)}}{\mu_2^{(k)}}\right\|_F^2 \right\} \tag{7.36}$$

To solve this subproblem, we can employ a linearized augmented Lagrangian multiplier with the singular value threshold (Cai et al., 2010). Thereby, $\boldsymbol{C}^{(k+1)}$ can be updated by

$$\boldsymbol{C}^{(k+1)} = \Omega_{\frac{1}{\kappa_{\boldsymbol{C}}^{(k)}}}\left\{\boldsymbol{C}^{(k)} - \frac{P_{\boldsymbol{C}}^{(k)}}{\kappa_{\boldsymbol{C}}^{(k)}}\right\} \tag{7.37}$$

where $\kappa_{\boldsymbol{C}}^{(k)} = (\mu_1^{(k)} + \mu_2^{(k)})\frac{\tau_C}{2}$, $\tau_C > \sigma(\boldsymbol{A}\boldsymbol{A}^T)$, and $P_{\boldsymbol{C}}^{(k)} = \boldsymbol{A}^{(k)}(\mu_1^{(k)} + \mu_2^{(k)})\boldsymbol{A}^{(k)} - \mu_1^{(k)}(\boldsymbol{B}^{(k)} - \boldsymbol{E}^{(k)}) - \boldsymbol{Z}_1^{(k)} + \mu_2^{(k)}(\boldsymbol{C}^{(k)} - \boldsymbol{Q}^{(k)}) + \boldsymbol{Z}_2^{(k)}$.

Again, to update $\boldsymbol{Q}$, we keep $\boldsymbol{A}$, $\boldsymbol{E}$, $\boldsymbol{C}$, and $\boldsymbol{\Delta\tau}$ as constants, and $\boldsymbol{Q}^{(k+1)}$ can then be determined by

$$\boldsymbol{Q}^{(k+1)} = \underset{\boldsymbol{Q}}{\operatorname{argmin}} \mathcal{L}\left\{\boldsymbol{A}^{(k+1)}, \boldsymbol{E}^{(k+1)}, \boldsymbol{C}^{(k+1)}, \boldsymbol{Q}, \boldsymbol{\Delta\tau}^{(k)}\right\} \tag{7.38}$$

By ignoring all of the irrelevant terms, Eq. (7.38) can be simplified as

$$\boldsymbol{Q}^{(k+1)} = \underset{\boldsymbol{Q}}{\operatorname{argmin}} \mathcal{L}\left\{\begin{array}{l} \lambda_1 \|\boldsymbol{Q}\|_{2,1} \\ + \frac{\mu_2^{(k)}}{2}\left\|\boldsymbol{C}^{(k)} - \boldsymbol{Q} + \frac{\boldsymbol{Z}_2^{(k)}}{\mu_2^{(k)}}\right\|_F^2 \end{array}\right\} \tag{7.39}$$

Again, by using lemma in Yang et al. (2009), the update of the ith column of $\boldsymbol{Q}^{(k+1)}$, $\boldsymbol{Q}_i^{(k+1)}$, is given by

$$Q_i^{(k+1)} = \begin{cases} \frac{\left\|P_i^{(k)}\right\|_2 - \frac{\lambda_1}{\mu_2^{(k)}}}{\left\|P_i^{(k)}\right\|_2} P_i^{(k)}, & \text{if } \left\|P_i^{(k)}\right\|_2 \geq \frac{\lambda_1}{\mu_2^{(k)}} \\ 0, & \text{otherwise} \end{cases} \tag{7.40}$$

where $\boldsymbol{P}^{(k)} = (\boldsymbol{C}^{(k+1)} + \frac{\boldsymbol{Z}_2^{(k)}}{\mu_2^{(k)}})$. Lastly, to get an update of $\boldsymbol{\Delta\tau}$, we keep $\boldsymbol{A}$, $\boldsymbol{E}$, $\boldsymbol{C}$, and $\boldsymbol{Q}$ as constants, and $\boldsymbol{\Delta\tau}^{(k+1)}$ can be determined by

$$\boldsymbol{\Delta\tau}^{(k+1)} = \underset{\boldsymbol{\Delta\tau}}{\operatorname{argmin}} \mathcal{L}\left\{\boldsymbol{A}^{(k+1)}, \boldsymbol{E}^{(k+1)}, \boldsymbol{C}^{(k+1)}, \boldsymbol{\Delta\tau}, \boldsymbol{Q}^{(k+1)}\right\} \tag{7.41}$$

By ignoring all irrelevant terms of $\boldsymbol{\Delta\tau}$, we can obtain

$$\boldsymbol{\Delta\tau}^{(k+1)} = \underset{\boldsymbol{\Delta\tau}}{\operatorname{argmin}} \mathcal{L}\left\{\frac{\mu_1^{(k)}}{2}\left\|\boldsymbol{B}^{(k)} - \boldsymbol{A}^{(k+1)}\boldsymbol{C}^{(k+1)} - \boldsymbol{E}^{(k+1)} + \frac{\boldsymbol{Z}_1^{(k)}}{\mu_1^{(k)}}\right\|_F^2\right\} \tag{7.42}$$

Solving (7.42) with the threshold operators (Peng et al., 2012; Chen et al., 2016), we can get an update of $\boldsymbol{\Delta\tau}^{(k+1)}$ as

$$\boldsymbol{\Delta\tau}^{(k+1)} = \sum_{i=1}^{n} \boldsymbol{J}_i^{+}\left(\boldsymbol{A}^{(k+1)}\boldsymbol{C}^{(k+1)} + \boldsymbol{E}^{(k+1)} - \boldsymbol{M}_{\boldsymbol{o\tau}} - \frac{\boldsymbol{Z}_1^{(k)}}{\mu_1^{(k)}}\right)\boldsymbol{v}_i\boldsymbol{v}_i^T \tag{7.43}$$

where $\boldsymbol{J}_i^{+}$ denotes the Moores-Penroses pseudoinverse of $\boldsymbol{J}_i$ (Courrieu, 2008). Following the same steps as the above, the Lagrangian multipliers $\boldsymbol{Z}_1$ and $\boldsymbol{Z}_2$ are updated by

$$\boldsymbol{Z}_1^{(k+1)} = \boldsymbol{Z}_1^{(k)} + \mu_1^{(k+1)}\left\{\boldsymbol{B}^{(k)} - \boldsymbol{A}^{(k+1)}\boldsymbol{C}^{(k+1)} - \boldsymbol{E}^{(k+1)}\right\} \tag{7.44}$$

$$\text{and } \boldsymbol{Z}_2^{(k+1)} = \boldsymbol{Z}_2^{(k)} + \mu_2^{(k+1)}\left\{\boldsymbol{C}^{(k+1)} - \boldsymbol{Q}^{(k+1)}\right\} \tag{7.45}$$

Likewise, the regularization parameters μ_1 and μ_2 are updated, respectively, by

$$\mu_1^{(k+1)} = min\left\{\mu_{max}, \rho\mu_1^{(k)}\right\} \tag{7.46}$$

$$\text{and} \quad \mu_2^{(k+1)} = min\left\{\mu_{max}, \rho\mu_2^{(k)}\right\} \tag{7.47}$$

where ρ is a properly chosen constant and μ_{max} is a tunable parameter adjusting the convergence of the proposed method. The updating equations progress in a round-robin fashion until convergence is achieved. The efficacy of RPCA with AT + $L_{2,1}$ norm is validated through validation using retinal image enhancement, as depicted in Fig. 7.3 and summarized in Table 7.2.

7.3.3 Uniqueness of Parameter Estimation

This section considers the convergence characteristics of the updating equations addressed in the previous section. Two theorems are established to address this issue.

Theorem 7.3.1 *If $\left\{\mu_1^{(k)}\right\}$ is nondecreasing and upper bounded by $\tau_{\boldsymbol{A}} > \sigma(\boldsymbol{C}\boldsymbol{C}^T)$, then the sequences $\{\boldsymbol{A}^{(k)}\}$, $\{\boldsymbol{E}^{(k)}\}$, and $\left\{\mathbf{Z}_1^{(k)}\right\}$ by ADMM converge to a Karush-Kuhn-Tucker (KKT) point of (7.44) and (7.45).*

Theorem 7.3.2 *If $\left\{\mu_1^{(k)}\right\}$ and $\left\{\mu_2^{(k)}\right\}$ are nondecreasing and upper bounded by $\tau_C > \sigma(\boldsymbol{A}\boldsymbol{A}^T)$, then the sequences $\{\boldsymbol{C}^{(k)}\}$, $\{\boldsymbol{Q}^{(k)}\}$, $\{\boldsymbol{\Delta\tau}^{(k)}\}$, $\{\mathbf{Z}_1{}^{(k)}\}$, $\{\mathbf{Z}_2{}^{(k)}\}$ generated by ADMM converge to a KKT point of (7.46) and (7.47).*

The proofs of both theorems can be readily available in Likassa et al. (2019); Liang et al. (2022).

Theorem 7.3.1 implies that the variables $\boldsymbol{A}^{(k)}$ and $\boldsymbol{E}^{(k)}$ are guaranteed to converge to the global optimum with an appropriate choice of the Lagrange multipliers $\left\{\boldsymbol{Z}_1^{(k)}\right\}$ and $\left\{\boldsymbol{Z}_2^{(k)}\right\}$ and sufficiently large penalty parameters $\left\{\mu_1^{(k)}\right\}$. Meanwhile, Theorem 7.3.2 shows that the variables $\boldsymbol{C}^{(k)}$, $\boldsymbol{Q}^{(k)}$, and $\boldsymbol{\Delta\tau}^{(k)}$ are guaranteed to converge to the global optimum with an appropriate choice of the Lagrange multipliers $\left\{\boldsymbol{Z}_1^{(k)}\right\}$ and $\left\{\boldsymbol{Z}_2^{(k)}\right\}$ and sufficiently large penalty parameters $\left\{\mu_1^{(k)}\right\}$ and $\left\{\mu_2^{(k)}\right\}$. The proof of this entire theorem is provided in Likassa et al. (2019); Liang et al. (2022). To make the proposed method easy to understand, the pseudo-code is summarized in Algorithm 7.2.

Algorithm 7.2: Robust PCA with AT + $L_{2,1}$ norms

Input: Data Matrix $\boldsymbol{M} \in \Re^{m\times n}$, $\boldsymbol{A}^0 \in \Re^{m\times n}$, $\boldsymbol{C}^0 \in \Re^{n\times n}$, $\boldsymbol{E}^0 \in \Re^{m\times n}$, $\boldsymbol{\Delta\tau}^0 \in \Re^{p\times n}$,$\lambda$, ρ
While not converged **Do**
$\boldsymbol{A}^{(k+1)}$ updated by (31)
$\boldsymbol{E}^{(k+1)}$ updated by (34)
$\boldsymbol{C}^{(k+1)}$ updated by (37) $\boldsymbol{Q}^{(k+1)}$ updated by (40)
$\boldsymbol{\Delta\tau}^{(k+1)}$ updated by (43)
$\mathbf{Z}_1{}^{(k+1)}$ updated by (44)
$\mathbf{Z}_2{}^{(k+1)}$ updated by (45)
$\boldsymbol{\mu}_1{}^{(k+1)}$ updated by (46)
$\boldsymbol{\mu}_2{}^{(k+1)}$ updated by (47)
End while
Outputs:$\boldsymbol{A}, \boldsymbol{E}, \boldsymbol{C}, \boldsymbol{Q}, \boldsymbol{\Delta\tau}, z_1, z_2$

7.4 Tensor RPCA with AF + $L_{2,1}$ Norm

The RPCA with AT + $L_{2,1}$ norms fails to well perform by detecting the little disturbance of blood vessels for a long retinal fundus image serial. To address this issue, Sect. 7.4.2 introduces the $L_{2,1}$ norms into the problem formulation in multi-array data, aiming to mitigate this drawback. Tensor RPCA model is used to detect the serial change and variation which extends matrix decomposition like RPCA with AT + $L_{2,1}$ norms to a tensor-based retinal image decomposition and preserves the domain-specific prior knowledge of the retinal fundus images.

7.4.1 *The Tensor AF + $L_{2,1}$ Norm Method*

For the given retinal images, the matrix representation is shown as RPCA with AT $L_{2,1}$ norms is obtained by vectorizing each image, and the whole serial image becomes an image matrix. The tensor representation takes each retinal image as a matrix slice in a tensor volume. Hence, the whole retinal image is represented as a third-order tensor images written in the form of images: $\boldsymbol{I} = [I^1, I^2, \ldots I^d]$. Each slice $I^i \in \Re^{w \times h}$ in tensor I is the ith retinal images. The tensor volume I can be written in the form of data matrix $\boldsymbol{D}^{n_1 \times n_2 \times n_3}$ to which it can be further decomposed as the sum of the background volume or low-rank component represented by $\boldsymbol{Z}^{n_1 \times n_2 \times n_3}$ and the dynamic volume (He et al., 2016; Liang et al., 2022; Zhang et al., 2021; Yaman et al., 2019), denoted by $\boldsymbol{S}^{n_1 \times n_2 \times n_3}$, denoted by $\boldsymbol{D} = \boldsymbol{Z} + \boldsymbol{S}$ (Fu et al., 2020; Peng et al., 2012). To consider in multiple subspace parameter estimation as in Dong et al. (2018), $\boldsymbol{D} = \boldsymbol{ZC} + \boldsymbol{S}$, where we assumed that the subspaces may not be independent from each other, or the data are contaminated by large noise, so the low-rank component lies in a union of subspaces, in which $\boldsymbol{Z} \in \Re^{n_1 \times n_2 \times n_3}$ is a clean low-rank dictionary, $\boldsymbol{C} \in \Re^{n_3 \times n_3}$ is a coefficient matrix as the low-rank representation by $\mathbf{Z}$, and $\boldsymbol{S} \in \Re^{n_1 \times n_2 \times n_3}$ denotes a sparse error matrix incurred by outliers or corruptions.

In practice, $\boldsymbol{I}_i^0$ are generally not well aligned, entailing the above low-rank plus sparse decomposition to be imprecise. To take account of this, inspired by Likassa et al. (2019) we apply affine transformations $\boldsymbol{\tau}_i$ to the potentially misaligned input three-way tensor images $\boldsymbol{I}_i^0$ to get a collection of transformed three-way tensor images $\boldsymbol{I}_i = \boldsymbol{I}_i^0 o \boldsymbol{\tau}_i$, where the operator o indicates the transformation. We can then stack these aligned three-way tensor images into a matrix and obtain $\boldsymbol{D_{o\tau}} = [vec(\mathbf{I}_1) \mid vec(\mathbf{I}_2) \mid \ldots \mid vec(\mathbf{I}_n)] \in \Re^{n_3 \times n_1 \times n_2}$. The aligned images can be treated as samples taken from a union of low-dimensional subspaces, which, if well aligned, should exhibit a low-rank subspace structure as the rank of the transformed three-way tensor images is as small as possible, up to some outliers and heavy sparse errors. Solving for the variables corresponding to the constraints $\boldsymbol{D_{o\tau}} = \boldsymbol{ZC} + \boldsymbol{S}$ is intractable due to its nonlinearity. To avoid the influence of corruption on recovery accuracy (Zhang et al., 2021; Liang et al., 2022), a tensor robust principal component analysis model is developed to decompose the raw

Table 7.1 Comparison of the proposed approach with other related state of the art of the works in terms of the objective function and constraints

Methods	Objective function	Constraints
Candès et al. (2011)	$\min_{A,E} \|A\|_* + \lambda \|E\|_1$	$M = A + E$
Chen et al. (2016); Zhang et al. (2017)	$\min_{A,E} \|A\|_* + \lambda \|E\|_1$	$M_{o\tau} + \sum_{i=1}^{n} J_i \Delta\tau v_i v_i^T = A + E$
Lerman and Maunu (2018)	$\min_{C,E,Q} \|C\|_* + \lambda \|E\|_{2,1}$	$M = AC + E, C = Q$
Ours	$\min_{Z,S,C,Q,\Delta\tau} \|Z\|_* + \|C\|_* + \alpha_1 \|Q\|_{2,1} + \alpha_2 \|S\|_{2,1}$	$D_{o\tau} + \sum_{i=1}^{n} J_i \Delta\tau\omega_i\omega_i^T = ZC + S, C = Q, Q \succeq 0$

data tensor into a low-rank normal data tensor and a sparse error tensor (Liang et al., 2022), but yet the issue of misalignment is not resolved. To resolve this dilemma, we assume that the change produced by these affine transformations τ_i is small and an initial of τ_i is known. We can then linearize $D_{o\tau}$ by using the first-order Taylor approximation as $D_{o(\tau+\Delta\tau)} \approx D_{o\tau} + \sum_{i=1}^{n_1 \times n_2 \times n_3} J_i \Delta\tau\omega_i\omega_i^T$, where $D_{o\tau} \in \Re^{n_1 \times n_3 \times n_2}$ is the transformed image, $\Delta\tau \in \Re^{p \times n}$ with p being the number of variables, $J_i = \frac{\partial vec(I_i o\tau_i)}{\partial \tau_i} \in \Re^{n_3 \times p}$ denotes the Jacobian of the ith image with respect to τ_i, and v_i is the standard basis for $\Re^n$. In this way, we obtain approximate transformations to recover the low-rank component from the underlying subspaces (Table 7.1).

To make the new approach more resilient to outliers and heavy sparse noise, the $L_{2,1}$ norm, which combines the advantages of the L_1 and L_2 norms, is used here. The $L_{2,1}$ regularizer is considered as the rotational invariant of the L_1 norm and can effectively handle outliers (Ding et al., 2006; Liu et al., 2018). Also, as observed in Likassa et al. (2019), the $L_{2,1}$ regularizer can also achieve better sparsity promotion than the L_1 norm. The L_1 norm may yield a biased estimation as it ignores the extreme values and cannot handle the collinearity of features. In contrast, the $L_{2,1}$ norm is more stable and has the ability to better preserve the spatial information than the L_1 regularizer, as demonstrated in Ding et al. (2006), Li et al. (2018). Invoked by Tang et al. (2018), we propose a new Tensor RPCA via AT + $L_{2,1}$ norms. To make the low-rank approximation more robust, Wang et al. (2021) considered the $L_{2,1}$ norm, and Zhang et al. (2017) used a new regularization term for sparse coefficients using Laplacian scale mixture model. Thus, the three-way tensor recovery has received a substantial amount of interest in high-dimensional three-way tensor images. Thereby, precise estimation of the three-way low-rank component is the major task of this work. The new developed robust tensor recovery also plays an instrumental role in robustifying tensor decompositions for multilinear data analysis against outliers, gross corruptions, and missing values and has a diverse array of applications. The overall problem can thus be posted as an optimization problem given by

Table 7.2 Performance comparisons on different databases in terms of PSNR and SSIM

Methods	PSNR	SSIM
Singh et al. (2019) HET	14.60	0.39
RPCA with AT + RPI	20.33	0.76
Singh et al. (2022) 2LIM + DNN	17.02	0.41
RPCA with AT + $L_{2,1}$ Norms	20.26	0.67
Xian et al. (2023) NHM	19.78	0.76
Tensor RPCA with AT + $L_{2,1}$ Norms	26.87	0.78

$$\min_{\boldsymbol{Z},\boldsymbol{S},\boldsymbol{C},\boldsymbol{Q},\boldsymbol{\Delta\tau}} \|\boldsymbol{Z}\|_* + \|\boldsymbol{C}\|_* + \lambda_1 \|\boldsymbol{Q}\|_{2,1} + \lambda_2 \|\boldsymbol{S}\|_{2,1}$$

$$\text{s.t } \boldsymbol{D_{o\tau}} + \sum_{i=1}^{n} \boldsymbol{J}_i \boldsymbol{\Delta\tau}\boldsymbol{\omega}_i\boldsymbol{\omega}_i^T = \boldsymbol{ZC} + \boldsymbol{S}, \boldsymbol{C} = \boldsymbol{Q}, \boldsymbol{Q} \succeq \boldsymbol{0} \tag{7.48}$$

where $\|\boldsymbol{Z}\|_* = \sum_{i=1}^{min(n_1,n_2,n_3)} \sigma_i(\boldsymbol{Z})$ denotes the nuclear norm of $\boldsymbol{Z}$, in which $\sigma_i(\boldsymbol{Z})$ indicates the singular values of $\boldsymbol{Z}$, λ_1 and λ_2 are the regularization parameters, and $\|\boldsymbol{E}\|_{2,1} = \sum_{i=1}^{n}(\sum_{j=1}^{m} \boldsymbol{E}_{ji}^2)^{1/2}$ denotes the $L_{2,1}$ norm of $\boldsymbol{E}$. In this chapter, two novel ideas are taken into account: the first is affine transformation, while the second one is the $L_{2,1}$ norm (Li et al., 2017). Vaswani et al. (2018) proposed online Robust Low-Rank Tensor Learning to deal with the issue of distorted outliers and heavy sparse noises to process the big data; however $L_{2,1}$ norm is not considered in the work. The first nuclear norm term in (7.48) enforces the dictionary $\boldsymbol{Z}$ to lie in low-dimensional subspaces. The second and the third terms constrain the representation to be low rank plus sparse. The fourth term regularizes the error $\boldsymbol{E}$ to be sparse. The new robust tensor PCA is mainly used to decompose high-dimensional tensor images into the tensor low-rank and sparse components. For easy reference, a comparison of the proposed approach with other related methods is furnished in Table 7.2.

7.4.2 Parameter Estimation

To solve the optimization problem in (7.48), we use the augmented Lagrangian multiplier technique and rewrite (7.48) as

$$\mathcal{L}\big(\boldsymbol{Z}, \boldsymbol{C}, \boldsymbol{S}, \boldsymbol{Q}, \boldsymbol{\Delta\tau}\big) = \|\boldsymbol{Z}\|_* + \|\boldsymbol{C}\|_* + \alpha_1 \|\boldsymbol{Q}\|_{2,1} + \alpha_2 \|\boldsymbol{S}\|_{2,1}$$

$$+ \langle \boldsymbol{\Gamma}_1, \boldsymbol{F} - \boldsymbol{ZC} - \boldsymbol{S}\rangle + \frac{\mu_1}{2} \|\boldsymbol{F} - \boldsymbol{ZC} - \boldsymbol{S}\|_F^2$$

$$+ \langle \boldsymbol{\Gamma}_2, \boldsymbol{C} - \boldsymbol{Q}\rangle + \frac{\mu_2}{2} \|\boldsymbol{C} - \boldsymbol{Q}\|_F^2 \tag{7.49}$$

where $\boldsymbol{\Gamma}_1 \in \Re^{n_1\times n_2\times n_3}$ and $\boldsymbol{\Gamma}_2 \in \Re^{n_3\times n_3}$ are the Lagrangian multipliers, μ_1 and μ_2 are the penalty parameters, $\langle \boldsymbol{X}, \boldsymbol{Y}\rangle = Trace(\boldsymbol{X}^T\boldsymbol{Y})$, $\|\cdot\|_F$ denotes the Frobenius norm, and $\boldsymbol{F} = \boldsymbol{D_{o\tau}} + \sum_{i=1}^{n} \boldsymbol{J}_i \boldsymbol{\Delta\tau}\boldsymbol{\omega}_i\boldsymbol{\omega}_i^T$. By using augmented Lagrange multiplier with adaptive penalty (Boyd & Vandenberghe, 2004), (7.49) can be rewritten as

$$\mathcal{L}\left(\boldsymbol{Z}, \boldsymbol{C}, \boldsymbol{S}, \boldsymbol{Q}, \boldsymbol{\Delta\tau}\right) = \|\boldsymbol{Z}\|_* + \|\boldsymbol{C}\|_* + \alpha_2 \|\boldsymbol{S}\|_{2,1} + \alpha_1 \|\boldsymbol{Q}\|_{2,1} + \frac{\mu_1}{2}\left\|\boldsymbol{F} - \boldsymbol{ZC} - \boldsymbol{S} + \frac{\boldsymbol{\Gamma}_1}{\mu_1}\right\|_F^2 + \frac{\mu_2}{2}\left\|\boldsymbol{C} - \boldsymbol{Q} + \frac{\boldsymbol{\Gamma}_2}{\mu_2}\right\|_F^2 \tag{7.50}$$

Solving (7.50) directly is computationally prohibitive; thereby we consider to iteratively update the variables alternatively via ADMM (Boyd & Vandenberghe, 2004), which decomposes the original problem into a set of subproblems. In each step, we update just one variable while keeping the other variables unchanged. So the above terms like $\|\boldsymbol{F} - \boldsymbol{ZC} - \boldsymbol{S}\|_F$ are convex even if it involves the matrix factorization term $\boldsymbol{ZC}$ (Zhang et al., 2017).

Firstly, to update the tensor low-rank component $\boldsymbol{Z}$, we fix $\boldsymbol{S}$, $\boldsymbol{Q}$, $\boldsymbol{C}$, and $\boldsymbol{\Delta\tau}$, so $\boldsymbol{Z}^{(k+1)}$ can be determined by

$$\boldsymbol{Z}^{(k+1)} = \underset{\boldsymbol{Z}}{\operatorname{argmin}} \mathcal{L}\left\{\boldsymbol{Z}, \boldsymbol{S}^{(k)}, \boldsymbol{C}^{(k)}, \boldsymbol{Q}^{(k)}, \boldsymbol{\Delta\tau}^{(k)}\right\} \tag{7.51}$$

where k is the iteration index. By ignoring all irrelevant terms of the tensor low-rank component $\boldsymbol{Z}$, Eq. (7.51) can be simplified as

$$\boldsymbol{Z}^{(k+1)} = \underset{\boldsymbol{Z}}{\operatorname{argmin}} \mathcal{L}\left\{ \|\boldsymbol{Z}\|_* + \frac{\mu_1^{(k)}}{2}\left\|\boldsymbol{F}^{(k)} - \boldsymbol{Z}\boldsymbol{C}^{(k)} - \boldsymbol{S}^{(k)} + \frac{\boldsymbol{\Gamma}_1^{(k)}}{\mu_1^{(k)}}\right\|_F^2 \right\} \tag{7.52}$$

We can then use the linear augmented direction method with the soft shrinkage operator as mentioned in Cai et al. (2010) and update the tensor low-rank component $\boldsymbol{Z}^{(k+1)}$ by

$$\boldsymbol{Z}^{(k+1)} = \Omega_{\frac{1}{\kappa_{\mathbf{Z}}^{(k)}}}\left\{\boldsymbol{Z}^{(k)} - \frac{P_{\mathbf{Z}}^{(k)}}{\kappa_{\mathbf{Z}}^{(k)}}\right\} \tag{7.53}$$

where Ω is the singular value threshold, $P_{\mathbf{Z}}^{(k)} = (\mu_1^{(k)})(\boldsymbol{Z}^{(k)})^T\boldsymbol{C}^{(k)} - \mu_1^{(k)}(\boldsymbol{F}^{(k)} - \boldsymbol{S}^{(k)}) - (\boldsymbol{\Gamma}_1^{(k)} + \boldsymbol{\Gamma}_2^{(k)})(\boldsymbol{C}^{(k)})^T$, $\kappa_{\mathbf{Z}}^{(k)} = (\mu_1^{(k)})\frac{\tau_{\mathbf{Z}}}{2}$, $\tau_{\mathbf{Z}} > \sigma(\boldsymbol{C}^T\boldsymbol{C})$ is the proximal parameter, in which $\sigma(\boldsymbol{C}^T\boldsymbol{C})$ denotes the spectral radius of $\boldsymbol{C}^T\boldsymbol{C}$.

Secondly, to update $\boldsymbol{S}$, we keep $\boldsymbol{Z}$, $\boldsymbol{Q}$, $\boldsymbol{C}$, and $\boldsymbol{\Delta\tau}$ as constants, so $\boldsymbol{S}^{(k+1)}$ can be determined by

$$\boldsymbol{S}^{(k+1)} = \underset{\boldsymbol{S}}{\operatorname{argmin}} \mathcal{L}\left\{\boldsymbol{Z}^{(k+1)}, \boldsymbol{S}, \boldsymbol{C}^{(k)}, \boldsymbol{Q}^{(k)}, \boldsymbol{\Delta\tau}^{(k)}\right\} \tag{7.54}$$

Again, by ignoring all irrelevant terms of $\boldsymbol{S}$, Eq. (7.54) can be simplified as

$$S^{(k+1)} = \underset{E}{\text{argmin}}\left\{\alpha_2 \|S\|_{2,1} + \frac{\mu_1^{(k)}}{2}\left\| F^{(k)} - Z^{(k)}C^{(k)} - S + \frac{\Gamma_1^{(k)}}{\mu_1^{(k)}} \right\|_F^2 \right\} \quad (7.55)$$

By using lemma shown in Yang et al. (2009), the update of the ith column of $S^{(k+1)}$, $S_i^{(k+1)}$, is given by

$$S_i^{(k+1)} = \begin{cases} \dfrac{\left\|U_i^{(k)}\right\|_2 - \frac{\alpha_2}{\mu_1^{(k)}}}{\left\|U_i^{(k)}\right\|_2} U_i^{(k)}, & \text{if } \left\|U_i^{(k)}\right\|_2 \geq \frac{\alpha_2}{\mu_1^{(k)}} \\ 0, & \text{otherwise} \end{cases} \quad (7.56)$$

where $\|.\|_2$ denotes the Euclidean norm and $U^{(k)} = (F^{(k)} - Z^{(k)}C^{(k)} + \frac{\Gamma_1^{(k)}}{\mu_1^{(k)}})$

Thirdly, to find an update of C, we keep Z, S, Q, and $\Delta\tau$ as constants, and thus $C^{(k+1)}$ can be determined by

$$C^{(k+1)} = \underset{C}{\text{argmin}}\mathcal{L}\left\{Z^{(k+1)}, S^{(k+1)}, C, Q^{(k)}, \Delta\tau^{(k)}\right\} \quad (7.57)$$

By ignoring all irrelevant terms of C, Eq. (7.57) can be simplified as

$$C^{(k+1)} = \underset{C}{\text{argmin}}\left\{ \|C\|_* + \frac{\mu_1^{(k)}}{2}\left\| F^{(k)} - Z^{(k)}C - S^{(k)} + \frac{\Gamma_1^{(k)}}{\mu_1^{(k)}} \right\|_F^2 + \frac{\mu_2}{2}\left\| C - Q^{(k)} + \frac{\Gamma_2^{(k)}}{\mu_2^{(k)}} \right\|_F^2 \right\} \quad (7.58)$$

To solve this subproblem, we can employ a linearized augmented Lagrangian multiplier with the singular value threshold (Cai et al., 2010). Thereby, $C^{(k+1)}$ can be updated by

$$C^{(k+1)} = \Omega_{\frac{1}{\kappa_C^{(k)}}}\left\{C^{(k)} - \frac{P_C^{(k)}}{\kappa_C^{(k)}}\right\} \quad (7.59)$$

where $\kappa_C^{(k)} = (\mu_1^{(k)} + \mu_2^{(k)})\frac{\tau_C}{2}$, $\tau_C > \sigma(ZZ^T)$, and $P_C^{(k)} = Z^{(k)}(\mu_1^{(k)} + \mu_2^{(k)})Z^{(k)} - \mu_1^{(k)}(F^{(k)} - S^{(k)}) - \Gamma_1^{(k)} + \mu_2^{(k)}(C^{(k)} - Q^{(k)}) + \Gamma_2^{(k)}$.

Again, to update Q, we keep Z, S, C, and $\Delta\tau$ as constants, and $Q^{(k+1)}$ can then be determined by

$$Q^{(k+1)} = \underset{Q}{\text{argmin}}\mathcal{L}\left\{Z^{(k+1)}, E^{(k+1)}, C^{(k+1)}, Q, \Delta\tau^{(k)}\right\} \quad (7.60)$$

By ignoring all of the irrelevant terms, Eq. (7.60) can be simplified as

$$Q^{(k+1)} = \underset{Q}{\operatorname{argmin}} \left\{ \begin{array}{l} \alpha_1 \| Q \|_{2,1} \\ + \frac{\mu_2^{(k)}}{2} \left\| C^{(k)} - Q + \frac{\Gamma_2^{(k)}}{\mu_2^{(k)}} \right\|_F^2 \end{array} \right\} \tag{7.61}$$

Again, by using lemma in Yang et al. (2009), the update of the ith column of $Q^{(k+1)}$, $Q_i^{(k+1)}$, is given by

$$Q_i^{(k+1)} = \begin{cases} \frac{\left\| P_i^{(k)} \right\|_2 - \frac{\alpha_1}{\mu_2^{(k)}}}{\left\| P_i^{(k)} \right\|_2} P_i^{(k)}, & \text{if } \left\| P_i^{(k)} \right\|_2 \geq \frac{\alpha_1}{\mu_2^{(k)}} \\ 0, & \text{otherwise} \end{cases} \tag{7.62}$$

where $P^{(k)} = (C^{(k+1)} + \frac{\Gamma_2^{(k)}}{\mu_2^{(k)}})$.

Lastly, to get an update of $\Delta\tau$, we keep Z, S, C, and Q as constants, and $\Delta\tau^{(k+1)}$ can be determined by

$$\Delta\tau^{(k+1)} = \underset{\Delta\tau}{\operatorname{argmin}} \mathcal{L} \left\{ Z^{(k+1)}, S^{(k+1)}, C^{(k+1)}, \Delta\tau, Q^{(k+1)} \right\} \tag{7.63}$$

By ignoring all irrelevant terms of $\Delta\tau$, we can obtain

$$\Delta\tau^{(k+1)} = \underset{\Delta\tau}{\operatorname{argmin}} \left\{ \frac{\mu_1^{(k)}}{2} \left\| F^{(k)} - Z^{(k+1)} C^{(k+1)} - S^{(k+1)} + \frac{\Gamma_1^{(k)}}{\mu_1^{(k)}} \right\|_F^2 \right\} \tag{7.64}$$

Solving (7.64) with the threshold operators (Peng et al., 2012; Chen et al., 2016), we can get an update of $\Delta\tau^{(k+1)}$ as

$$\Delta\tau^{(k+1)} = \sum_{i=1}^{n} J_i^{+} \left(Z^{(k+1)} C^{(k+1)} + S^{(k+1)} - D_{o\tau} - \frac{\Gamma_1^{(k)}}{\mu_1^{(k)}} \right) \omega_i \omega_i^T \tag{7.65}$$

where J_i^{+} denotes the Moores-Penroses pseudoinverse of J_i (Courrieu, 2008).

Following the same steps as the above, the Lagrangian multipliers Γ_1 and Γ_2 are updated by

$$\Gamma_1^{(k+1)} = \Gamma_1^{(k)} + \mu_1^{(k+1)} \left\{ {}^{(k)} - Z^{(k+1)} C^{(k+1)} - S^{(k+1)} \right\} \tag{7.66}$$

$$\text{and } \Gamma_2^{(k+1)} = \Gamma_2^{(k)} + \mu_2^{(k+1)} \left\{ C^{(k+1)} - Q^{(k+1)} \right\} \tag{7.67}$$

Likewise, the regularization parameters μ_1 and μ_2 are updated, respectively, by

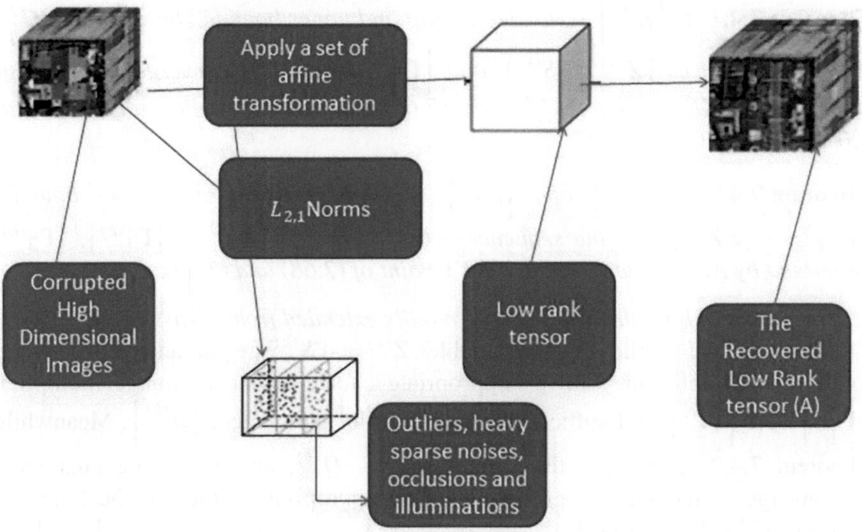

Fig. 7.1 First we consider the original tensor datasets. Then following this, we employ both AT + $L_{2,1}$ norms to correct the distorted tensor images. After this, in high-dimensional images as it is highly impacted by the extreme values, we additionally employ the $L_{2,1}$ norms to the sparse noises and the subspace parameters, see (1). By this process, we decompose the original tensor datasets as the low-rank tensor and sparse noises. To boost the performance of the new method with novel ideas of AT + $L_{2,1}$ norms into the existing methods (Likassa et al., 2019)

$$\mu_1^{(k+1)} = min\left\{\mu_{max}, \rho\mu_1^{(k)}\right\} \tag{7.68}$$

and $$\mu_2^{(k+1)} = min\left\{\mu_{max}, \rho\mu_2^{(k)}\right\} \tag{7.69}$$

where ρ is a properly chosen constant and μ_{max} is a tunable parameter adjusting the convergence of the proposed method. The overall structure how the parameters are interacting to one another through incorporating AT + $L_{2,1}$ norms is shown in Fig. 7.1. The overall updating equations proceed in a round-robin manner until convergence. The effectiveness of the proposed method is checked using the retinal image enhancement as shown in Fig. 7.4 and Table 7.2.

7.4.3 Uniqueness of Parameter Estimation

This section considers the convergence characteristics of the updating equations addressed in the previous section. Two theorems are established to address this issue.

Theorem 7.4.1 *If* $\left\{\mu_1^{(k)}\right\}$ *is nondecreasing and upper bounded by* $\tau_Z > \sigma(\boldsymbol{C}\boldsymbol{C}^T)$, *then the sequences* $\left\{\mathbf{Z}^{(k)}\right\}$, $\left\{\boldsymbol{S}^{(k)}\right\}$, *and* $\left\{\boldsymbol{\Gamma}_1^{(k)}\right\}$ *by ADMM converge to a Karush-Kuhn-Tucker (KKT) point of (7.66) and (7.67). The proof is similar to Likassa et al. (2019), Liang et al. (2022).*

Theorem 7.4.2 *If* $\left\{\mu_1^{(k)}\right\}$ *and* $\left\{\mu_2^{(k)}\right\}$ *are nondecreasing and upper bounded by* $\tau_C > \sigma(\boldsymbol{Z}\boldsymbol{Z}^T)$, *then the sequences* $\left\{\boldsymbol{C}^{(k)}\right\}$,$\left\{\boldsymbol{Q}^{(k)}\right\}$, $\left\{\boldsymbol{\Delta\tau}^{(k)}\right\}$, $\left\{\boldsymbol{\Gamma_1}^{(k)}\right\}$, $\left\{\boldsymbol{\Gamma_2}^{(k)}\right\}$ *generated by ADMM converge to a KKT point of (7.68) and (7.69).*

The proofs of both theorems can be readily extended from Likassa et al. (2019).

Theorem 7.4.1 implies that the variables $\boldsymbol{Z}^{(k)}$ and $\boldsymbol{S}^{(k)}$ are guaranteed to converge to the global optimum with an appropriate choice of the Lagrange multipliers $\left\{\boldsymbol{\Gamma}_1^{(k)}\right\}$ and $\left\{\boldsymbol{\Gamma}_2^{(k)}\right\}$ and sufficiently large penalty parameters $\left\{\mu_1^{(k)}\right\}$. Meanwhile, Theorem 7.4.2 shows that the variables $\boldsymbol{C}^{(k)}$, $\boldsymbol{Q}^{(k)}$, and $\boldsymbol{\Delta\tau}^{(k)}$ are guaranteed to converge to the global optimum with an appropriate choice of the Lagrange multipliers $\left\{\boldsymbol{\Gamma}_1^{(k)}\right\}$ and $\left\{\boldsymbol{\Gamma}_2^{(k)}\right\}$ and sufficiently large penalty parameters $\left\{\mu_1^{(k)}\right\}$ and $\left\{\mu_2^{(k)}\right\}$. Tensor RPCA is applicable in the areas of retinal image enhancement and breast cancer detection. For instance, one of the potential applications of the retinal image enhancement is shown in Fig. 7.4. To make the proposed method easy to understand, the pseudo-code is summarized in Algorithm 7.3.

Algorithm 7.3: Tensor RPCA with AT + $L_{2,1}$ norms

```
Input:Data Matrix D ∈ ℜ^{n1×n2×n3}, Z ∈ ℜ^{n1×n2×n3}, C^0 ∈ ℜ^{n1×n2}, S^0 ∈ ℜ^{n1×n2×n3},
  Δτ^0 ∈ ℜ^{n1×n2×n3}, α1, α2, ρ
While not converged Do
Z^(k+1) updated by (53)
S^(k+1) updated by (56)
C^(k+1) updated by (62)
Q^(k+1) updated by (62)
Δτ^(k+1) updated by (65)
Γ1^(k+1) updated by (66)
Γ2^(k+1) updated by (67)
μ1^(k+1) updated by (68)
μ2^(k+1) updated by (69)
End while
Outputs:Z, S, C, Q, Δτ, Γ1, Γ2
```

7.5 Retinal Image Analysis

This section describes the retinal image dataset utilized in the analysis conducted by the proposed methods. Initially, we provide an overview of the dataset's characteristics and evaluation criterion, followed by simulation results along with subsequent discussions. To assess the efficacy of our proposed method, we compared it with several existing approaches. Specifically, we considered HET by Singh et al. (2019), 2LIM + DNN by Singh et al. (2022), and NHM by Xian et al. (2023). In the following subsections, we will elaborate on the datasets used, the numerical evaluation criteria employed, and the results of our medical image analyses.

7.5.1 Dataset

Eye-Quality (EyeQ) Assessment Dataset is a re-annotation subset from the Eye-PACS dataset for fundus image quality assessment used for various purposes in the fields of ophthalmology to diagnosis eye diseases, monitoring disease progression, and evaluating the effectiveness of treatment methods in biomedical image analysis. It typically consists of high-resolution images of the retina, including images of the optic nerve, macula, and blood vessels. The three experiments predominantly focus on retinal image enhancement from the degraded images. The three simulations consider three true color degraded retinal images with a size of 256×256 pixels from the testing set to assess the performance of the proposed method through visualization and numerical analysis. The EyeQ dataset also used in Fu et al. (2019) consists of 40 retinal images, from which three distorted retinal images are considered for medical image analysis. We conduct an extensive simulation study to investigate performance of the proposed methods in enhancing retinal image enhancement through visualization and numerical analysis. After the visualization performance evaluation, the performance of the proposed method is justified through the numerical analysis. Those images are distorted due to various variation, outliers, and noises. To verify the effectiveness of the proposed method with also conducted a simulation on more retinal images taking ten images from the EyeQ dataset.

7.5.2 Evaluation Criterion

In this chapter, two popular evaluation criterions mainly the PSNR (Peak Signal-to-Noise Ratio) (Gravel et al., 2004) and SSIM (Structural Similarity Index Measure) (Sara et al., 2019) are used as quantitative analysis evaluation indicators from which the PSNR is given by

$$\mathrm{PSNR}(f, \hat{f}) = 10log_{10}^{\frac{255^2}{\frac{1}{m\times n}\sum_{i=1}^{m}\sum_{i=1}^{n}(f_{ij}-\hat{f}_{ij})^2}} \tag{7.70}$$

where both the ground truth f and the enhanced image $\hat{f}$ are of size $m \times n$. The quality of retinal image enhancement by the proposed method is verified using SSIM (Sara et al., 2019) to measure the similarity between two images and given by

$$\mathrm{SSIM}(f, \hat{f}) = \frac{(2\mu_f \mu_{\hat{f}} + C_1)((2\sigma_f \sigma_{\hat{f}} + C_2))}{(\mu_f^2 + \mu_{\hat{f}}^2 + C_1)(\sigma_f^2 + \sigma_{\hat{f}}^2 + C_2)} \tag{7.71}$$

where f is the enhanced retinal images and $\hat{f}$ is denoting the ground truth with size $m \times n$, and μ_f, $\mu_{\hat{f}}$, σ_f^2, $\sigma_{\hat{f}}^2$ are denoting the mean and variance of the ground truth and enhanced retinal images. The largest PSNR and SSIM is the better the performance of the proposed method.

The performance of RPCA with AT + RPI, RPCA with AT $+L_{2,1}$ norms, and Tensor RPCA with AT $+L_{2,1}$ norms are evaluated using a publicly EyeQ retinal dataset. The simulation results for each proposed method are given in both through image visualization and numerical analysis.

7.5.3 Results from RPCA with AT + RPI

The performance of RPCA with AT + RPI is evaluated using three retinal images selected from 40 retinal images as in Fu et al. (2019). First, the degraded retinal images are considered to examine how the proposed method is enhancing using AT + RPI through retinal image visualization. Then, the enhanced image by the proposed method is compared with the ground truth using the PSNR and SSIM. Furthermore, in the context of medical image analysis utilizing rank prior information, our method's performance is compared to both ground truth and degraded retinal images, demonstrating its closer alignment with ground truth as compared by Singh et al. (2019), as illustrated in Fig. 7.2. These findings are further supported by numerical results, as presented in Table 7.2, from which we learnt that the proposed method outperforms the approach described in Singh et al. (2019). The PSNR for ten different retinal images is also illustrated in Fig. 7.5 from which we confirmed that the proposed method is better as compared with the existing method (Singh et al., 2019).

7.5.4 Results from RPCA with AT + $L_{2,1}$ Norms

In this section, we evaluate the performance of the proposed method, which incorporates AT + $L_{2,1}$ norms, for enhancing medical retinal images. First, we conducted retinal image enhancement analysis from the degraded one and then compared it with the ground truth using PSNR and SSIM. Then, we compare the RPCA incorporating AT + $L_{2,1}$ norms with Singh et al. (2022) 2LIM + DNN

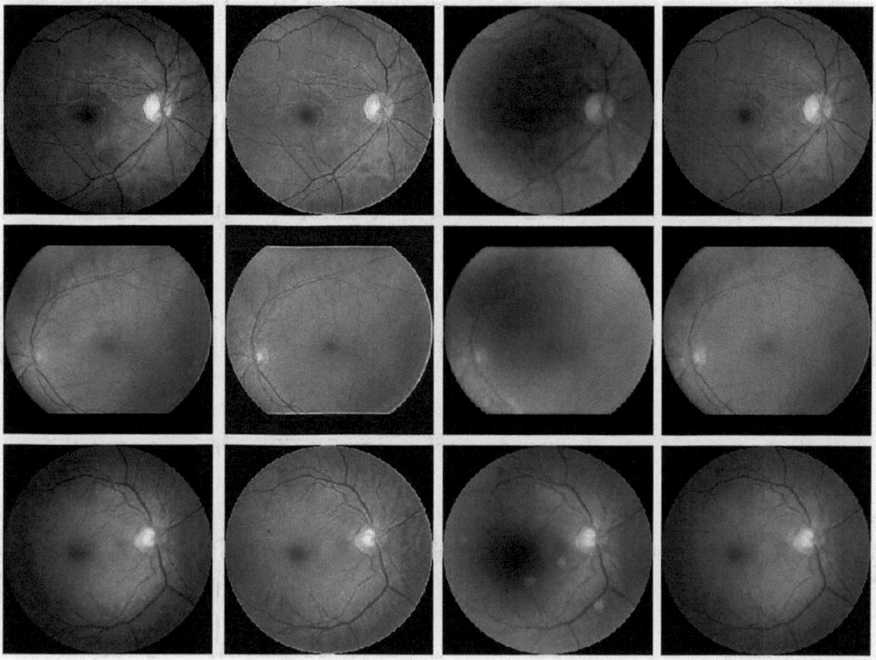

Fig. 7.2 The first column is the Retinal Medical Image Enhanced by Singh et al. (2019), (**b**) the second column is by the proposed method, and (**c**) the third column is the degraded image and the fourth column is the ground truth

through retinal image visualization. Figure 7.3 illustrates image enhanced by the proposed method (shown in second column) is closer to the ground truth (as shown in third column) and far from the degraded image (shown in fourth column) than the state of the art of the work (Singh et al., 2022). Table 7.2 justifies the result shown in Fig. 7.3. This is due to incorporating AT $+L_{2,1}$ norms. The PSNR for ten different retinal images is also illustrated in Fig. 7.5 from which we confirmed that the proposed method is better as compared with the existing method (Singh et al., 2022).

7.5.5 *Results from Tensor RPCA with AT + $L_{2,1}$ Norms*

This section assesses the performance of the proposed method compared with Xian et al. (2023). To examine the performance of the proposed method, three degraded retinal images shown in the fourth column of Fig. 7.4 are considered, from which the performance of the proposed method is better as compared by Xian et al. (2023).

This enhanced robustness can be attributed to the incorporation of affine transformations and the utilization of $L_{2,1}$ norms, enabling the simultaneous alignment

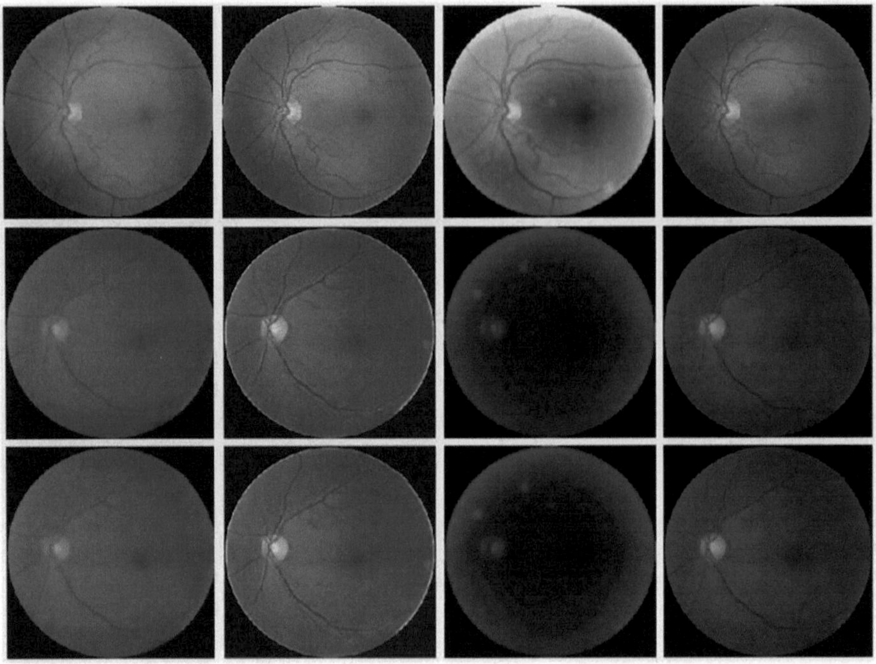

Fig. 7.3 The first column is Retinal Medical Image Enhanced by Singh et al. (2022), (**b**) the second column is by the proposed method, and (**c**) the third column is the degraded image and the fourth column is the ground truth

and recovery of retinal images. Furthermore, numerical simulations also verify the efficacy of the tensor proposed method compared to existing approaches, as evidenced in Table 7.2. The PSNR for ten different retinal images is also illustrated in Fig. 7.5 from which we confirmed that the proposed method is better as compared with the existing method (Xian et al., 2023).

The PSNRs based on the individual retinal images are illustrated and shown in Fig. 7.5, from which we noted that the proposed methods are better compared with existing methods based on the individual retinal images. This improvement is attributed due to the incorporation of affine transformation, $L_{2,1}$ norms, and incorporation of affine transformation to each proposed method which is unseen in the previous methods. The result of Fig. 7.6 shows the tensor RPCA with $L_{2,1}$ norms and affine transformation over boosts as compared with the state-of-the-art methods.

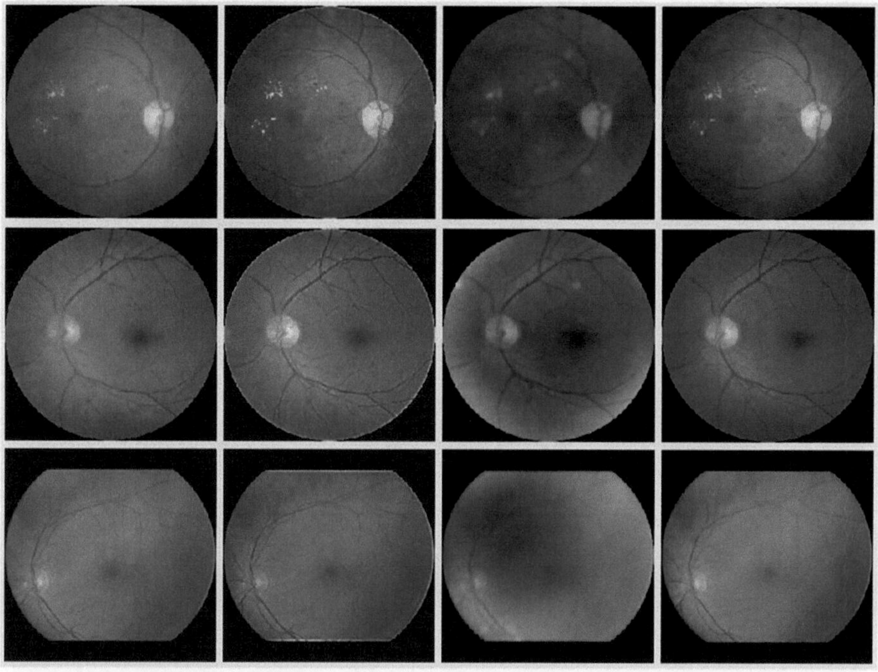

Fig. 7.4 The first column is Retinal Medical Image Enhanced by Xian et al. (2023), (**b**) the second column is by the proposed method, (**c**) the third column is the degraded image and the fourth column is the ground truth

7.6 Discussions and Conclusions

This chapter is dedicated to the enhancement of existing RPCA method (Candès et al., 2011) through the incorporation of AT, RPI, and $L_{2,1}$ norms, aimed at improving their robustness. The development of these approaches represents a significant contribution to the field of mathematical and statistical modeling, particularly in the realm of high-dimensional medical images. This work introduces three independent methods, each focusing on the integration of AT, RPI, and $L_{2,1}$ norms. Existing methods, as referenced in Zheng et al. (2019), Liu et al. (2022), often lack robustness in the presence of gross errors and outliers within high-dimensional retinal images. In response to this challenge, this chapter presents three distinct approaches designed to address these issues head-on.

First, we highlighted the drawbacks of PCA and then shifted our focus to the development of RPCA with AT + RPI for high-dimensional image processing. Following this, we delved into the benefits of incorporating AT + RPI. To achieve this, an additional term is introduced in the data matrix decomposition, enhancing the method's resilience to errors, outliers, and occlusions. The problem is formulated as a constrained optimization problem, which is subsequently solved using a

Fig. 7.5 The PSNRs for different retinal images by baselines and the three methods

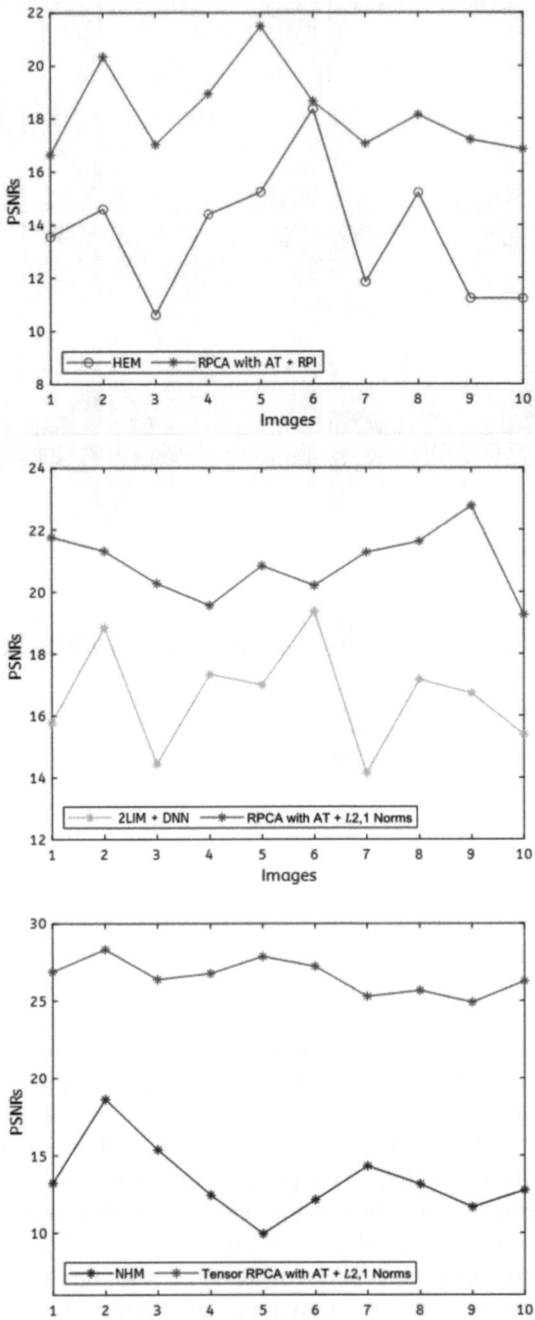

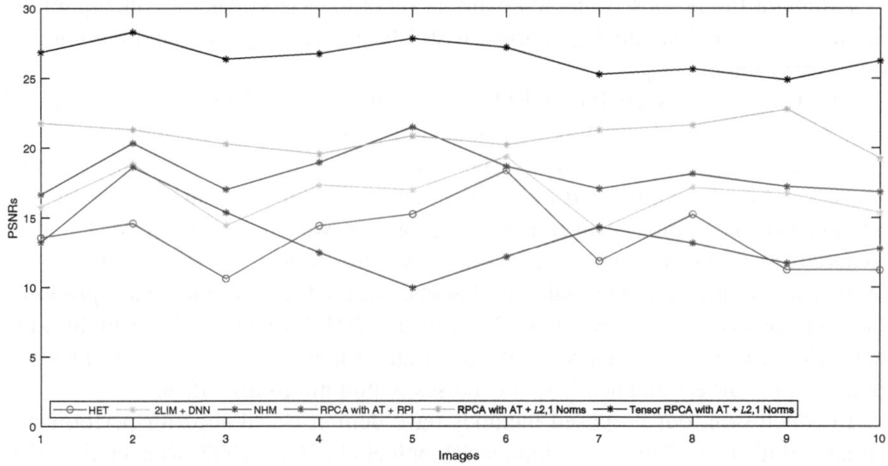

Fig. 7.6 The PSNRs for different retinal images by methods

convex program. Furthermore, a new set of equations is derived to iteratively update the involved variables in a round-robin manner. This chapter underscores the advantages of considering rank prior information to enhance performance, particularly in accurately identifying the true underlying objects within distorted high-dimensional images. However, a limitation of this convex optimization method is its consideration of the low-rank component solely within a single subspace.

Secondly, we describe the limitations of RPCA when AT and RPI are incorporated and then proposed a novel approach incorporating $L_{2,1}$ norm to enhance the quality of retinal fundus images via convex optimization techniques. Initially, affine transformation is applied in Candès et al. (2011) to mitigate potential distortions, updating the warp using Taylor series expansion and Jacobian transformation. Subsequently, the $L_{2,1}$ norm is introduced to address sparse components in the objective function, reducing correlated samples within retinal images. Parameter updating is approached iteratively, drawing on optimization techniques in a round-robin fashion, demonstrating superior performance compared to existing methods on public datasets.

To mitigate various adverse effects like occlusions, outliers, and sparse noise, the proposed method integrates affine transformations with low-rank plus sparse decomposition. The low-rank component spans disjoint subspaces, rectifying distorted or misaligned images for a more accurate representation. Additionally, the $L_{2,1}$ norm aids in removing correlated samples across images, enhancing resilience against outliers and significant image variations. The determination of parameters and affine transformations is framed as a convex optimization problem, with the ADMM method used to iteratively update optimization variables and affine transformations, thus improving computational efficiency.

Although the proposed method exhibits superior performance by incorporating affine transformation and $L_{2,1}$ norms, it still faces challenges in handling noise in multi-array data.

Thirdly, we introduce Tensor RPCA augmented with affine transformation and $L_{2,1}$ norms, with a specific focus on enhancing its performance for multi-array data by incorporating these techniques. The determination of both variables and affine transformations is formulated as a convex optimization problem. To mitigate the computational complexity inherent in our approach, we employ the ADMM method to iteratively update optimization variables and affine transformations, resulting in a more efficient process. Through simulations, we confirm that the tensor proposed method outperforms the baseline (Xian et al., 2023) when handling multi-array data. Consequently, our approach demonstrates superiority over existing methods in detecting outliers and heavy sparse noises within multi-array data.

In conclusion, our proposed methods have demonstrated superior performance compared to state-of-the-art techniques (Singh et al., 2019, 2022; Xian et al., 2023) using a publicly available retinal image dataset. The Tensor RPCA with affine transformation and $L_{2,1}$ norms perform better as compared with the other two counter proposed methods. Therefore, the authors suggest considering the methods in the detection of eye cataracts and cancer.

Acknowledgments This work is partially supported by South Africa National Research Foundation (NRF) and South Africa Medical Research Council (SAMRC) (South Africa DST-NRF-SAMRC SARChI Research Chair in Biostatistics, Grant Number 114613). Opinions expressed and conclusions arrived at are those of the author and are not necessarily to be attributed to the NRF and SAMRC.

References

Abidi, M. A., Gribok, A. V., & Paik, J. (2016). *Optimization techniques in computer vision*. Springer.

Alimanov, A., & Islam, M. B. (2023) . Denoising diffusion probabilistic model for retinal image generation and segmentation. In *2023 IEEE International Conference on Computational Photography (ICCP)* (pp. 1–12). IEEE

Bertsekas, D. (2015). *Convex optimization algorithms*. Athena Scientific.

Boyd, S. P., & Vandenberghe, L. (2004). *Convex optimization*. Cambridge University Press.

Cai, J.-F., Candès, E. J., & Shen, Z. (2010). A singular value thresholding algorithm for matrix completion. *SIAM Journal on Optimization, 20*(4), 1956–1982.

Candès, E. J., Li, X., Ma, Y., & Wright, J. (2011). Robust principal component analysis? *Journal of the ACM (JACM), 58*(3), 1–37.

Cao, W., Wang, Y., Sun, J., Meng, D., Yang, C., Cichocki, A., & Xu, Z. (2016). Total variation regularized tensor RPCA for background subtraction from compressive measurements. *IEEE Transactions on Image Processing, 25*(9), 4075–4090.

Celebi, M. E., Celiker, F., & Kingravi, H. A. (2011). On Euclidean norm approximations, *Pattern Recognition, 44*(2), 278–283.

Chen, X., Han, Z., Wang, Y., Tang, Y., & Yu, H. (2016). Nonconvex plus quadratic penalized low-rank and sparse decomposition for noisy image alignment. *Science China Information Sciences, 59*(5), 052107–1.

Courrieu, P. (2008). Fast computation of Moore-Penrose inverse matrices. arXiv preprint arXiv:0804.4809.

De Cheveigné, A., & Simon, J. Z. (2007). Denoising based on time-shift PCA. *Journal of Neuroscience Methods, 165*(2), 297–305.

Dhara, A., & Dutta, J. (2011). *Optimality conditions in convex optimization: A finite-dimensional view*. CRC Press.

Ding, C., Zhou, D., He, X., & Zha, H. (2006). R1-PCA: Rotational invariant L_1-norm principal component analysis for robust subspace factorization. In *Proceedings of the 23rd International Conference on Machine Learning* (pp. 281–288).

Dong, W., Huang, T., Shi, G., Ma, Y., & Li, X. (2018). Robust tensor approximation with Laplacian scale mixture modeling for multiframe image and video denoising. *IEEE Journal of Selected Topics in Signal Processing, 12*(6), 1435–1448.

Fu, H., Wang, B., Shen, J., Cui, S., Xu, Y., Liu, J., & Shao, L. (2019). Evaluation of retinal image quality assessment networks in different color-spaces. In *Medical Image Computing and Computer Assisted Intervention–MICCAI 2019: 22nd International Conference, Shenzhen, China, October 13–17, 2019, Proceedings, Part I 22* (pp. 48–56). Springer

Fu, Y., Wang, Y., Zhong, Y., Fu, D., & Peng, Q. (2020). Change detection based on tensor RPCA for longitudinal retinal fundus images. *Neurocomputing, 387*, 1–12.

Gao, Y., Lin, T., Zhang, Y., Luo, S., & Nie, F. (2021). Robust principal component analysis based on discriminant information. *IEEE Transactions on Knowledge and Data Engineering, 35*, 1991–2003.

Gravel, P., Beaudoin, G., & De Guise, J. A. (2004). A method for modeling noise in medical images. *IEEE Transactions on Medical Imaging, 23*(10), 1221–1232.

He, J., Liu, Q., Christodoulou, A. G., Ma, C., Lam, F., & Liang, Z.-P. (2016). Accelerated high-dimensional MR imaging with sparse sampling using low-rank tensors. *IEEE Transactions on Medical Imaging, 35*(9), 2119–2129.

He, J., Zhang, D., Balzano, L., & Tao, T. (2014). Iterative Grassmannian optimization for robust image alignment. *Image and Vision Computing, 32*(10), 800–813.

Hu, Z., Nie, F., Tian, L., & Li, X. (2018). A comprehensive survey for low rank regularization. arXiv preprint arXiv:1808.04521.

Jain, P., Kar, P. et al. (2017). Non-convex optimization for machine learning. *Foundations and Trends® in Machine Learning, 10*(3–4), 142–363.

Jiang, Y., Wang, Y., Li, S., Zhang, Y., Zhao, M., & Gao, Y. (2023). Event-based low-illumination image enhancement. *IEEE Transactions on Multimedia, 26*, 1920–1931.

Kasten, J., Lazeyras, F., & Van De Ville, D. (2013). Data-driven MRSI spectral localization via low-rank component analysis. *IEEE Transactions on Medical Imaging, 32*(10), 1853–1863.

Kong, D., Ding, C., & Huang, H. (2011). Robust nonnegative matrix factorization using l21-norm. In *Proceedings of the 20th ACM International Conference on Information and Knowledge Management* (pp. 673–682).

Lerman, G., & Maunu, T. (2018). An overview of robust subspace recovery. *Proceedings of the IEEE, 106*(8), 1380–1410.

Li, P., Feng, J., Jin, X., Zhang, L., Xu, X., & Yan, S. (2017). Online robust low-rank tensor learning. In *IJCAI* (pp. 2180–2186).

Li, R., Wang, X., Lei, L., & Song, Y. (2018). *l*_{21}-norm based loss function and regularization extreme learning machine. *IEEE Access, 7*, 6575–6586.

Li, Y., Chen, C., Yang, F., & Huang, J. (2015). Deep sparse representation for robust image registration. In *Proceedings of the IEEE Conference on Computer Vision and Pattern Recognition* (pp. 4894–4901).

Liang, P., Likassa, H. T., Zhang, C., & Guo, J. (2021). New robust PCA for outliers and heavy sparse noises' detection via affine transformation, the l_,w and l_2,1 norms, and spatial weight matrix in high-dimensional images: From the perspective of signal processing, *International Journal of Mathematics and Mathematical Sciences, 2021*, 1–9.

Liang, P., Zhang, C., Likassa, H. T., & Guo, J. (2022). New robust tensor PCA via affine transformations and [formula: see text] norms for exact tubal low-rank recovery from highly corrupted and correlated images in signal processing. *Mathematical Problems in Engineering (Web), 2022.*

Likassa, H. T. (2020). New robust principal component analysis for joint image alignment and recovery via affine transformations and Frobenius and l_2,1 norms. *International Journal of Mathematics and Mathematical Sciences, 2020*, 1–9.

Likassa, H. T., & Fang, W.-H. (2018) . Robust regression for image alignment via subspace recovery techniques. In *Proceedings of the 2018 VII International Conference on Network, Communication and Computing* (pp. 288–293).

Likassa, H. T., Fang, W.-H., & Chuang, Y.-A. (2018). Modified robust image alignment by sparse and low rank decomposition for highly linearly correlated data. In *2018 3rd International Conference on Intelligent Green Building and Smart Grid (IGBSG)* (pp. 1–4). IEEE

Likassa, H. T., Fang, W.-H., & Leu, J.-S. (2019). Robust image recovery via affine transformation and *l*_{2, 1} norm. *IEEE Access, 7*, 125011–125021.

Likassa, H. T., Xia, Y., Gotu, B. et al. (2022). An efficient new robust PCA method for joint image alignment and reconstruction via the norms and affine transformation. *Scientific Programming, 2022.*

Lin, Z., Chen, M., & Ma, Y. (2010). The augmented Lagrange multiplier method for exact recovery of corrupted low-rank matrices. arXiv preprint arXiv:1009.5055.

Liu, H., Li, H., Fu, H., Xiao, R., Gao, Y., Hu, Y., & Liu, J. (2022). Degradation-invariant enhancement of fundus images via pyramid constraint network. In *International Conference on Medical Image Computing and Computer-Assisted Intervention* (pp. 507–516). Springer

Liu, Y., Chen, L., & Zhu, C. (2018). Improved robust tensor principal component analysis via low-rank core matrix. *IEEE Journal of Selected Topics in Signal Processing, 12*(6), 1378–1389.

Lu, C., Feng, J., Chen, Y., Liu, W., Lin, Z., & Yan, S. (2016). Tensor robust principal component analysis: Exact recovery of corrupted low-rank tensors via convex optimization. In *Proceedings of the IEEE Conference on Computer Vision and Pattern Recognition* (pp. 5249–5257).

Lu, C., Feng, J., Chen, Y., Liu, W., Lin, Z., & Yan, S. (2019). Tensor robust principal component analysis with a new tensor nuclear norm. *IEEE Transactions on Pattern Analysis and Machine Intelligence, 42*(4), 925–938.

Peng, Y., Ganesh, A., Wright, J., Xu, W., & Ma, Y. (2012). RASL: Robust alignment by sparse and low-rank decomposition for linearly correlated images. *IEEE Transactions on Pattern Analysis and Machine Intelligence, 34*(11), 2233–2246.

Prasad, K. M., & Bapat, R. (1992). The generalized Moore-Penrose inverse. *Linear Algebra and Its Applications, 165*, 59–69.

Rahmani, M., & Atia, G. K. (2015). Randomized subspace learning approach for high dimensional low rank plus sparse matrix decomposition. In *2015 49th Asilomar Conference on Signals, Systems and Computers* (pp. 1796–1800). IEEE

Rosas-Romero, R., Martínez-Carballido, J., Hernández-Capistrán, J., & Uribe-Valencia, L. J. (2015). A method to assist in the diagnosis of early diabetic retinopathy: Image processing applied to detection of microaneurysms in fundus images. *Computerized Medical Imaging and Graphics, 44*, 41–53.

Rublee, M. R., & Cohen, A. (2018). Nuclear norms in global governance: A progressive research agenda. *Contemporary Security Policy, 39*(3), 317–340.

Santosh, N. K., & Barpanda, S. S. (2022). Wavelet and PCA-based glaucoma classification through novel methodological enhanced retinal images. *Machine Vision and Applications, 33*(1), 11.

Sara, U., Akter, M., & Uddin, M. S. (2019). Image quality assessment through FSIM, SSIM, MSE and PSNR—a comparative study. *Journal of Computer and Communications, 7*(3), 8–18.

Shen, Y., Sheng, B., Fang, R., Li, H., Dai, L., Stolte, S., Qin, J., Jia, W., & Shen, D. (2020). Domain-invariant interpretable fundus image quality assessment. *Medical Image Analysis, 61*, 101654.

Singh, A., Chougule, A., Narang, P., Chamola, V., & Yu, F. R. (2022). Low-light image enhancement for UAVs with multi-feature fusion deep neural networks. *IEEE Geoscience and Remote Sensing Letters, 19*, 1–5.

Singh, N., Kaur, L., & Singh, K. (2019). Histogram equalization techniques for enhancement of low radiance retinal images for early detection of diabetic retinopathy. *Engineering Science and Technology, an International Journal, 22*(3), 736–745.

Solomon, O., Cohen, R., Zhang, Y., Yang, Y., He, Q., Luo, J., van Sloun, R. J., & Eldar, Y. C. (2019). Deep unfolded robust PCA with application to clutter suppression in ultrasound. *IEEE Transactions on Medical Imaging, 39*(4), 1051–1063.

Tang, Z., Chen, L., Zhang, X., & Zhang, S. (2018). Robust image hashing with tensor decomposition. *IEEE Transactions on Knowledge and Data Engineering, 31*(3), 549–560.

Vaswani, N., Bouwmans, T., Javed, S., & Narayanamurthy, P. (2018). Robust subspace learning: Robust PCA, robust subspace tracking, and robust subspace recovery. *IEEE Signal Processing Magazine, 35*(4), 32–55.

Vidal, R., Ma, Y., & Sastry, S. (2005). Generalized principal component analysis (GPCA). *IEEE Transactions on Pattern Analysis and Machine Intelligence, 27*(12), 1945–1959.

Wall, M. E., Rechtsteiner, A., & Rocha, L. M. (2003). Singular value decomposition and principal component analysis. In *A practical approach to microarray data analysis* (pp. 91–109). Springer

Wang, Y., Li, T., Chen, L., Yu, Y., Zhao, Y., & Zhou, J. (2021). Tensor-based robust principal component analysis with locality preserving graph and frontal slice sparsity for hyperspectral image classification. *IEEE Transactions on Geoscience and Remote Sensing, 60*, 1–19.

Wei, X., Li, Y., Shen, H., Xiang, W., & Murphey, Y. L. (2017). Joint learning sparsifying linear transformation for low-resolution image synthesis and recognition. *Pattern Recognition, 66*, 412–424.

Wen, F., Adhikari, L., Pei, L., Marcia, R. F., Liu, P., & Qiu, R. C. (2017). Nonconvex regularization-based sparse recovery and demixing with application to color image inpainting. *IEEE Access, 5*, 11513–11527.

Wen, F., Chu, L., Liu, P., & Qiu, R. C. (2018). A survey on nonconvex regularization-based sparse and low-rank recovery in signal processing, statistics, and machine learning. *IEEE Access, 6*, 69883–69906.

Wu, Y., Zhang, Z., Huang, T. S., & Lin, J. Y. (2001). Multibody grouping via orthogonal subspace decomposition. In *Proceedings of the 2001 IEEE Computer Society Conference on Computer Vision and Pattern Recognition. CVPR 2001* (Vol. 2, pp. II–II). IEEE

Xian, Y., Zhao, G., Wang, C., Chen, X., & Dai, Y. (2023). A novel hybrid retinal blood vessel segmentation algorithm for enlarging the measuring range of dual-wavelength retinal oximetry. In *Photonics* (Vol. 10, p. 722). Multidisciplinary Digital Publishing Institute.

Yaman, B., Weingärtner, S., Kargas, N., Sidiropoulos, N. D., & Akçakaya, M. (2019). Low-rank tensor models for improved multidimensional MRI: Application to dynamic cardiac t_1 mapping. *IEEE Transactions on Computational Imaging, 6*, 194–207.

Yang, J., Yin, W., Zhang, Y., & Wang, Y. (2009). A fast algorithm for edge-preserving variational multichannel image restoration. *SIAM Journal on Imaging Sciences, 2*(2), 569–592.

Zhang, C., Likassa, H. T., Liang, P., & Guo, J. (2021). New robust part-based model with affine transformations for facial landmark localization and detection in big data. *Modelling and Simulation in Engineering, 2021*, 1–11.

Zhang, F., & Yang, J. (2011). A linear subspace learning approach via low rank decomposition. In *2011 Second International Conference on Innovations in Bio-inspired Computing and Applications* (pp. 81–84). IEEE

Zhang, T., & Lerman, G. (2014). A novel m-estimator for robust PCA. *The Journal of Machine Learning Research, 15*(1), 749–808.

Zhang, X., He, J., Li, Y., Chi, Y., & Zhou, Y. (2021). Recovery of corrupted data in wireless sensor networks using tensor robust principal component analysis. *IEEE Communications Letters, 25*(10), 3389–3393.

Zhang, Y., Shi, D., Gao, J., & Cheng, D. (2017). Low-rank-sparse subspace representation for robust regression. In *Proceedings of the IEEE Conference on Computer Vision and Pattern Recognition* (pp. 7445–7454).

Zhao, H., Yuen, P. C., & Kwok, J. T. (2006). A novel incremental principal component analysis and its application for face recognition. *IEEE Transactions on Systems, Man, and Cybernetics, Part B (Cybernetics), 36*(4), 873–886.

Zhao, X., An, G., Cen, Y., Wang, H., & Zhao, R. (2019). Robust discriminant low-rank representation for subspace clustering. *Soft Computing, 23*, 7005–7013.

Zheng, Q., Wang, Y., & Heng, P. A. (2019). Online subspace learning from gradient orientations for robust image alignment. *IEEE Transactions on Image Processing, 28*(7), 3383–3394.

Zhu, W., Qiu, P., Farazi, M., Nandakumar, K., Dumitrascu, O. M., & Wang, Y. (2023). Optimal transport guided unsupervised learning for enhancing low-quality retinal images. arXiv preprint arXiv:2302.02991.

Part III
Public Health Applications

Chapter 8
SEIRD Mathematical Modeling of Malaria Transmission Dynamics in Ethiopia

Denekew Bitew Belay, Ding-Geng Chen, and Sintayehu Agegnehu Matintu

8.1 Introduction

Malaria is a leading cause of morbidity and mortality in developing countries, and it is one of the most severe public health problems worldwide. Nearly half the world's population lives in areas at risk of malaria transmission in only 87 countries and territories. Although there has been a significant decline in the new infection and death of malaria since 2000, it continues to be a global health threat and the decline stalled due to the COVID-19 outbreak, as shown in Fig. 8.1 adopted from WHO (2022) and from Fig. 8.2 taken from ISGlobal Barcelona Institute for Global Health (2023). According to the latest report in 2022, there were an estimated 249 million malaria cases and 608,000 malaria deaths only in 85 countries, staying significantly higher than the 2019 pre-pandemic levels. While a steady pipeline of innovative tools for malaria prevention and control is in place, the malaria financing gap has widened with a 3.7 billion USD deficit in 2022. Malaria epidemic in the WHO African region carries a disproportionately high share of the global malaria disease burden as compared to other regions which comprise 94% of malaria cases (233 million) and 95% (580,000) of malaria deaths. Only four African countries

D. B. Belay (✉)
Department of Statistics, Bahir Dar University, Bahir Dar, Ethiopia

Department of Statistics, University of Pretoria, Pretoria, South Africa

D. -G. Chen
Department of Statistics, University of Pretoria, Pretoria, South Africa

College of Health Solutions, Arizona State University, Tempe, AZ, USA
e-mail: Ding-Geng.Chen@asu.edu

S. A. Matintu
Department of Mathematics, Injibara University, Injibara, Ethiopia

D.-G. Chen, C. A. Coelho (eds.), *Biostatistics Modeling and Public Health Applications*, Emerging Topics in Statistics and Biostatistics,
https://doi.org/10.1007/978-3-031-69690-9_8

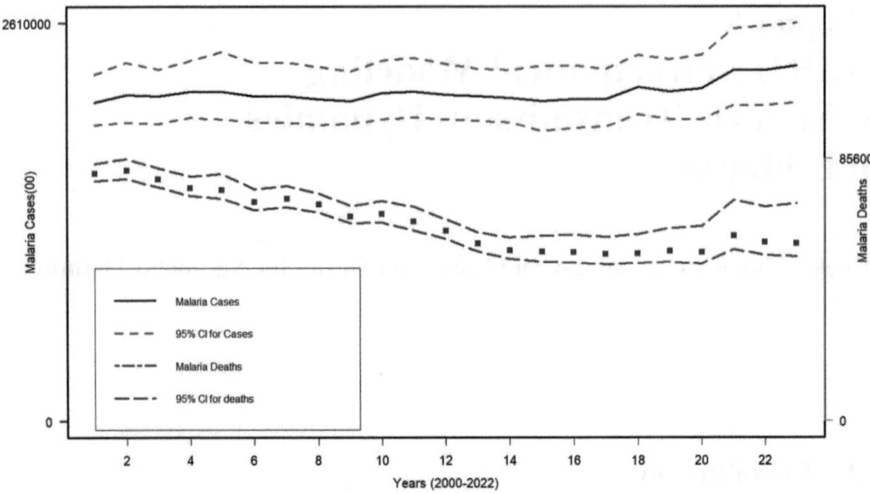

Fig. 8.1 Estimated malaria cases (00) and deaths are shown with 95% upper and lower confidence intervals from 2000 to 2022. (Adopted from WHO, 2023)

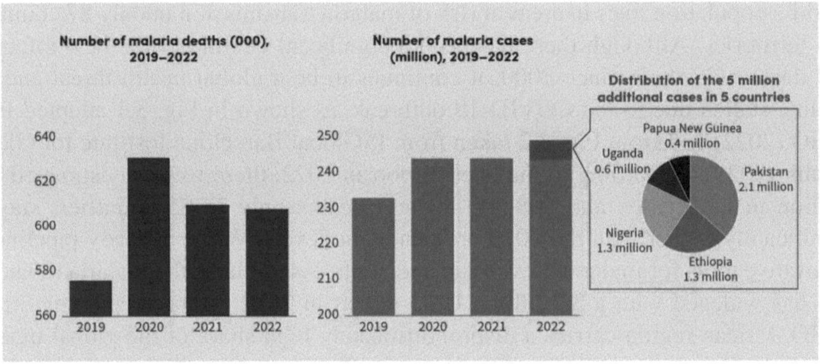

Fig. 8.2 Stalled progress against malaria meets a cocktail of threats. (Taken from ISGlobal Barcelona Institute for Global Health, 2023)

accounted for just over half of all malaria deaths worldwide: Nigeria (26.8%), the Democratic Republic of the Congo (12.3%), Uganda (5.1%) and Mozambique (4.2%). The distribution of the death count is much higher for under-five children, which accounts for about 78% of all malaria deaths in the Region. About 95% of all malaria cases occurred in sub-Saharan Africa and five countries (Pakistan, Ethiopia, Nigeria, Uganda and Papua New Guinea) shouldered most of the burden of the global rise in malaria cases (Kendie et al., 2021; WHO, 2022; ISGlobal Barcelona Institute for Global Health, 2023).

In Ethiopia, the distribution of malaria varies from place to place depending on extreme weather events, rainfall patterns, altitude, humanitarian crises and converging biological threats. In Ethiopia, 68% of the populations living in areas below 2000 meters of altitude are at risk of malaria, and there is approximately an average of 5 million cases a year (Belay et al., 2017; Hakizimana, 2020; Hawaria et al., 2021; Kendie et al., 2021; Nigussie et al., 2022b). In poor countries like Ethiopia, scarce resources and socioeconomic instability have hindered efficient malaria control activities, and local weather conditions often allow transmission to occur year-round during specific seasons. This disease was one of the leading health problems in Ethiopia which were even worst during the early years, and there were about 9.5 million cases per year between 2001 and 2005 (Legesse et al., 2007; Barofsky et al., 2011; WHO, 2015a, b, 2022; Hawaria et al., 2021; Yalew, 2022; ISGlobal Barcelona Institute for Global Health, 2023).

Although Ethiopia has shown successive malaria morbidity and mortality decline in the effort in the success of Millennium Development Goals (MDGs), there are still 9% and 8% of the global *Plasmodium vivax* cases that occurred in 2017 and 2018, respectively. Additionally, districts in the Amhara regional state have substantial malaria incidence variations, under lower transmission settings (Bugssa & Tedla, 2020; Hawaria et al., 2021; Nigussie et al., 2022a).

Malaria transmission, disease progression and associated risk factors are studied mostly using statistical models. These statistical models are usually applied for identifying the clinical, sociodemographic risk factors and spatial aspects to see the hot spot areas and distribution of the disease across the country and the region (Nigussie et al., 2022a, b). In the Amhara regional state, mathematical models like SEIRD, SEIRDS models of malaria dynamics are not frequently applied in the existing literature to see the changing aspects of the disease transmission in the region. Thus, the exposed, susceptible and infected proportion of the population in the region is not clearly known for policymakers and for appropriate interventions. Therefore, to get reliable approximation about the proportion of each compartment, mathematical models are crucial to know each compartment/population, and it is important for malaria control strategies and eventually eliminating malaria infection to reach the Sustainable Development Goals of UN2030 (World Bank, 2012a, b; WHO, 2015a, b, 2022; World Bank, 2016; WHO, 2023).

For better understanding of the disease transmission rate and for appropriate intervention, modeling the transmission of malaria disease is crucial. The general objective of this study is to explore malaria transmission using different mathematical modeling approaches. In this study, we applied susceptible-exposed-infected-recovered-death (SEIRD) model which is an extension of the classical susceptible-infected-recovered (SIR) and susceptible-exposed-infected-recovered (SEIR) epidemiological mathematical model to include E and D (hereafter referred to as model I) (Huang et al., 2010; Rodrigues, 2016; Carcione et al., 2020; Das et al., 2021a). To further analyze the malaria data in the Amhara regional state, Ethiopia, we extend the above SEIRD model in the sense that the infected population will recover from the disease and then again become susceptible and named as SEIRDS model, which can be described as susceptible-exposed-infected-recovered-death-susceptible model (hereafter referred to as model II). Both mode I and model II are further explored by considering the dynamic population approach which we called

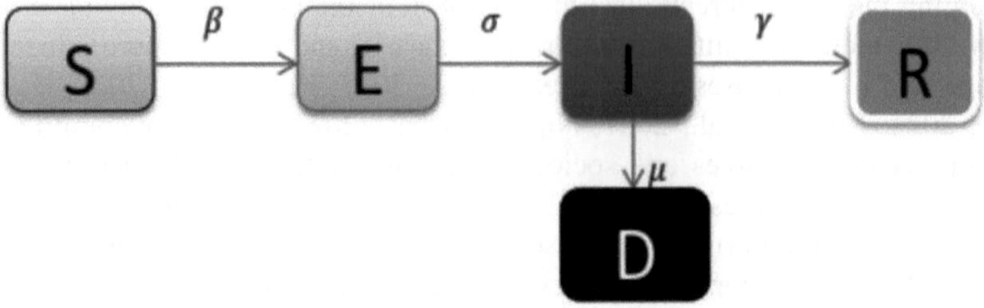

Fig. 8.3 Diagram of malaria transmission using SEIRD model

SEIRD and SEIRDS models with dynamic demography due to births and natural deaths (hereafter referred to as models III and IV) which are the extensions of the above two models (model I and model II) (Shah & Gupta, 2013; Biswas et al., 2014; Yan et al., 2016; Mojeeb et al., 2017; Das et al., 2021b; Melo, 2022).

8.2 Mathematical Disease Modeling

In this study, we used the Amhara regional state malaria cases reports, the yearly World Health Organization's malaria report and the Amhara regional state population. Then we classified these reports, obtained from various sources, into five groups or compartments based on their conditions related to the disease, in order to estimate the model parameters for our malaria disease modeling approaches. We described the above four extended SEIR models in details along with the data by applying two different scenarios in our malaria transmission mathematical modeling.

8.2.1 Mathematical Model I

In this first model, we assumed the SEIRD mathematical model approach which is an extension of SIR, usually groups of people who have recovered and died into a single statistic and SEIR models which includes E in the model, and the diagram for this model SEIRD is described in the below diagram (Kermack & McKendrick, 1927; Kamrujjaman et al., 2020) as shown in Fig. 8.3, where S represents susceptible population who are vulnerable to the disease but do not currently have it; E stands for exposed populations, I for infected population, or those who have the disease and can spread it to susceptible, R for recovered individuals or people who have had the disease but are now free of it and D for dead individuals. As it is indicated in the above diagram, the assumption in this mathematical model is that the infected population goes to the recovered population and never goes back to the S class, susceptible population.

In this model, we assume a constant population so that

$$N = S + E + I + R + D.$$

The parameters in the model are as follows: β is called the infectious contact rate, σ is the incubation rate, γ is the recovery rate and μ is mortality rate due to malaria infection.

The following first-order ordinary differential equation system can be used to characterize the malaria transmission mechanism:

$$\frac{dS}{dt} = -\frac{\beta SI}{N} \tag{8.1}$$

$$\frac{dE}{dt} = \frac{\beta SI}{N} - \sigma E \tag{8.2}$$

$$\frac{dI}{dt} = \sigma E - (\gamma + \mu) I \tag{8.3}$$

$$\frac{dR}{dt} = \gamma I \tag{8.4}$$

$$\frac{dD}{dt} = \mu I \tag{8.5}$$

With the initial conditions $S(0) > 0$, $E(0) \geq 0$, $I(0) \geq 0$, $R(0) \geq 0$, $D(0) \geq 0$.

8.2.2 *Mathematical Model II*

Some infectious diseases like malaria confer only temporary immunity, causing a flow of individuals from the R class to go back to the S class. These are referred to as SEIRDS disease model (model II) which we applied in this study by assuming that the recovered population goes back to the S class, susceptible population, and we introduced the rate at which the recovered individuals return to the susceptible population due to loss of immunity as α, and the model diagram is depicted in Fig. 8.4.

In this model, we assumed the individuals in the R class go back to the S class; the foregoing first-order ordinary differential equation system can be modified as follows:

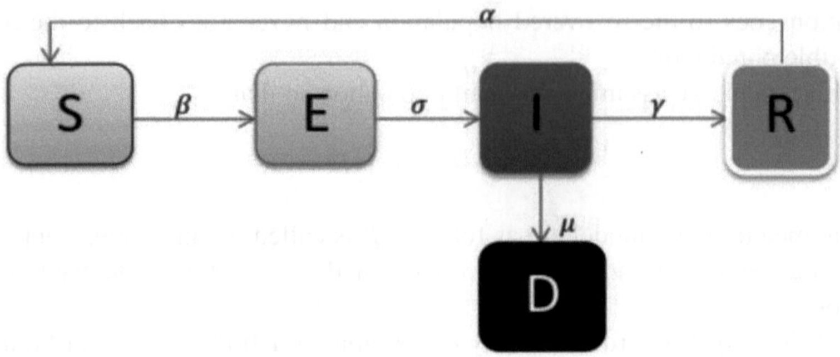

Fig. 8.4 Diagram of malaria transmission using SEIRDS model

$$\frac{dS}{dt} = \frac{-\beta SI}{N} + \alpha R \tag{8.6}$$

$$\frac{dE}{dt} = \frac{\beta SI}{N} - \sigma E \tag{8.7}$$

$$\frac{dI}{dt} = \sigma E - (\gamma + \mu) I \tag{8.8}$$

$$\frac{dR}{dt} = \gamma I - \alpha R \tag{8.9}$$

$$\frac{dD}{dt} = \mu I \tag{8.10}$$

With the initial conditions, $S(0) > 0$, $E(0) \geq 0$, $I(0) \geq 0$, $R(0) \geq 0$, $D(0) \geq 0$.

8.2.3 Mathematical Model III

In this model, we formulated the mathematical disease model assuming the dynamic demography by considering the existence of birth rate λ , which flows to the susceptible populations, and natural death rate δ , which is simultaneously deducted from each compartment, causing each proportion of the population to vary over time as depicted in Fig. 8.5.

In this model, we assumed that the *R* class does not go back into the *S* class, susceptible population, and the foregoing first-order ordinary differential equation system can be modified as follows:

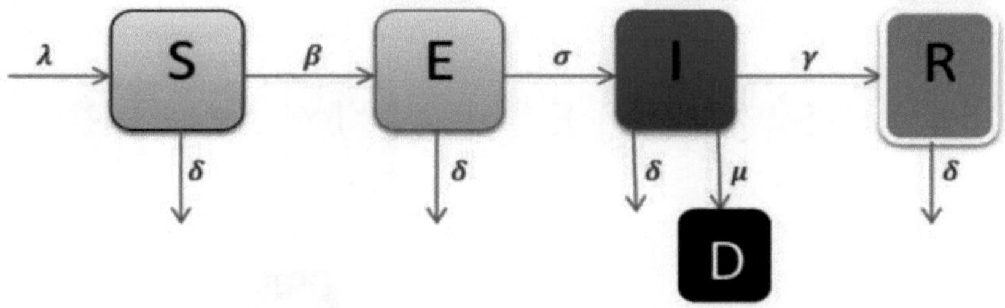

Fig. 8.5 Diagram of malaria transmission using SEIRD model with dynamic population

$$\frac{dS}{dt} = \lambda N - \frac{\beta SI}{N} - \delta S \tag{8.11}$$

$$\frac{dE}{dt} = \frac{\beta SI}{N} - (\sigma + \delta)\, E \tag{8.12}$$

$$\frac{dI}{dt} = \sigma E - (\gamma + \mu + \delta)\, I \tag{8.13}$$

$$\frac{dR}{dt} = \gamma I - \delta R \tag{8.14}$$

$$\frac{dD}{dt} = \mu I \tag{8.15}$$

With the initial conditions, $S(0) > 0$, $E(0) \geq 0$, $I(0) \geq 0$, $R(0) \geq 0$, $D(0) \geq 0$.

We now present the following theorem concerning the boundedness of the solutions.

Theorem All solutions $(S(t), E(t), I(t))$ of the model system equations (11–15) with nonnegative initial condition (S_0, E_0, I_0) are bounded and positively invariant in the region

$$\Gamma = \left\{ (S, E, I) \mid S + E + I \leq \frac{\lambda N}{\delta}, S > 0, E \geq 0, I \geq 0 \right\}.$$

Proof Since the variables R and D of the system equations (11–15) do not appear in the first three equations in the analysis, we only consider the first three equations of the system. Adding these equations to the system gives

$$\frac{d\,(S + E + I)}{dt} = \lambda N - \delta\,(S + E + I) - (\gamma + \mu)\, I \leq \lambda N - \delta\,(S + E + I)$$

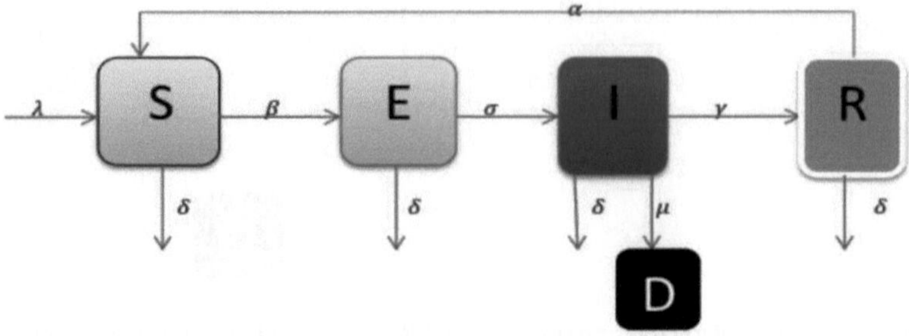

Fig. 8.6 Diagram of malaria transmission using SEIRDS model with dynamic population

By applying integration by part and evaluating the result as $t \to \infty$, we find that

$$S + E + I \leq \frac{\lambda N}{\delta}.$$

Therefore, the solutions of the model are bounded and positively invariant in the region Γ.

8.2.4 *Mathematical Model IV*

In this model, we formulated a mathematical disease model with demographic changes in the population by considering the birth rate and natural death rate of the population, and we also induce the assumption that the recovered population will return back to the susceptible populations. The diagram for this proposed mathematical model is described in Fig. 8.6.

By assuming that the R class, recovered population, goes back into the S class, susceptible population, the foregoing first-order ordinary differential equation system can be modified as follows:

$$\frac{dS}{dt} = \lambda N - \frac{\beta SI}{N} + \alpha R - \delta S \tag{8.16}$$

$$\frac{dE}{dt} = \frac{\beta SI}{N} - (\sigma + \delta) E \tag{8.17}$$

$$\frac{dI}{dt} = \sigma E - (\gamma + \mu + \delta) I \tag{8.18}$$

$$\frac{dR}{dt} = \gamma I - (\delta + \alpha) R \tag{8.19}$$

$$\frac{dD}{dt} = \mu I \tag{8.20}$$

With the initial conditions $S(0) > 0$, $E(0) \geq 0$, $I(0) \geq 0$, $R(0) \geq 0$, $D(0) \geq 0$. we can also present the following theorem concerning the boundedness of the solutions for model IV as follows:

Theorem All solutions $(S(t), E(t), I(t), R(t))$ of the model system equations $(16 - 20)$ with nonnegative initial condition (S_0, E_0, I_0) are bounded and positively invariant in the region

$$\Gamma = \left\{ (S, E, I, R) \mid S + E + I + R \leq \frac{\lambda N}{\delta}, S > 0, E \geq 0, I \geq 0, R \geq 0 \right\}.$$

Proof Since variable D of the system $(16 - 20)$ does not appear in the first four equations in the analysis, we only consider the first four equations of the system. Adding these equations of the system gives

$$\frac{d\,(S+E+I+R)}{dt} = \lambda N - \delta\,(S + E + I + R) - \mu I \leq \lambda N - \delta\,(S + E + I + R)$$

By applying integration by part and evaluating the result as $t \to \infty$, we find that

$$S + E + I + R \leq \frac{\lambda N}{\delta}.$$

Therefore, the solutions of the model are bounded and positively invariant in the region Γ. We implemented all the above four models using two scenarios or assumptions; the first scenario is without any intervention and the second scenario is the induction of any kind of intervention which helps to reduce disease transmission and deaths.

8.2.5 Calculation of Basic Reproduction Number (R_0)

In infectious disease modeling, it is important to estimate the basic reproduction number (R_0), and it is used to determine if the emerging disease can spread in a population and decide what proportion of the population should be immunized or vaccinated to eradicate the disease from the population. To understand the progression of the disease for all four models, we calculated the basic reproduction number (R_0), and the detailed algebra is explained in the next subsection for all four models (Mohajan & Mohajan, 2022).

R_0 in Mathematical Models I and II

Let

$$F_1(E, I) = \frac{\beta SI}{N},\ F_2(E, I) = \sigma E \text{ and } V_1(E, I) = \sigma E,\ V_2(\mathrm{E}, \mathrm{I}) = (\gamma + \mu) I$$

then ***SEIRD*** and ***SEIRDS*** models have a unique disease-free equilibrium, namely $(S^*, E^*, I^*, R^*, D^*) = (N, 0, 0, 0, 0)$, which can be obtained by setting all equations in model I and model II equal to zero. Thus, we determine the matrices F and V with components $F = \frac{\partial F_i}{\partial x_j}$ and $V = \frac{\partial V_i}{\partial x_j}$, for $i, j = 1, 2$, (where $x_1 = E$ and $x_2 = I$), and this can be defined as

$$F(S, E, I, R, D) = \begin{bmatrix} 0 & \frac{\beta S}{N} \\ \sigma & 0 \end{bmatrix}, \text{ implies that } F(N, 0, 0, 0, 0) = \begin{bmatrix} 0 & \beta \\ \sigma & 0 \end{bmatrix}$$

and

$$V(N, 0, 0, 0, 0) = \begin{bmatrix} \sigma & 0 \\ 0 & \gamma + \mu \end{bmatrix}$$

respectively. The next-generation matrix is defined to be $K = FV^{-1}$. Thus, the basic matrix multiplication yields

$$K = \begin{bmatrix} 0 & \beta \\ \sigma & 0 \end{bmatrix} \frac{1}{\sigma(\gamma + \mu)} \begin{bmatrix} \gamma + \mu & 0 \\ 0 & \sigma \end{bmatrix} = \begin{bmatrix} 0 & \frac{\beta}{\mu + \lambda} \\ 1 & 0 \end{bmatrix}.$$

Mathematically, the basic reproduction number, R_0, for model I and model II is known to be the largest spectral radius of the next-generation matrix K, and its eigenvalues are obtained as $\mathcal{R}_0^2 = \frac{\beta}{(\gamma + \mu)}$, where $\mathcal{R}$ is an eigenvalue of K. Thus, the basic reproductive number is taken to be the highest value of $\mathcal{R}$ and is simplified to be

$$R_0 = \sqrt{\frac{\beta}{(\gamma + \mu)}}. \tag{8.21}$$

R_0 in Mathematical Models III and IV

Let

$$\mathrm{P}_1(E, I) = \frac{\beta SI}{N},\ \mathrm{P}_2(E, I) = \sigma E$$

and

$$Q_1(E, I) = (\sigma + \delta) E, \; Q_2(\mathrm{E}, \mathrm{I}) = (\gamma + \mu + \delta) I.$$

Now, our **SEIRD** or **SEIRDS** model with dynamic population has a unique disease-free equilibrium, namely $(S^*, E^*, I^*, R^*, D^*) = \left(\frac{\lambda N}{\delta}, 0, 0, 0, 0\right)$. This disease-free equilibrium has been obtained by setting all equations in model III and model IV equal to zero. Thus, we determine the matrices P and Q with components $P = \frac{\partial F_i}{\partial x_j}$ and $Q = \frac{\partial V_i}{\partial x_j}$, for $i, j = 1, 2$, (where $x_1 = E, x_2 = I$), and this can be defined as

$$P(S, E, I, R, D) = \begin{bmatrix} 0 & \frac{\beta S}{N} \\ \sigma & 0 \end{bmatrix}, \text{ implies that } P\left(\frac{\lambda N}{\delta}, 0, 0, 0, 0\right) = \begin{bmatrix} 0 & \frac{\beta\lambda}{\delta} \\ \sigma & 0 \end{bmatrix}$$

and

$$Q\left(\frac{\lambda N}{\delta}, 0, 0, 0, 0\right) = \begin{bmatrix} \sigma + \delta & 0 \\ 0 & \gamma + \mu + \delta \end{bmatrix}$$

respectively. The next-generation matrix is defined to be $M = PQ^{-1}$. Thus, basic matrix multiplication yields

$$M = \begin{bmatrix} 0 & \frac{\beta\lambda}{\delta} \\ \sigma & 0 \end{bmatrix} \frac{1}{(\sigma + \delta)(\gamma + \mu + \delta)} \begin{bmatrix} \gamma + \mu + \delta & 0 \\ 0 & \sigma + \delta \end{bmatrix}$$

$$= \frac{1}{(\sigma + \delta)(\gamma + \mu + \delta)} \begin{bmatrix} 0 & \frac{\beta\lambda}{\delta(\sigma+\delta)} \\ \sigma(\gamma + \mu + \delta) & 0 \end{bmatrix} = \begin{bmatrix} 0 & \frac{\beta\lambda}{\delta(\gamma+\mu+\delta)} \\ \frac{\sigma}{(\sigma+\delta)} & 0 \end{bmatrix}.$$

As defined in section the basic reproduction number, R_0, for model III and model IV is also known to be the largest spectral radius of the next-generation matrix M, and it is calculated as $\mathcal{R}_0^2 = \frac{\beta\lambda\sigma}{\delta(\sigma+\delta)(\gamma+\mu+\delta)}$, where $\mathcal{R}$ is an eigenvalue of M. Thus, the basic reproductive number is assumed to be the maximum value of $\mathcal{R}$ and is simplified as

$$R_0 = \sqrt{\frac{\beta\lambda\sigma}{\delta(\sigma + \delta)(\gamma + \mu + \delta)}}. \tag{8.22}$$

8.2.6 The Estimation

In this study, we first estimated the model parameters using the observed malaria monthly time series data from the Amhara regional state, Ethiopia. In the above system of ordinary differential equation of four models, each compartment indicates the rate at which each compartment/population changes with a function of time and the corresponding rate of change; the parameters are estimated using the adaptation of the inversion methods to the available malaria data which is recommended by Taghizadeh & Mohammad-Djafari (2022) using differencing methods. The observed malaria data has 96 months' time series data and used for estimating the parameters β, σ *and* γ. Additionally, the rate at which the recovered individuals go back to the susceptible compartment (α) is estimated using the observed monthly malaria data by using the proportion of the recovered and susceptible for 96 months' time series malaria data. The other three parameters such as μ, λ and δ are estimated using the data from the WHO death report in 2013 and World Bank reports (World Bank, 2012a, b; WHO, 2013). The approximation method used for the above four mathematical models is the classic Runge-Kutta method, which is widely known as fourth-order Runge-Kutta (RK4) method to approximate numerically for the differential equations using MATLAB software with the given initial values for each population/compartment, and the procedure used to implement RK4 to the SEIRD and SEIRDS model can be found in Melo (2022).

8.3 Results

8.3.1 Mathematical Model I—SEIRD Model Parameter Estimation

We first estimated the parameters used in our SEIRD and SEIRDS malaria transmission models using available data obtained from different sources. The parameter used in SEIRD and SEIRDS malaria transmission models for both fixed and dynamic populations is (β, σ, γ, μ, α, λ and δ) with initial values $S(0)$, $E(0)$, $I(0)$, $R(0)$ and $D(0)$. We first estimated the three model parameters (β, σ and γ) using an adaptation of the inversion methods by using available data using a 96 months' time series observed malaria data as proposed by Taghizadeh & Mohammad-Djafari (2022), and the rate at which the recovered individuals go back to the susceptible compartment (α) is estimated using the ratio of the recovered and susceptible populations from observed malaria data. As recommended by Taghizadeh & Mohammad-Djafari (2022), we used the 96-month observed monthly time series malaria data for estimating these parameters using differencing methods.

The other parameters for this study, such as the rate of transition from infectious population to the death compartment (μ), natural death rate (δ) and birth rate (λ) are obtained from World Bank (2012a, b), and WHO (2013) to know the transmission rate from each respective compartment. The estimated parameters and initial values are presented in Table 8.1. We also assumed the susceptible population for malaria in the Amhara region to be 68% of the total populations in the region in 2012 as suggested by Taffese, Hemming-Schroeder et al. (2018). We obtained the number

Table 8.1 Parameter values estimated from observed data and initial values used for the prediction of malaria transmission for the proposed four models

Parameters	Estimates	Remarks
Beta (β)	0.239	Transmission rate of malaria disease
Sigma (σ)	0.041	The rate of the latent individual becoming infectious
Gamma (γ)	0.055	Recovery rate from the disease
Mu (μ)	0.003	The rate at which the infected individual goes to death compartment
Alpha (α)	0.0035	The rate at which recovered population goes back to susceptible populations
Birth rate (λ)	0.035	The birth rate which is added to the susceptible compartment
Death rate (δ)	0.008	The natural death rate which comes out from each compartment at this rate
Initial value for each compartment		
$S(0)$	13,256,842.6	The initial susceptible population in Amhara regional state which is 68 % of the population in 2012
E(0)	6,175,141.17	The initial exposed population in Amhara regional state in 2012
I(0)	63,373	The initial observed number of malaria cases in July 2012
R(0)	0	Assumed initial recovered population
D(0)	0	Assumed initial dead population due to malaria

of observed malaria cases from the Amhara Regional Public Health Institute, and the other compartments are calculated using these observed data.

8.3.2 Mathematical Model I Without Intervention

For this SEIRD disease model which we call it model I, we assumed the constant population with two scenarios, and in this section, we made a prediction by assuming without any intervention the scenario during the prediction period. For this SEIRD disease model which we call it model I, we assumed the constant population with two scenarios, and in this section, we made a prediction by assuming without any intervention scenario during the prediction period. As presented in Table 8.2 and Fig. 8.7, the prediction using model I shows that, out of the total susceptible population, approximately 469,027.54 individuals will not become infected by the end of the prediction period. At the peak of the infection period, a total population of 3,906,694.86 were simultaneously infectious. From the total infection period, a total population of 14, 991, 652.36 (76.9%) recovered by the end of the prediction period. From this prediction, to the utmost 817,726.49 population were assumed to be died during this epidemic period, for the total of 96 months. This shows that about 284 lives lost due to malaria every day which is a red line that victory over this epidemic is still a long way off. The fact that so many people are dying from vector-borne diseases or mosquito bites is one of the greatest tragedies of the twenty-first century. We also understood that the infection peak time occurred at the 46th month during the modeling period.

Table 8.2 Prediction without intervention scenario and some of the statistics using model I

	S	E	I	R	D
Max	13256842.60	6270345.92	3906694.86	14991652.36	817726.49
Min	469027.54	1414114.61	63373.00	0	0
Mean	4557575.94	4498243.93	2848790.97	7198121.13	392624.79
Median	2672204.19	5344937.52	3033758.51	7186745.08	392004.28
Std	4257622.75	1624353.67	932037.34	4988435.33	272096.47

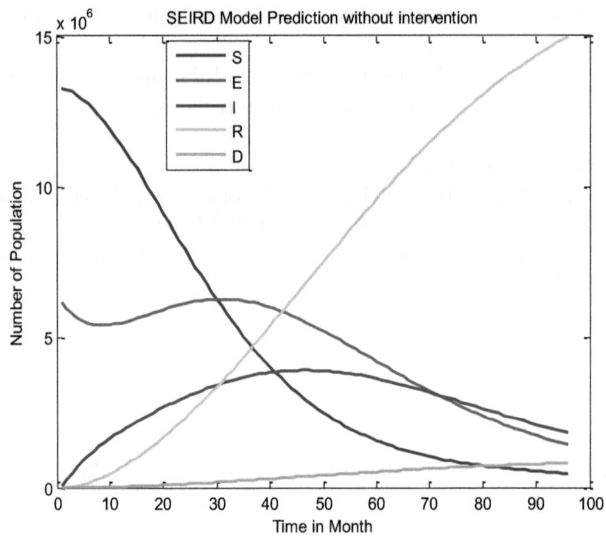

Fig. 8.7 Prediction of malaria infection using SEIRD model without any intervention and with constant population ($S = 13{,}256{,}842.6$, $E = 6{,}175{,}141.17$, $I = 633{,}73$, $R = 0$, $D = 0$, $\beta = 0.239$, $\sigma = 0.041$, $\gamma = 0.055$, $\mu = 0.003$)

8.3.3 *Mathematical Model I with Intervention*

If we employed our utmost potential for the reduction of the transmission of this malaria epidemic and apply the anticipated intervention to decrease the rate of transmission by 50%, by halving the rate of disease transmission, from 0.239 to 0.1195 and keeping other parameters the same as the above first scenario, we got a decreased number of infected populations and mortality using the SEIRD mathematical model. The expected reduction of the disease transmission rate can be achieved by using different intervention mechanisms like distribution of long-lasting insecticide net (LLIN), a campaign for proper usage of the available LLIN, advancement of indoor residual spraying (IRS) for as many as possible households and adequate drainage of pond to prevent mosquito development which is based on vector reduction/control mechanism by increasing the budgets from different budget sources to bring the disease under control. From this prediction as it is

Table 8.3 Prediction with intervention scenario and some of the statistics using model I

	S	E	I	R	D
Max	13256842.60	6175141.17	2752575.16	11733723.97	640021.31
Min	3585210.88	1801417.56	63373.00	0	0
Mean	7689182.77	3610162.59	2231422.86	5656075.34	308513.20
Median	7038246.47	3728422.78	2396983.22	5681540.31	309902.20
SD	3147303.46	1036152.56	568421.76	3772024.95	205746.82

depicted in Table 8.3 and Fig. 8.8, the total number of malaria infections can be decreased by 16% as compared to the first scenario (without intervention). The total number of deaths using this scenario decreased from 817,726.49 to 640,021.31 as compared to the first scenario. We can also understand from this model that from the total susceptible population, about 3,585,210.88 were not ever infected at any time during the malaria infection period. This shows that the total uninfected population is increased because of the presumed intervention as compared to the model without intervention. The total uninfected susceptible population has increased from 469,027.54 to 3,585,210.88. This implied that in a constant population, we can increase the total number of uninfected populations from 2.4% to 18.4%, which shows a big improvement with an increased healthy population if we applied the proposed intervention properly. About 3,116,183 of the susceptible population can be saved from malaria infection, which is 15.98% of the total population, if we impose the proposed interventions properly. We can also save the lives of many people by applying this intervention and can save about 177,705.2 lives from death.

8.3.4 *Mathematical Model I Short-Term Predictions Without Intervention*

We have also made a short-term prediction of malaria transmission to see the SEIRD model prediction consistency using the 48-month time period which is half of the long period. Using our short period SEIRD prediction without having any interventions, we can see from the result, out of the total susceptible population about 2,736,026.26 did not ever infected with malaria till the end of the prediction period. When we compare this prediction with our full-time prediction with the same time period, it is almost the same prediction which is about 2,736,053.36 susceptible populations as it is shown in Fig. 8.7. The total number of deaths at the end of the prediction period is 386,157.22, which is almost the same as the predicted deaths for half of the full-time period prediction with the same parameter settings (Table 8.4 and Fig. 8.9).

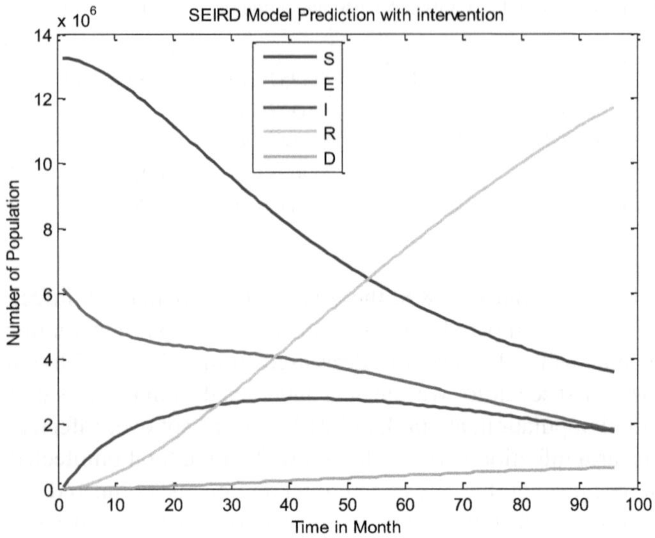

Fig. 8.8 Prediction of malaria infection using SEIRD model by applying the intended intervention ($S = 13{,}256{,}842.6$, $E = 6{,}175{,}141.17$, $I = 63{,}373$, $R = 0$, $D = 0$, $\beta = 0.1195$, $\sigma = 0.041$, $\gamma = 0.055$ and $\mu = 0.003$)

Table 8.4 Prediction without intervention scenario for a short period and some of the statistics using model I

	S	E	I	R	D
Max	13256842.60	6270292.25	3906835.24	7079548.97	386157.22
Min	2736026.26	5390631.95	63373.00	0	0
Mean	7978170.73	5865317.84	2722521.28	2777828.98	151517.94
Median	7798475.37	5894563.13	3044873.75	2381199.68	129883.62
SD	3516741.68	305076.85	1127678.10	2235354.37	121928.42

8.3.5 *Mathematical Model I Short-Term Predictions with Intervention*

In this case, we have made a short-period prediction using a presumed intervention to compare the SEIRD model prediction with the above corresponding model using the 48-month time period. In this short period, SEIRD prediction with interventions, out of the total susceptible population about 7,097,221.79, was not ever infected, which shows a great improvement in decreasing the infected populations. As compared to Fig. 8.8's similar full-period model and with the same prediction time period, the total uninfected population is almost the same with this short period prediction, which is a population of 7,097,293.02, and the results can be found in Table 8.5 and Fig. 8.10.

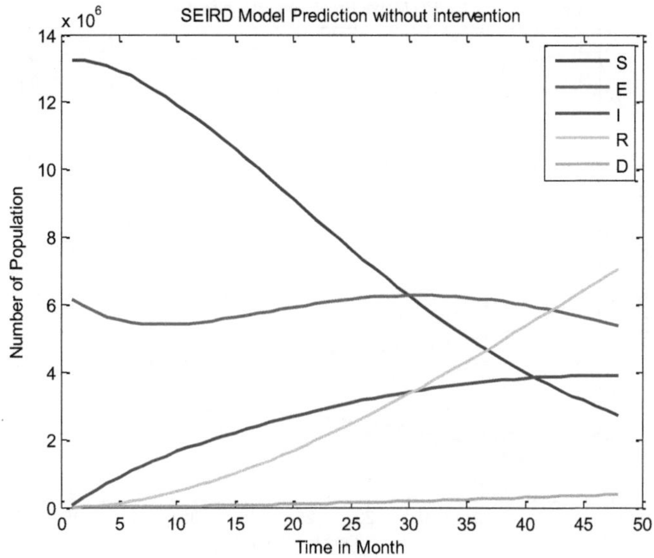

Fig. 8.9 Prediction of malaria infection using SEIRD model without intervention using a 48-month prediction period ($S = 13256842.6$, $E = 6175141.17$, $I = 63373$, $R = 0$, $D = 0$, $\beta = 0.239$, $\sigma = 0.041$, $\gamma = 0.055$ and $\mu = 0.003$)

Table 8.5 Prediction with intervention scenario for short period and some of the statistics using model I

	S	E	I	R	D
Max	13256842.60	6175141.17	2752660.74	5606280.53	305797.12
Min	7097221.79	3745810.52	63373.00	0	0
Mean	10400126.35	4468018.69	2152353.10	2346848.70	128009.93
Median	10445099.62	4316659.28	2477713.59	2139200.61	116683.67
SD	1998896.22	572263.91	736769.98	1780489.16	97117.59

8.3.6 Mathematical Model II Without Intervention

In this mathematical model (model II), we assumed the recovered population goes back to the susceptible population with the rate $\alpha = 0.0035$. When we compare this model (model II) with model I, there is a significant difference in the predicted compartments. As displayed in Table 8.6 and Fig. 8.11, the predicted infected population, which is 3,941,188.26 in model II, is higher than the infected population in model I, which is 3,906,694.86. This might be due to the additional flow of susceptible population from recovered population with the rate of 0.0035 which causes an increment of exposed populations, which can be used as a source of infectious population. On the other hand, the estimated recovered population in model II is less than the estimated recovered population in model I. This is due to an instant reduction of the recovered population which goes to the susceptible

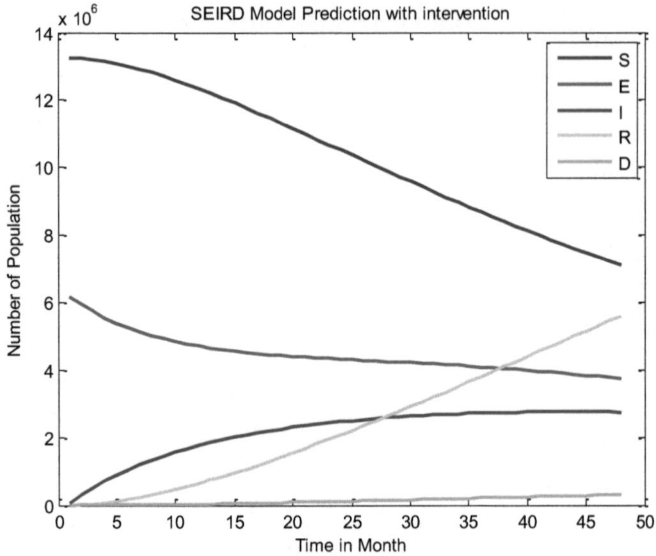

Fig. 8.10 Prediction of malaria infection using SEIRD model by assuming the intended intervention using a 48-month prediction period ($S = 13256842.6$, $E = 6175141.17$, $I = 63373$, $R = 0$, $D = 0$, $\beta = 0.1195$, $\sigma = 0.041$, $\gamma = 0.055$ and $\mu = 0.003$)

Table 8.6 Prediction and some statistical results of scenario one (without intervention) using model II

	S	E	I	R	D
Max	13256842.60	6298820.22	3941188.26	13214849.75	840529.59
Min	1371405.65	1929415.94	63373.00	0	0
Mean	4883489.47	4683971.51	2929428.81	6601203.01	397263.98
Median	2925996.39	5405944.17	3134616.98	6759931.92	393084.29
SD	4018482.03	1450385.95	924366.12	4443668.96	277607.80

population with a rate of 0.0035. The predicted death population in model II is greater than in model I. This is due to the existence of a more susceptible population due to loss of immunity which goes to the infectious population which causes an increase in death. In general, if a population is more vulnerable, there will be more infection and death unless intervention methods are implemented.

8.3.7 *Mathematical Model II with Intervention*

We also made a prediction with an intervention scenario for this model to see the changes in model II as compared to the first scenario. If we halved the disease transmission rate ($\beta = 0.1195$), we get a reduction of the infected population, and

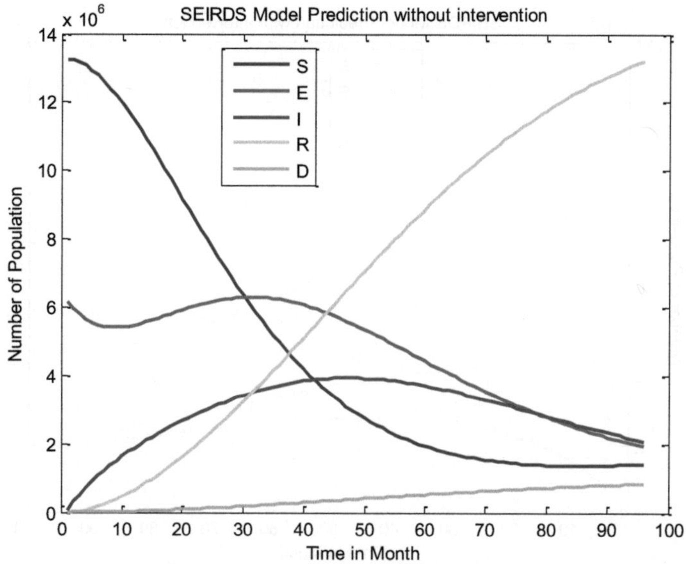

Fig. 8.11 Prediction of malaria infection using SEIRDS model by assuming without any intervention and with a constant population ($S = 13256842.6$, $E = 6175141.17$, $I = 63373$, $R = 0$, $D = 0$, $\beta = 0.239$, $\sigma = 0.041$, $\gamma = 0.055$, $\mu = 0.003$ and $\alpha = 0.0035$)

Table 8.7 Prediction and some statistical results of scenario two (with intervention) using model II

	S	E	I	R	D
Max	13256842.60	6175141.17	2763331.13	10212579.45	650410.23
Min	4680258.76	2077532.18	63373.00	0	0
Mean	8071175.82	3698099.79	2268225.37	5147317.90	310537.89
Median	7335384.56	3782944.34	2436983.40	5313372.47	310349.41
SD	2832995.61	951767.91	566108.98	3312246.11	208176.95

we also can save many young lives. As depicted in Table 8.7 and Fig. 8.12, the total number of malaria infections can be minimized by 17% as compared to model II without intervention as shown in Table 8.6. The total number of deaths using this scenario is decreased from 840,529.59 to 650,410.23 as compared to the above scenario which is predicted without any presumed intervention. The total uninfected susceptible population is increased from 1,371,405.65 to 4,680,258.76. This implied that in a constant population, the total number of uninfected susceptible population has been increased from 7% to 24%, which showed a big improvement with an increased healthy population, if we applied the proposed intervention properly. About 3,308,853 of the population can be saved from malaria infection, which is 17% of the total population, if we imposed the proposed interventions properly.

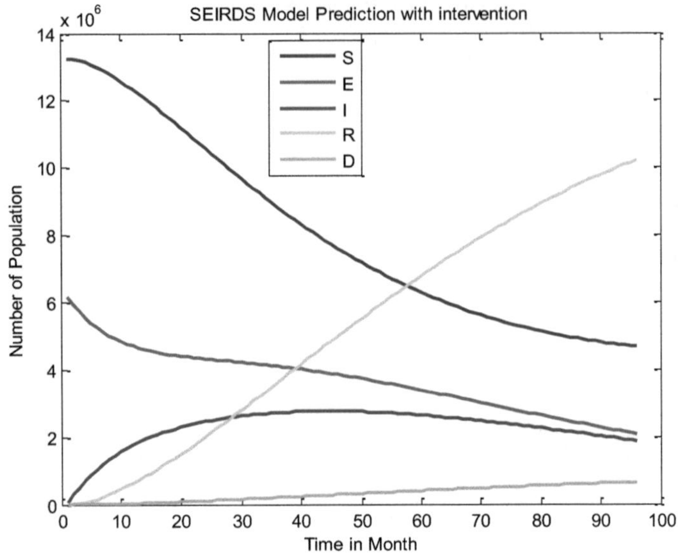

Fig. 8.12 Prediction of malaria infection using SEIRDS model without any intervention and with a fixed population ($S = 13256842.6$, $E = 6175141.17$, $I = 63373$, $R = 0$, $D = 0$, $\beta = 0.1195$, $\sigma = 0.041$, $\gamma = 0.055$, $\mu = 0.003$ and $\alpha = 0.0035$)

8.3.8 Mathematical Models III and IV

In this study, we have also made predictions using two additional extended models (model III and model IV). In model III, we assumed the existence of dynamic demography which includes birth and natural death rates and applied it for malaria disease prediction. We induce the Ethiopian birth rate and natural death rate which alters the assumptions of constant populations from which we obtained the estimated parameters from the report (World Bank, 2012a, b; WHO, 2013). The total number of infections in this model is relatively high since there is a new source of susceptible population from natural birth rates, and this contributes to an increase in the exposed population which contributes to be able to have an increased infection of malaria. Similarly, a reduction in malaria infection and deaths is observed when we applied the anticipated interventions using this model. We have also implemented a prediction using model IV by assuming that the recovered population goes back to the susceptible population and added to it in addition to the assumption included in model III. The predicted infected individuals using this model showed a big hump in the susceptible population which shows a large number of susceptible populations accumulated at the beginning of the infection period and the exposed population starts to decrease at the beginning of the prediction period of the infection then starts to build up and continues its increment and vice versa for the susceptible population. The position of these two compartments/populations exchanges around

Table 8.8 Estimated malaria case from the observed data and predicted malaria cases for each model without intervention

Observed malaria cases	Model I (SEIRD)	Model II (SEIRDS)	Model III (SEIRD) with dynamic demography	Model IV (SEIRDS) with dynamic demography
4,541,310	3,906,694.86	3,941,188.26	9,288,624.17	9,619,508.47

the 40th month of the prediction period. The result for these models is not displayed in this chapter.

8.3.9 Model Comparison

In this study, we made a comparison of our proposed four mathematical models using the predicted infected population and our observed malaria cases as described in Table 8.8, and we found that model II has a close approximation with the observed malaria cases, and it is the best model compared to other models based on the predicted malaria cases.

8.3.10 Malaria Disease Transmissibility and Basic Reproduction Number (R_0)

In epidemiological study, the basic reproductive number (R_0) is the key measure in estimating the ability of a disease to spread in the population, which is defined as the average number of secondary transmissions from one infected person. When the reproductive number, R_0, is greater than 1, the disease is spreading to the population and when R_0 is less than 1, the disease is dying out (Melo, 2022). In this study, we used the next-generation matrix method to obtain the basic reproduction number. And this estimated value, R_0, has an important implication for disease intervention and for bringing a disease under control by using different intervention mechanisms which may include long lasting insecticide net (LLIN) distribution, indoor residual spraying (IRS) and adequate drainage of pond to prevent mosquito development. Using the above methods which explain how to calculate the reproduction number in section "R_0 in Mathematical models I and II" Eq. 8.21, we found that the estimated basic reproduction number for model I and model II is 2.03, which shows that malaria will continue spreading in the population. Moreover, the basic reproduction number as explained in section "R_0 in Mathematical Models III and IV" in Eq. 8.22 for model III and model IV is 3.641. Similarly, this shows us the epidemic will continue spreading in the community unless strict intervention mechanisms take place in the region to bring the disease under control (Chaudhry, 2022).

8.4 Conclusion

In this study, we proposed four mathematical models, and for each of the four models, a prediction is made using the two scenarios referred to as "without intervention" and "with intervention." The two scenarios, without intervention and with intervention, are applied and prediction is made for each four models. To assess the model's predictive performance, we first estimated the model parameters from the observed Ethiopian malaria data. Then we used these estimated model parameters for our prediction. The four models applied in this study are SEIRD and SEIRDS with constant population and SEIRD and SEIRDS with dynamic population to see their prediction performance. From these four models, model II without intervention has predicted malaria infection, and it is similar with the observed malaria cases which we used for parameter estimation. Despite the fact that model III and model IV, respectively, have better parameter considerations which accommodate the natural death rate and birth rate, model II best predicted the malaria disease transmission as compared to the observed malaria cases. In this study, we used 68% of the total population of Amhara region as the susceptible population as recommended by Taffese, Hemming-Schroeder et al. (2018). The only observed data in our parameter estimation is monthly malaria cases, and the other data are taken from different literatures (World Bank, 2012a, b; WHO, 2013; Taffese et al., 2018). In this study, we found that the basic reproduction number (R_0) is greater than one, and it showed that malaria will continue as a public health threat. Based on this study, it is recommended that governmental and different national and international organizations continue their effort in the eradication of this epidemic by applying strict intervention mechanisms. The intervention mechanisms are long lasting insecticide net (LLIN) distribution, a campaign for proper usage of the available LLIN, an advancement of indoor residual spraying (IRS) for households and adequate drainage of ponds to prevent mosquito development which is based on vector reduction/control mechanism that can reduce the transmission of the disease, eventually making the epidemic no longer to be a public health threat.

Acknowledgments This work is partially based upon research supported by the South Africa Department of Research and Innovation (DSI), National Research Foundation (NRF) and South Africa Medical Research Council (SAMRC) (South Africa DSI-NRF-SAMRC SARChI Research Chair in Biostatistics, Grant number 114613). Opinions expressed and conclusions arrived at are those of the author and are not necessarily to be attributed to the NRF and SAMRC.

Appendices

A. MATLAB Code for Model I

A1. Without Intervention Scenario

```
function dydt = sinden(t,y,N,beta,sigma,gamma,mu)
dydt = [-beta*y(1)*y(3)./N;beta*y(1)*y(3)./N-sigma*y(2);sigma*y(2)-
(gamma+mu)*y(3);gamma*y(3);mu*y(3)];
end
time = 1:1:96;
y0 = [13256842.6;6175141.17;63373;0;0];%initial conditions for
S,E,I,R,D
N=19495356.77;
beta=0.239;
sigma=0.041;
gamma=0.055;
mu = 0.003;
ode = @(t,y) sinden(t,y,N,beta,sigma,gamma,mu);
[t,y] = ode45(ode, time, y0);

plot(t,y(:,1),'b',t,y(:,2),'m',t,y(:,3),'r',t,y(:,4),'c',t,y(:,5),'g','linewi
dth',2)

legend('S','E','I','R','D')
xlabel('Time in Month')
ylabel('Number of Population')
title('SEIRD Model Prediction without intervention')
%y(1)=S, y(2)=E, y(3)=I, y(4)=R, y(5)=D
```

A2. With Intervention Scenario

```
function dydt = sinden(t,y,N,beta,sigma,gamma,mu)
dydt = [-beta*y(1)*y(3)./N;beta*y(1)*y(3)./N-sigma*y(2);sigma*y(2)-
(gamma+mu)*y(3);gamma*y(3);mu*y(3)];
end
time = 1:1:96;
y0 = [13256842.6;6175141.17;63373;0;0];%initial conditions for
S,E,I,R,D
N=19495356.77;
beta=0.1195;
sigma=0.041;
gamma=0.055;
mu = 0.003;
ode = @(t,y) sinden(t,y,N,beta,sigma,gamma,mu);
[t,y] = ode45(ode, time, y0);

plot(t,y(:,1),'b',t,y(:,2),'m',t,y(:,3),'r',t,y(:,4),'c',t,y(:,5),'g','linewi
dth',2)

legend('S','E','I','R','D')
xlabel('Time in Month')
ylabel('Number of Population')
title('SEIRD Model Prediction with intervention')
%y(1)=S, y(2)=E, y(3)=I, y(4)=R, y(5)=D
```

B. MATLAB Code for Short-Period Prediction Using Model I

B1. Without Intervention Scenario for Short-Period Prediction

```
function dydt = sinden(t,y,N,beta,sigma,gamma,mu)
dydt = [-beta*y(1)*y(3)./N;beta*y(1)*y(3)./N-sigma*y(2);sigma*y(2)-
(gamma+mu)*y(3);gamma*y(3);mu*y(3)];
end
time = 1:1:48;
y0 = [13256842.6;6175141.17;63373;0;0];%initial conditions for
S,E,I,R,D
N=19495356.77;
beta=0.239;
sigma=0.041;
gamma=0.055;
mu = 0.003;
ode = @(t,y) sinden(t,y,N,beta,sigma,gamma,mu);
[t,y] = ode45(ode, time, y0);

plot(t,y(:,1),'b',t,y(:,2),'m',t,y(:,3),'r',t,y(:,4),'c',t,y(:,5),'g','linewi
dth',2)

legend('S','E','I','R','D')
xlabel('Time in Month')
ylabel('Number of Population')
title('SEIRD Model Prediction without intervention')
%y(1)=S, y(2)=E, y(3)=I, y(4)=R, y(5)=D
```

B2. With Intervention Scenario for Short-Period Prediction

```
function dydt = sinden(t,y,N,beta,sigma,gamma,mu)
dydt = [-beta*y(1)*y(3)./N;beta*y(1)*y(3)./N-sigma*y(2);sigma*y(2)-
(gamma+mu)*y(3);gamma*y(3);mu*y(3)];
end
time = 1:1:48;
y0 = [13256842.6;6175141.17;63373;0;0];%initial conditions for
S,E,I,R,D
N=19495356.77;
beta=0.1195;
sigma=0.041;
gamma=0.055;
mu = 0.003;
ode = @(t,y) sinden(t,y,N,beta,sigma,gamma,mu);
[t,y] = ode45(ode, time, y0);

plot(t,y(:,1),'b',t,y(:,2),'m',t,y(:,3),'r',t,y(:,4),'c',t,y(:,5),'g','linewi
dth',2)

legend('S','E','I','R','D')
xlabel('Time in Month')
ylabel('Number of Population')
title('SEIRD Model Prediction with intervention')
%y(1)=S, y(2)=E, y(3)=I, y(4)=R, y(5)=D
```

C. MATLAB Code for Model II

C1. Without Intervention Scenario

```
function dydt = sinden(t,y,N,beta,sigma,gamma,mu,alpha)
dydt = [-beta*y(1)*y(3)./N+alpha*y(4);beta*y(1)*y(3)./N-
sigma*y(2);sigma*y(2)-(gamma+mu)*y(3);gamma*y(3)-alpha*y(4);mu*y(3)];
end

time = 1:1:96;
y0 = [13256842.6;6175141.17;63373;0;0];%initial conditions for
S,E,I,R,D
N=19495356.77; % N=S+E+I+R+D
alpha=0.0035;
beta=0.239;
sigma=0.041;
gamma=0.055;
mu = 0.003;
ode = @(t,y) sinden(t,y,N,beta,sigma,gamma,mu,alpha);
[t,y] = ode45(ode, time, y0);

% Plot solution
plot(t,y(:,1),'b',t,y(:,2),'m',t,y(:,3),'r',t,y(:,4),'c',t,y(:,5),'g','linewi
dth',2)

legend('S','E','I','R','D')
xlabel('Time in Month')
ylabel('Number of Population')
title('SEIRDS Model Prediction without intervention')
%y(1)=S, y(2)=E, y(3)=I, y(4)=R, y(5)=D
```

C2. With Intervention Scenario

```
function dydt = sinden(t,y,N,beta,sigma,gamma,mu,alpha)
dydt = [-beta*y(1)*y(3)./N+alpha*y(4);beta*y(1)*y(3)./N-
sigma*y(2);sigma*y(2)-(gamma+mu)*y(3);gamma*y(3)-alpha*y(4);mu*y(3)];
end

time = 1:1:96;
y0 = [13256842.6;6175141.17;63373;0;0];%initial conditions for
S,E,I,R,D
N=19495356.77; % N=S+E+I+R+D
alpha=0.0035;
beta=0.1195;
sigma=0.041;
gamma=0.055;
mu = 0.003;
ode = @(t,y) sinden(t,y,N,beta,sigma,gamma,mu,alpha);
[t,y] = ode45(ode, time, y0);

% Plot solution
plot(t,y(:,1),'b',t,y(:,2),'m',t,y(:,3),'r',t,y(:,4),'c',t,y(:,5),'g','linewi
dth',2)

legend('S','E','I','R','D')
xlabel('Time in Month')
ylabel('Number of Population')
title('SEIRDS Model Prediction with intervention')
%y(1)=S, y(2)=E, y(3)=I, y(4)=R, y(5)=D
```

References

Barofsky, J., Chase, C., Anekwe, T. & Farzadfar, F. (2011). The economic effects of malaria eradication: Evidence from an intervention in Uganda (70).
Belay, D. B., Kifle, Y. G., Goshu, A. T., Gran, J. M., Yewhalaw, D., Duchateau, L., & Frigessi, A. (2017). Joint Bayesian modeling of time to malaria and mosquito abundance in Ethiopia. *BMC Infectious Diseases, 17*, 1–12.
Biswas, M. H. A., Paiva, L. T., & de Pinho, M. D. R. (2014). A SEIR model for control of infectious diseases with constraints. *Mathematical Biosciences and Engineering, 11*(4), 761–784.
Bugssa, G., & Tedla, K. (2020). Feasibility of malaria elimination in Ethiopia. *Ethiopian Journal of Health Sciences, 30*(4), 607.
Carcione, J. M., Santos, J. E., Bagaini, C., & Ba, J. (2020). A simulation of a COVID-19 epidemic based on a deterministic SEIR model. *Frontiers in public health, 8*, 230.
Chaudhry, M. R. A. (2022). Coronavirus infection outbreak: comparison with other viral infection outbreak. *Coronavirus Disease*. Academic Press, 47–57.
Das, K., Murthy, B., Samad, S. A., & Biswas, M. H. A. (2021a). Mathematical transmission analysis of SEIR tuberculosis disease model. *Sensors International, 2*, 100120.
Das, T., Srivastava, P. K., & Kumar, A. (2021b). Nonlinear dynamical behavior of an SEIR mathematical model: Effect of information and saturated treatment. *Chaos: An Interdisciplinary Journal of Nonlinear Science, 31*(4), 043104.
Hakizimana, E. (2020). *Using seir-sei mathematical model to illustrate the dynamics of malaria transmission in Rwanda*. University of Rwanda Digital repository. http://dr.ur.ac.rw/handle/123456789/1228
Hawaria, D., Kibret, S., Demissew, A., Tsegaye, A., Bitew, D., Yan, G., & Yewhalaw, D. (2021). Survivorship of Anopheles gambiae sensu lato in irrigated sugarcane plantation scheme in Ethiopia. *Parasites & Vectors, 14*, 1–10.
Huang, G., Takeuchi, Y., Ma, W., & Wei, D. (2010). Global stability for delay SIR and SEIR epidemic models with nonlinear incidence rate. *Bulletin of Mathematical Biology, 72*, 1192–1207.
ISGlobal Barcelona Institute for Global Health. (2023). World Malaria report 2023 highlights the climate change and health nexus.
Kamrujjaman, M., Saha, P., Islam, M. S., & Ghosh, U. (2022). Dynamics of SEIR model: A case study of COVID-19 in Italy. *Results in Control and Optimization, 7*, 100119.
Kendie, F. A., W/kiros, T. H., Semegn, E. N., & Ferede, M. W. (2021). Prevalence of malaria among adults in Ethiopia: a systematic review and meta-analysis. *Journal of Tropical Medicine, 2021*, 1–9.
Kermack, W. O., & McKendrick, A. G. (1927). A contribution to the mathematical theory of epidemics. *Proceedings of the Royal Society of London Series A: Containing Papers of a Mathematical and Physical Character, 115*(772), 700–721.
Legesse, Y., Tegegn, A., Belachew, T., & Tushune, K. (2007). Knowledge, attitude and practice about malaria transmission and its preventive measures among households in urban areas of Assosa Zone, Western Ethiopia. *Ethiopian Journal of Health Development, 21*(2), 157–165.
Melo, L. (2022). Modeling COVID-19 spread through the SEIRD epidemic model and optimal control. *Proceedings of GREAT Day, 2021*(1), 19.
Mohajan, D., & Mohajan, H. K. (2022). Mathematical analysis of SEIR model to prevent COVID-19 pandemic. *Journal of Economic Development, Environment and People, 11*(4), 5.
Mojeeb, A., Adu, I. K., & Yang, C. (2017). A simple seir mathematical model of malaria transmission. *Asian Research Journal of Mathematics, 7*, 1–22.
Nigussie, T. Z., Zewotir, T. T., & Muluneh, E. K. (2022a). Detection of temporal, spatial and spatiotemporal clustering of malaria incidence in northwest Ethiopia, 2012–2020. *Scientific Reports, 12*(1), 3635.
Nigussie, T. Z., Zewotir, T. T., & Muluneh, E. K. (2022b). Spatiotemporal trends and distributions of malaria incidence in the Northwest Ethiopia. *Journal of Tropical Medicine, 2022*, 6355481.

Rodrigues, H. S. (2016). Application of SIR epidemiological model: New trends. arXiv preprint arXiv:1611.02565.

Shah, N. H., & Gupta J. (2013). SEIR model and simulation for vector borne diseases.

Taffese, H. S., Hemming-Schroeder, E., Koepfli, C., Tesfaye, G., Lee, M.-C., Kazura, J., Yan, G.-Y., & Zhou, G.-F. (2018). Malaria epidemiology and interventions in Ethiopia from 2001 to 2016. *Infectious Diseases of Poverty, 7*(06), 1–9.

Taghizadeh, E., & Mohammad-Djafari, A. (2022). SEIR modeling, simulation, parameter estimation, and their application for COVID-19 epidemic prediction. Physical Sciences Forum, MDPI.

WHO. (2013). World malaria report 2013, Global Malaria Programme WHO report.

WHO. (2015a). *World malaria report 2014: Summary*. World Health Organization.

WHO. (2015b). *Global technical strategy for malaria 2016–2030*. World Health Organization.

WHO. (2022). *World malaria report 2022*. World Health Organization.

WHO. (2023). *World malaria report 2023*. World Health Organization.

World Bank. (2012a). https://data.worldbank.org/indicator/SP.DYN.CBRT.IN?locations=ET. Retrieved December 8.

World Bank. (2012b). https://www.macrotrends.net/countries/ETH/ethiopia/death-rate. Retrieved December 8, 2023.

World Bank. (2016). World development report 2016: Digital dividends.

Yalew, A. W. (2022). Achievements, gaps, and emerging challenges in controlling malaria in Ethiopia. *Frontiers in Tropical Diseases, 2*, 771030.

Yan, Q., Tang, S., Gabriele, S., & Wu, J. (2016). Media coverage and hospital notifications: Correlation analysis and optimal media impact duration to manage a pandemic. *Journal of Theoretical Biology, 390*, 1–13.

Chapter 9
Variable Selection in Generalized Semiparametric Longitudinal Models

Mohammad Arashi and Samuel Manda

9.1 Introduction

Predictive modeling in biomedical research is the utilization of statistical learning approaches to forecast diverse outcomes associated with disease infection, treatment response, disease progression, and epidemiological patterns. These models are essential in providing information in public health policies, enhancing clinical management, and enhancing the quality of life in patients. Since time dependency for disease progression, generalized longitudinal predictive modeling has become more important in recent years. With special focus on statistical learning techniques for predictive modeling, readers are referred to Wang et al (2005), Wang and Fan (2011), Wang (2017), Wang et al. (2018), and Taavoni et al. (2023).

Parametric learning ensures the accuracy of predictive modeling by requiring that important explanatory variables are regressed on the response variable and that the underlying assumptions for regression closely align with the data. For example, in HIV studies, the interest often focuses on modeling trajectories of CD4 count data as a component of the actual data analysis. Figure 9.1 exhibits a nearly nonlinear relationship between the duration of time and the CD4 response variable. Therefore,

M. Arashi (✉)
Department of Statistics, Faculty of Mathematical Sciences, Ferdowsi University of Mashhad, Mashhad, Iran

Department of Statistics, Faculty of Natural and Agricultural Sciences, University of Pretoria, Pretoria, South Africa
e-mail: arashi@um.ac.ir

S. Manda
Department of Statistics, Faculty of Natural and Agricultural Sciences, University of Pretoria, Pretoria, South Africa
e-mail: samuel.manda@up.ac.za

D.-G. Chen, C. A. Coelho (eds.), *Biostatistics Modeling and Public Health Applications*, Emerging Topics in Statistics and Biostatistics,
https://doi.org/10.1007/978-3-031-69690-9_9

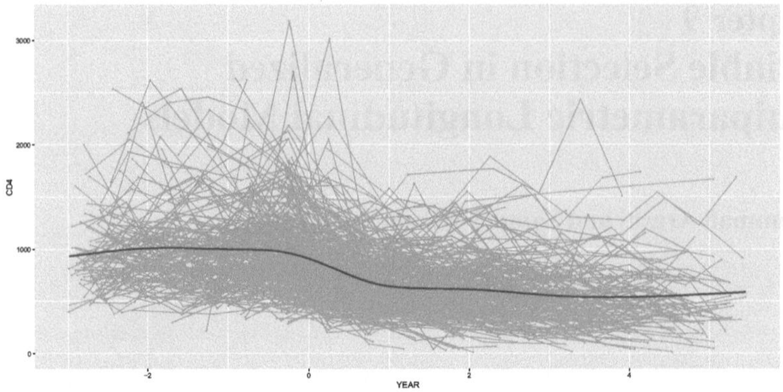

Fig. 9.1 Trajectory plot for the observed evolution (in gray) of CD4 cell counts for 369 men against time (in YEAR). Solid (in thick blue) line shows the smoothed mean profile of men

when it comes to predictive modeling, it is necessary to consider the characteristics of a partially linear model, also known as a semiparametric model, to accurately represent the true connection between the explanatory and response variables.

In the case of CD4 predictive modeling, additional concern arises with the distribution of the CD4 response variable. The primary investigations Wang et al (2005), Huang et al. (2007), and Ma et al. (2013) analyze the CD4 numbers after applying a square root transformation. This transformation is performed to approximate a Gaussian distribution for the data. Nevertheless, to account for the characteristics of the data and ensure accuracy, it is necessary to employ a discrete regression model. Therefore, it is necessary to take into account a generalized linear model (GLM) that incorporates a suitable link function to establish a linear relationship with the predictors. The linear predictor link function is limiting when considering the nonlinear trend shown in Fig. 9.1. The generalized semiparametric longitudinal model allows for both parametric and nonparametric relationships between the average response and the predictors. We cite the works of Roozbeh (2015), Roozbeh (2016), Roozbeh (2018), and Roozbeh et al. (2020) as reliable sources for comprehensive studies on semiparametric modeling.

This chapter examines the process of selecting important variables in predictive generalized longitudinal modeling, with a specific emphasis on parametric learning. For the application to modeling CD4 count data in HIV studies, we incorporate a semiparametric predictor component that accommodates both linear and nonlinear predictors in the nonnormal longitudinal model. Thus, we have combined the marginal mean model and addressed the correlation between repeated measurements. The organization of the rest of this chapter is as follows. Section 9.2 contains a detailed description of the semiparametric longitudinal model with LASSO for selecting relevant variables. This section primarily focuses on the methodological exploration. Section 9.3 presents our empirical application to the modeling of CD4 count data in HIV studies. The conclusions and future directions are provided in Sect. 9.4.

9.2 Model Specification and LASSO

Assume there are n subjects and the ith subject has n_i observations over time with $i = 1, \ldots, n$ and $j = 1, \ldots, n_i$. Let $N = \sum_{i=1}^{n} n_i$. Denote the set of explanatory fixed-effect and response variables by $\{(\boldsymbol{X}_{ij}, y_{ij}), i = 1, \ldots, n, j = 1, \ldots, n_i\}$ with the assumption $\mathrm{E}(y_{ij}) = \mu_{ij}$ and $\mathrm{Var}(y_{ij}) = \phi\nu(\mu_{ij})$, where ϕ is a scale parameter and $\nu(.)$ is a known variance function. For the generalized semiparametric longitudinal model (GSLM), we further assume the marginal mean μ_{ij} is given by

$$\eta_{ij} = g(\mu_{ij}) = \boldsymbol{X}_{ij}^{\top}\boldsymbol{\beta} + f(t_{ij}), \tag{9.1}$$

where $\mu_{ij} = g^{-1}(\eta_{ij})$, $\boldsymbol{\beta} = (\beta_1, \ldots, \beta_p)^{\top}$ is the regression coefficient vector, $\boldsymbol{X}_{ij}$ are the fixed-effect covariates, and $f(.)$ is an unknown smooth function. Further, $g(.)$ is a link function for the GSLM. We also assume independency between observations from different subjects. Finally, we assume t_{ij} are all scaled into the interval [0, 1].

Following Taavoni and Arashi (2021) and Taavoni et al. (2023), we approximate the smooth function by the polynomial spline as $f(t_{ij}) = \boldsymbol{B}^{\top}(t_{ij})\boldsymbol{\alpha}$, where $\boldsymbol{B}(t_{ij}) = \left(1, t_{ij}, \ldots, t_{ij}^{d}, (t_{ij} - t_i^{(1)})_{+}^{d}, \ldots, (t_{ij} - t_i^{(L_n)})_{+}^{d}\right)$ is a $h_n \times 1$ vector of basis functions, h_n is the number of basis functions used to approximate $f(t_{ij})$, $h_n = d+1+L_n$, d is the degree of the polynomial component, L_n is the number of interior knots, $(a)_+ = \max(0, a)$, and $\boldsymbol{\alpha}_n = (\alpha_0, \ldots, \alpha_d, \alpha_{d+1}, \ldots, \alpha_{d+1+L_n})^{\top}$ is the spline coefficients vector of dimension h_n. A small number of knots can provide satisfactory approximations. For the required number of knots, refer to Remark 1 of Taavoni et al. (2023).

This approach considers a nonparametric part as a linear relation with the basis functions as the pseudo-design variables. Therefore, this method linearizes our regression model (9.1) so that our GSLM becomes

$$\eta_{ij}(\boldsymbol{\theta}) = g(\mu_{ij}(\boldsymbol{\theta})) = \boldsymbol{X}_{ij}^{\top}\boldsymbol{\beta} + \boldsymbol{B}(t_{ij})^{\top}\boldsymbol{\alpha} = \boldsymbol{D}_{ij}^{\top}\boldsymbol{\theta}. \tag{9.2}$$

Here, the $(p + h_n) \times 1$ design matrix $\boldsymbol{D}_{ij} = \left(\boldsymbol{X}_{ij}^{\top}, \boldsymbol{B}(t_{ij})^{\top}\right)^{\top}$ blends the fixed and spline effects for the jth outcome of the ith subject. The combined regression coefficients $\boldsymbol{\theta} = (\boldsymbol{\beta}^{\top}, \boldsymbol{\alpha}^{\top})^{\top}$ have dimension $(p + h_n) \times 1$. Let $\boldsymbol{\mu}_i = (\mu_{i1}, \ldots, \mu_{in_i})^{\top}$, $\boldsymbol{Y}_i = (y_{i1}, \ldots, y_{in_i})^{\top}$, where $\mu_{ij} = g^{-1}(\boldsymbol{D}_{ij}^{\top}\boldsymbol{\theta})$, and $\boldsymbol{D}_i = (\boldsymbol{X}_i^{\top}, \boldsymbol{B}(\boldsymbol{t}_i)^{\top})^{\top}$.

9.2.1 Variable Selection

Our primary objective is to accurately estimate the vector parameter $\boldsymbol{\theta}$, which comprises the fixed-effect regression parameters as well as the spline coefficients. In sparse modeling scenarios, Tibshirani's least absolute shrinkage and selection operator (LASSO) can prove to be beneficial for variable selection. However, it is important to note that our method must only regularize the fixed-effect regression parameters $\boldsymbol{\beta}$ for variable selection. The proposed regularized technique of Taavoni et al. (2023) efficiently shrinks the vector parameter components using the ridge generalized estimating equation (GEE) procedure. Employing this approach requires us to first approximate LASSO. To achieve this, we use the local quadratic approximation (LQA) for LASSO. Similar approaches have been used in Oelker and Tutz (2017) and van der Wurp and Groll (2023).

For our purpose, denote the covariance matrix of $\boldsymbol{Y}_i$ by $\boldsymbol{V}_i$, where $\boldsymbol{V}_i = \boldsymbol{A}_i^{1/2}(\boldsymbol{\theta})\boldsymbol{R}(\boldsymbol{\tau})\boldsymbol{A}_i^{1/2}(\boldsymbol{\theta})$, with the finite-dimensional parameter $\boldsymbol{\tau}$, and $\boldsymbol{R}(\boldsymbol{\tau})$ is the working correlation matrix. Some commonly used working correlation structures include independence, autocorrelation (AR)-1, equally correlated, or unstructured correlation. For a given working correlation structure, $\boldsymbol{\tau}$ can be estimated using the residual-based moment method. The marginal density of Y_{ij} follows a canonical exponential family. Consequently, $\mu_{ij}(\boldsymbol{\theta}) = a(\theta_{ij})$ and $\sigma_{ij}^2(\boldsymbol{\theta}) = \phi a'(\theta_{ij})$, where $\theta_{ij} = \boldsymbol{D}_{ij}^\top\boldsymbol{\theta}$, for a differentiable function $a()$ and a scaling constant ϕ. Assume $\hat{\boldsymbol{R}}$ is the estimated working correlation matrix. For general purposes, one may assume $P_\lambda(|\boldsymbol{\beta}|) = (P_\lambda(|\beta_1|), \ldots, P_\lambda(|\beta_p|))^\top$ is the penalty term on the vector parameter $\boldsymbol{\beta}$ and λ is the tuning parameter. Then, using LQA, the approximated penalized GEE is given by

$$\begin{aligned}\boldsymbol{U}(\boldsymbol{\theta}) &= \boldsymbol{S}(\boldsymbol{\theta}) - q_\lambda(|\boldsymbol{\beta}|)\text{sgn}(\boldsymbol{\beta}) \\ &\propto \boldsymbol{S}(\boldsymbol{\theta}) - \boldsymbol{Q}\boldsymbol{\beta},\end{aligned} \tag{9.3}$$

where $q_\lambda(|\boldsymbol{\beta}|) = (q_\lambda(|\beta_1|), \ldots, q_\lambda(|\beta_p|))^\top$, $\text{sgn}(\boldsymbol{\beta}) = (\text{sgn}(\beta_1), \ldots, \text{sgn}(\beta_p))^\top$, $q_\lambda(x) = d/dx(P_\lambda(x))$, the first derivative,

$$\boldsymbol{Q} = \text{diag}\left(\frac{q_\lambda(|\beta_1^o|)}{|\beta_1^o|}, \ldots, \frac{q_\lambda(|\beta_p^o|)}{|\beta_p^o|}\right)$$

around the local point $\boldsymbol{\beta}^o = (\beta_1^o, \ldots, \beta_p^o)^\top$, and

$$\boldsymbol{S}(\boldsymbol{\theta}) = \frac{1}{n}\sum_{i=1}^{n} \boldsymbol{D}_i^\top \boldsymbol{A}_i^{1/2}(\boldsymbol{\theta})\hat{\boldsymbol{R}}^{-1}\boldsymbol{A}_i^{-1/2}(\boldsymbol{\theta})\big(\boldsymbol{Y}_i - \boldsymbol{\mu}_i(\boldsymbol{\theta})\big) \tag{9.4}$$

are the estimating functions defining the GEE. The penalized/regularized estimator $\hat{\boldsymbol{\beta}}_R$ is the solution to $\boldsymbol{U}(\boldsymbol{\theta}) = \boldsymbol{0}$. Since $\boldsymbol{U}(\boldsymbol{\theta})$ may contain discontinuous points, the equation $\boldsymbol{U}(\boldsymbol{\theta}) = \mathbf{0}$ may not have a solution, and hence we seek for an approximate solution, i.e., we find $\hat{\boldsymbol{\theta}}$ such that $\boldsymbol{U}(\hat{\boldsymbol{\theta}}) = o(a_n)$, with $a_n \to 0$. We use the Newton–Raphson algorithm along with (9.4), to get the following recursive solution:

$$\hat{\boldsymbol{\theta}}^{k+1} = \hat{\boldsymbol{\theta}}^{k} + \left[\boldsymbol{H}\left(\hat{\boldsymbol{\theta}}^{k}\right) + n\lambda \boldsymbol{E}\left(\hat{\boldsymbol{\theta}}^{k}\right)\right]^{-1} \times \left[\boldsymbol{S}\left(\hat{\boldsymbol{\theta}}^{k}\right) - n\lambda \boldsymbol{E}\left(\hat{\boldsymbol{\theta}}^{k}\right)\hat{\boldsymbol{\theta}}^{k}\right], \quad (9.5)$$

where

$$\boldsymbol{H}(\hat{\boldsymbol{\theta}}^{k}) = n^{-1}\sum_{i=1}^{n} \boldsymbol{D}_i^{\top} \boldsymbol{A}_i^{1/2}(\boldsymbol{\theta})\hat{\boldsymbol{R}}^{-1}\boldsymbol{A}_i^{-1/2}(\boldsymbol{\theta})\boldsymbol{D}_i$$

and

$$\boldsymbol{E}(\hat{\boldsymbol{\theta}}^{k}) = \text{diag}\left(\frac{q_\lambda(|\beta_1|)}{\epsilon + |\beta_1|}, \ldots, \frac{q_\lambda(|\beta_p|)}{\epsilon + |\beta_p|}, \mathbf{0}_{h_n}\right), \quad \epsilon = 10^{-6}$$

with $\mathbf{0}_{h_n}$ is an h_n-dimensional vector of zeros.

In this chapter, we focus on the LASSO for variable selection and compare its performance with the ridge of recent study Taavoni et al. (2023). Thus, for the LASSO, we have $P_\lambda(|\boldsymbol{\beta}|) = \lambda\sum_{j=1}^{p}|\beta_j|$, and consequently, $\boldsymbol{Q} = \lambda\text{diag}\left(\frac{1}{|\beta_1^o|}, \ldots, \frac{1}{|\beta_p^o|}\right)$. Furthermore, $\boldsymbol{E}(\hat{\boldsymbol{\theta}}^{k}) = \text{diag}\left(\lambda^{-1}\boldsymbol{Q}, \mathbf{0}_{h_n}\right)$. The suggested estimation approach can be implemented step by step, by combining the approximated penalized procedure into the Newton–Raphson iterative algorithm of GEE.

9.2.2 *Tuning Selection*

When selecting a tuning parameter λ, it is important to choose a value that will give you the results you are looking for in the selection process. While there are many methods for choosing the optimal tuning parameter, traditional model selection criteria like AIC and BIC have their limitations. To address this problem, Fan and Li (2001) suggested using generalized cross-validation (GCV), while Wang et al. (2007) proposed a Bayesian information criterion (BIC). For high-dimensional data, Wang et al. (2009) introduced a modified BIC to choose λ. Additionally, Li et al. (2011) expanded on the BIC information criterion. In our case, we will be using the recommended GCV method from Fan and Li (2001) to choose the tuning parameter λ. It is given by

$$\text{GCV}_\lambda = \frac{\frac{1}{n}\text{RSS}(\lambda_n)}{\left(1 - \frac{1}{n}d(\lambda_n)\right)^2},$$

where

$$\mathrm{RSS}(\lambda) = \frac{1}{n} \sum_{i=1}^{n} \big(y_i - \mu_i(\hat{\theta})\big)^{\top} \hat{V}_i^{-1} \big(y_i - \mu_i(\hat{\theta})\big)$$

is the residual sum of squares, and effective number is equal to

$$d(\lambda) = \mathrm{tr}\Big[\Big\{\boldsymbol{H}(\hat{\theta}) + n\mathrm{E}(\hat{\theta})\Big\}^{-1} \times \boldsymbol{H}_n(\hat{\theta})\Big].$$

The optimal parameter denoted by λ_{opt} is the minimizer of the GCV_{λ}. In practical implementation, one can use PGEE package of R software, where function CVfit computes cross-validated tuning parameter value for longitudinal data.

9.3 Modeling CD4 count data

In this section, to illustrate our method, we consider longitudinal CD4 count data of 369 men infected with the HIV virus. In total, there are 2376 observations of CD4 counts. Figure 9.2 (top-left) displays the CD4 trajectories of 369 men.

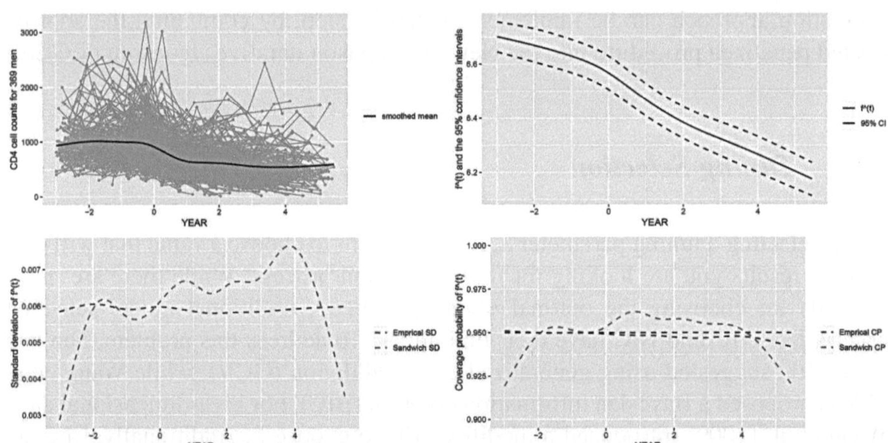

Fig. 9.2 Plots for estimated $f(t)$ for AIDS data based on LASSO and ridge. Plot top-left shows the trajectories plot for CD4 data. Observed evolution (in gray) of CD4 cell counts for 369 men against time (in YEAR). Solid (in thick blue) line shows the smoothed mean profile of men. Plot top-right shows the estimated baseline function $f(t)$ (in thick blue) in the selected model of P-GSLM and the 95% confidence interval (dashed line) corresponding to the robust confidence interval. Plots bottom-left and bottom-right, respectively, show the standard deviation and coverage probability rates for 95% confidence intervals based on empirical variance and sandwich formula

The primary goal of this analysis is to determine the average duration of CD4 decay in a population, taking into consideration additional predictor variables such as age, smoking status (measured in packs of cigarettes), drug use (yes, 1; no, 0), the number of sex partners, depression (as measured by the CESD scale, where larger values indicate more severe symptoms), and the effect of time since seroconversion (year). Incorporating a correlation structure into the estimation method is necessary due to the apparent positive correlation among responses from the same patient. According to Zeger and Diggle (1994), the data was reasonably well-fit by the compound symmetry covariance matrix.

For our research, we utilized a generalized semiparametric longitudinal model (GSLM) to fit the data. We did not transform the CD4 variable and instead employed Poisson regression. A significant statistical test, using the empirical Kolmogorov–Smirnov, confirmed the goodness of Poisson fit. In order to use the flexibility offered by partly linear models, we choose to represent the variable YEAR in a nonparametric manner, while the remaining variables are modeled parametrically. We conducted an analysis to determine if there are any interaction effects between the parametric covariates. To do this, we included all of these interactions in the parametric component of the study. We subsequently utilized the suggested methodology to choose noteworthy variables. We employed the LASSO penalty with a tuning parameter of $\lambda = 0.45$. In order to assess the effectiveness of our new approach (P-SLM) in comparison to two other existing scenarios, namely the unpenalized GSLM and the penalized GLM (P-GLM), we applied the sandwich method to determine the standard errors (SE) for all three methods. In order to determine the most suitable model based on the data, we leverage the Akaike information criterion (AIC) and the Bayesian information criterion (BIC). They are respectively given as $\text{AIC} = 2m - 2\ell_{\max}$ and $\text{BIC} = m \log n - 2\ell_{\max}$, where $\ell_{\max}$ is the maximized log-likelihood value and m is the number of free parameters in the model. Table 9.1 presents the summary of the fitting results including the values of standard errors, together with $\ell_{\max}$, AIC, and BIC under the three models.

Based on the data presented in Table 9.1, it can be observed that the P-GSLM generally has somewhat higher standard errors compared to both the GSLM and P-GLM. However, this difference is not particularly significant. Yet, the AIC and BIC values of our suggested model are lower than those of the other two competing models, indicating that the P-GSLM offers superior fitting performance. According to the P-GSLM model, the variables SMOKE, DRUGS, SEXP, $SOMKE*DRUG$, and $DRUG * SEXP$ are considered to be significant covariates. There is a modest variation in selection when P-GLM is employed, indicating that the variables $AGE * SMOKE$, $AGE * DRUG$, and $SMOKE * SEXP$ might also have a major impact. We have identified notable interactions between some factors that were ignored by Wang et al (2005) and Huang et al. (2007). The nonparametric curve estimates obtained using the P-GSLM estimators are visualized in Fig. 9.2 for the year $YEAR$. The display includes the estimated nonparametric function $f(t)$, its 95% point-wise confidence bands, standard deviation, and 95% coverage probability calculated using the empirical and sandwich formula variance. It is evident that the baseline function $f(t)$ has a diminishing impact as time progresses. Thus, it is

Table 9.1 Summary of parameter estimates along with standard errors (in parentheses) under the three fitted models for the HIV data

	GSLM	P-GLM	P-GSLM
Variables	$\widehat{\beta}$(SE)	$\widehat{\beta}$(SE)	$\widehat{\beta}$(SE)
AGE	0.073(0.039)	−0.092(0.051)	0(0)
$SMOKE$	0.188(0.179)	0.888(0.192)	0.079(0.045)
$DRUG$	0.130(0.143)	6.068(0.125)	0.142(0.074)
$SEXP$	−0.049(0.031)	0.672(0.030)	0.017(0.012)
$CESD$	−0.001(0.011)	0(0)	0(0)
$AGE * SMOKE$	0.002(0.014)	0.014(0.004)	0(0)
$AGE * DRUG$	−0.034(0.024)	0.032(0.035)	0(0)
$AGE * SEXP$	−0.009(0.003)	0(0)	0(0)
$AGE * CESD$	0.001(0.002)	0(0)	0(0)
$SMOKE * DRUG$	0.009(0.054)	−0.584(0.150)	−0.014(0.038)
$SMOKE * SEXP$	−0.010(0.012)	−0.034(0.010)	0(0)
$SMOKE * CESD$	−0.006(0.009)	0(0)	0(0)
$DRUG * SEXP$	−0.025(0.019)	−0.598(0.041)	−0.022(0.012)
$DRUG * CESD$	0.006(0.006)	0(0)	0(0)
$SEXP * CESD$	0.001(0.003)	0(0)	0(0)
$\ell_{\max}$	8463007	7529158	8624429
AIC	−16925983	−15058286	−17248827
BIC	−16925924	−15058228	−17248769

evident that placing it as a nonlinear component is a more rational choice. We see a discrepancy between the empirical standard deviation and the standard deviation calculated using the sandwich formula for the boundary positions. In cases when the sandwich formula standard deviations are smaller, the coverage probability decreases from 95

9.4 Remarks and Directions

We employed a generalized semiparametric longitudinal model (GSLM) and LASSO regression to address the issues of nonlinearity in the connection between the average response and variables, as well as the sparse significant estimation in the analysis of longitudinal data. The efficacy of our suggested approach diminishes as the interdependencies among the predictors of the model increased. The usefulness of our approach has been demonstrated by an analysis of CD4 count data among HIV positive men. By accurately identifying the response distribution in the GSLM, the variable selection strategy uncovered a significant interaction impact between the explanatory factors.

Although the LASSO has advantageous theoretical and computational qualities, it is associated with two drawbacks: (1) In high-dimensional scenarios, the LASSO approach is constrained to select a maximum number of variables that are equal to the sample size. This limitation restricts its effectiveness as a variable selection technique. (2) In the presence of a set of variables that are closely associated, the LASSO algorithm tends to choose only one variable from the group in an arbitrary manner. Therefore, in future investigations, our findings can be applied to scenarios involving group effects and employing alternative variable selection methods such as elastic-net or grouped LASSO. Another approach for expansion involves incorporating a random-effect element into the model and investigating a generalized semiparametric mixed-effect model for the analysis of HIV data.

Acknowledgments This work was based upon research supported in part by the National Research Foundation (NRF) of South Africa, Ref.: RA211204653274, grant No. 151035, the South African DST-NRF-MRC SARChI Research Chair in Biostatistics (Grant No. 114613) and STATOMET at the Department of Statistics at the University of Pretoria, South Africa. The opinions expressed and conclusions arrived at are those of the authors and are not necessarily to be attributed to the NRF. Mohammad Arashi's work is based on the research supported in part by the Iran National Science Foundation (INSF) grant No. 4015320.

References

Fan, J. Q., & Li, R. (2001). Variable selection via nonconcave penalized likelihood and its oracle properties. *Journal of the American Statistical Association, 96*, 1348–1360.

Huang, J. Z., Zhang, L., & Zhou, L. (2007). Efficient estimation in marginal partially linear models for longitudinal/clustered data using splines. *Scandinavian Journal of Statistics, 34*, 451–477.

Li, G. R., Peng, H., & Zhu, L. X. (2011). Nonconcave penalized M-estimation with a diverging number of parameters. *Statistica Sinica, 21*, 391–419.

Ma, S., Song, Q., & Wang, L. (2013). Simultaneous variable selection and estimation in semiparametric modeling of longitudinal/clustered data. *Bernoulli, 19*, 252–274.

Oelker, M. R., & Tutz, G. (2017). A uniform framework for the combination of penalties in generalized structured models. *Advances in Data Analysis and Classification, 11*, 97–120.

Roozbeh, M. (2015). Shrinkage ridge estimators in semiparametric regression models. *Journal of Multivariate Analysis, 136*, 56–74.

Roozbeh, M. (2016). Robust ridge estimator in restricted semiparametric regression models. *Journal of Multivariate Analysis, 147*, 127–144.

Roozbeh, M. (2018). Optimal QR-based estimation in partially linear regression models with correlated errors using GCV criterion. *Computational Statistics & Data Analysis, 117*, 45–61.

Roozbeh, M., Hesamian, G., & Akbari, M. G. (2020). Ridge estimation in semi-parametric regression models under the stochastic restriction and correlated elliptically contoured errors. *Journal of Computational and Applied Mathematics, 378*, 112940.

Taavoni, M., & Arashi, M. (2021). High-dimensional generalized semiparametric model for longitudinal data. *Statistics, 55*, 831–850.

Taavoni, M., Arashi, M., & Manda, S. (2023). Multicollinearity and linear predictor link function problems in regression modelling of longitudinal data. *Mathematics, 11*, 530.

van der Wurp, H., & Groll, A. (2023). Introducing LASSO-type penalisation to generalized joint regression modeling for count data. *AStA Advances in Statistical Analysis, 107*, 127–151.

Wang, W. L., & Fan, T. H. (2011). Estimation in multivariate t linear mixed models for multiple longitudinal data. *Statistica Sinica, 21*, 1857–1880.

Wang, W. L. (2017). Mixture of multivariate t linear mixed models for multi-outcome longitudinal data with heterogeneity. *Statistica Sinica, 27*, 733–760.

Wang, W. L., Lin, T. I., & Lachos, V. H. (2018). Extending multivariate-t linear mixed models for multiple longitudinal data with censored responses and heavy tails. *Statistical Methods in Medical Research., 27*, 48–64.

Wang, H. S., Li, B., & Leng, C. L. (2009). Shrinkage tuning parameter selection with a diverging number of parameters. *Journal of the Royal Statistical Society Series B, 71*, 671–683.

Wang, H. S., Li, R. Z., & Tcai C. L. (2007). Tuning parameter selectors for the smoothly clipped absolute deviation method. *Biometrika 94* 553–568.

Wang, N., Carroll, R., & Lin, X. H. (2005). Efficient semiparametric marginal estimation for longitudinal/clustered data. *Journal of the American Statistical Association, 100*, 147–157.

Zeger, S. L., & Diggle, P. J. (1994). Semi-parametric models for longitudinal data with application to CD4 cell numbers in HIV seroconverters. *Biometrics, 50*, 689–99.

Chapter 10
Geostatistical Analysis of Under-Five Children Mortality and Associated Factors Across Sub-Saharan African Countries

Haile Mekonnen Fenta, Ding-Geng Chen, and Temesgen T. Zewotir

10.1 Introduction

The under-five mortality (U5M) is the probability of a child dying before 5 years of age expressed per 1000 live births (Hug et al., 2020). One of the important Millennium Development Goals (MDGs) of the United Nations Sustainable Development Goals (SDGs) is to end preventable deaths of newborns and children under the age of five. It aims to reduce neonatal mortality at least as low as 12 per 1000 live births and under-five mortality at least as low as 25 per 1000 live births (United Nations, 2012; Resolution, 2015). Even if promising progress has been made in improving survival rates of children in Africa through the reduction of diseases and improved access to health facilities, sub-Saharan Africa (sSA) carried about half of the burden of the world's under-five deaths—three million in 2015 (United Nations, 2012). Children's survival prospects continue to be influenced by broad

H. M. Fenta (✉)
Department of Statistics, University of Pretoria, Pretoria, South Africa

Department of Statistics, Bahir Dar University, Bahir Dar, Ethiopia

D.-G. Chen
Department of Statistics, University of Pretoria, Pretoria, South Africa

College of Health Solutions, Arizona State University, Tempe, AZ, USA
e-mail: Ding-Geng.Chen@asu.edu

T. T. Zewotir
School of Mathematics, Statistics and Computer Science, College of Agriculture Engineering and Science, University of KwaZulu-Natal, Durban, South Africa
e-mail: zewotir@ukzn.ac.za

D.-G. Chen, C. A. Coelho (eds.), *Biostatistics Modeling and Public Health Applications*, Emerging Topics in Statistics and Biostatistics,
https://doi.org/10.1007/978-3-031-69690-9_10

geographical and socioeconomic variations (Fenta & Fenta, 2020; MacDonald et al., 2020; Bobo et al., 2022; Fisher et al., 2022). The sSA suffers the greatest burden of child mortality due to changing demography and other related factors (Fenta & Fenta, 2020; MacDonald et al., 2020).

The main aim of this chapter was to find a model that can explain variations in U5M across the sSA region. To achieve this goal, we employed three different statistical models like generalized linear mixed model (GLMM), generalized additive mixed model (GAMM), and generalized geo-additive mixed model (GGAMM). Specifically, linear statistical models were commonly employed in statistical analysis to examine the relationship between the outcome variable(s) and a set of predictor variables. However, first when the relationship between the variables is much complex, the generalized additive mixed model (GAMM) gives a flexible relationship (Hastie & Tibshirani, 1990; Wood, 2017) instead of the linear relationship. GAMMs have been used in count (Miaou et al., 2003) and binary (Khatab & Fahrmeir, 2008) outcome variables. Second, when the covariates are spatially indexed, both the spatial and nonspatial stationary regression give inadequate predictions due to ignoring the spatial dependences, and it will also lead to a poor estimation of parameters over study areas (Hastie & Tibshirani, 1990; Wood, 2017; Wand, 2003; Wand et al., 2011). The other challenge in classical linear models is how to adjust the spatial effect as well as provide measures of nonlinear effects of continuous variables and assess their impact on uncertainty. To address these challenges, in this chapter, we adopted a generalized geo-additive mixed model (GGAMM), which is a combination of the generalized additive mixed model (GAMM) and geo-statistics, for the big spatial data randomly distributed over regular/irregular areas. Moreover, the present study adopted the Bayesian techniques using the R integrated nested Laplace approximation (R-INLA) package (Lindgren & Rue, 2015; Van Niekerk et al., 2019), which has many advantages over frequentist approach in terms of inferring the model parameters of interest (Brunsdon et al., 2002; Assunçao, 2003; Cressie et al., 2009; Wheeler & Waller, 2009; Finley, 2011). The hierarchical Bayesian model was used to map the distribution of the outcome variable and confirmed that this model outperforms the other methods (linear models) in the smoothing effects as well as in the explanation of the different aspects of the patterns (Hu et al., 2011; Krainski et al., 2018; Fenta et al., 2021b).

In this chapter, three statistical models will be used, and their performance will be compared. The generalized linear mixed model (GLMM); the linear outcome variable is a linear function of the covariates plus some random error terms. The generalized additive mixed effects model; which is a generalization of the GLMM that incorporates the possible nonlinear effects of covariates; and the interest focuses on inference about the unknown smooth function. Hence, the parameter estimation and prior specification of the hyper-parameters will be discussed in detail. Moreover, the third model, the generalized geo-additive mixed effect model; a generalization of GAMM with structured and unstructured spatial effects. Finally, the child's mortality rate among under-five children across the sSA countries will be used for application purposes, and interpretation of the estimated parameter based on the selected model will be made.

10.2 Data Sources and Variables

The data for the analysis came from two sources: the first source was the Demographic and Health Survey (DHS), nationally representative surveys conducted mainly in low-income countries (https://dhsprogram.com). In DHS, the multistage sampling was used to select the sample for each survey in various countries. Hence, the first step of the sampling procedure involved the selection of clusters (enumeration areas (EAs)), followed by systematic household sampling within the selected EAs. The number of clusters is the first stage which is selected from the list of enumeration areas (EAs) created in recent population census of each country and the households which are randomly selected in each of EAs. From the selected households, women aged 15–49 years are selected for in-depth interview (Aliaga & Ren, 2006). Most of the recent DHS waves use global positioning systems (GPS) coordinates (latitude and longitude) of household clusters, which help to collect the geospatial information to identify the central point of each EA. The birth record files among under-five children from 33 sSA countries, which consist of data on the full birth history of all reproductive women interviewed and information on health indicators on fertility and mortality rates were used (Fig. 10.1, Fig. 10.2). Moreover, the geographical covariates were extracted from the DHS site and were linked to the original individual DHS datasets through the cluster identifying number (ID).

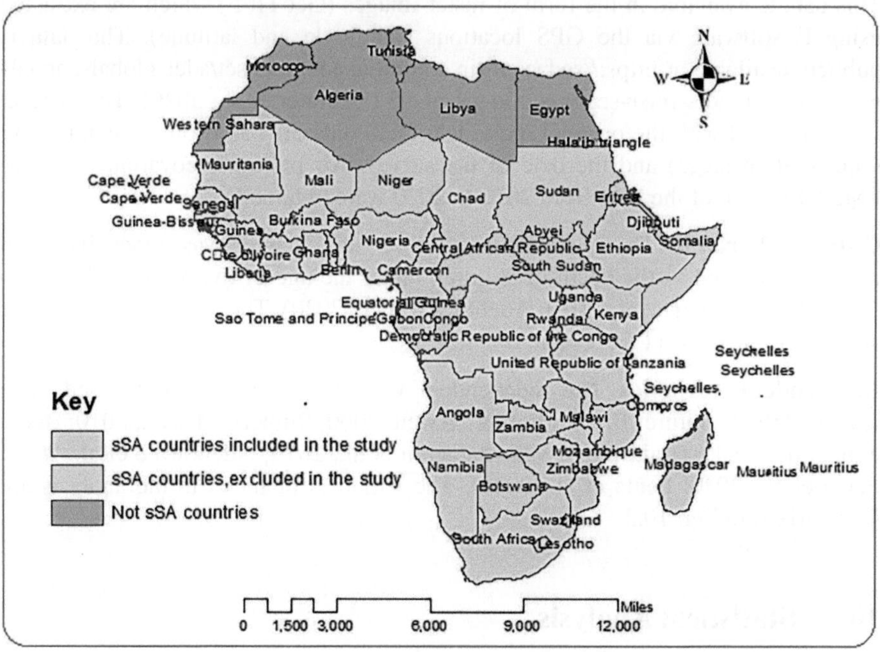

Fig. 10.1 Eligible sub-Saharan African countries included in the study

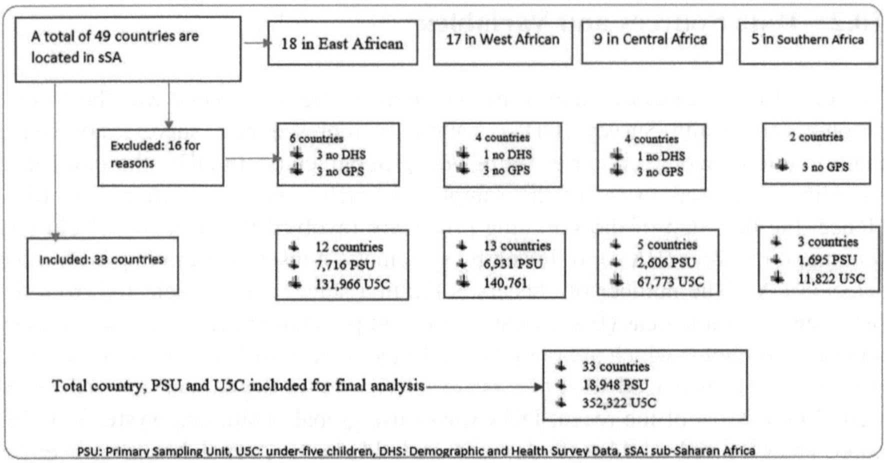

Fig. 10.2 Flowchart of participant selection for analysis using recent DHS reports from 2012 to 2022

The second data source is the National Aeronautics and Space Administration (NASA). From this source, the air pollution covariates such as global annual surface particulate matter (PM 2.5) concentration and nitrogen dioxide (NO_2) for 1998–2019 (v4.03) were estimated by the Atmospheric Composition Analysis Group. This data is available in the form of raster images (GeoTIFF) which are extracted using R software via the GPS locations (longitude and latitude). The data is publicly available at https://sedac.ciesin.columbia.edu/data/set/sdei-global-annual-gwr-pm2-5-modis-misr-seawifs-aod-v4-gl-03 (Hammer et al., 2020). This dataset was combined with the original individual DHS datasets based on the community (enumeration areas) and the date of the survey. Air pollution covariates such as PM2.5 for each of the EAs from 2012 to 2020 were obtained.

Outcome Variable The outcome variable for this chapter was under-five child mortality, defined as the death of children under the age of five years (Zike et al., 2018; Van Malderen et al., 2019; Adebowale et al., 2020). The values of the variable are dichotomized as (1 = yes and 0 = no).

Independent Variables The independent variables extracted were based on a review of the literature (Brockerhoff & Hewett, 2000; Rutherford et al., 2010; Bryce et al., 2013; Zike et al., 2018; Van Malderen et al., 2019; Adebowale et al., 2020; Fenta et al., 2020; Fenta et al., 2022). The variables included in the analysis are summarized in Fig. 10.3.

10.3 Statistical Analysis

The logistic regression was used to identify the potential independent variables for childhood mortality prior to the spatial analysis. According to the existing literature (Hosmer, Hosmer et al., 1997, Agresti, 2012), a significant level of 20% was taken as

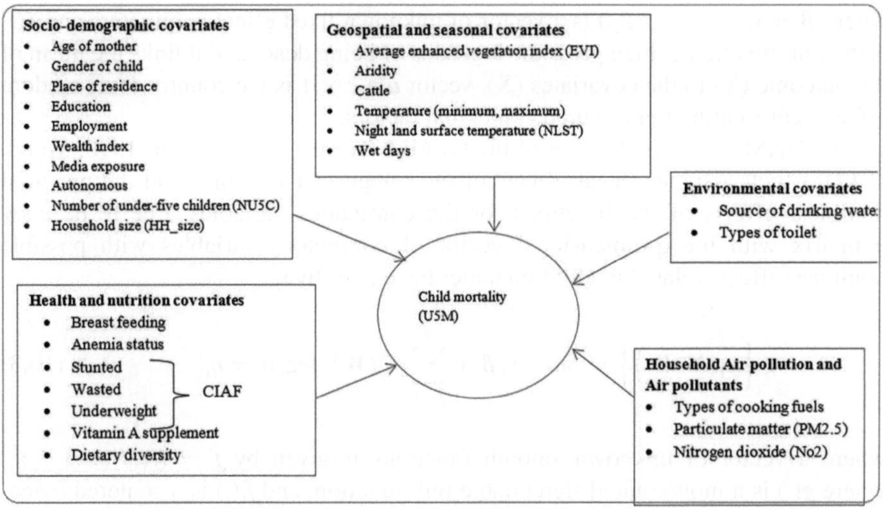

Fig. 10.3 Conceptual framework for variable description. Note: CIAF: composite index for anthropometric failure (Fenta et al., 2021a) and dietary diversity (Child, 2011; Fenta et al., 2021a)

a threshold for the selection of potential independent variables to be included in the further analysis of spatial modeling. After the selection of the potential covariates, three models namely generalized linear mixed model (GLMM), generalized additive mixed model (GAMM), and generalized geo-additive mixed model (GGAMM) were used to analyze the dataset.

10.3.1 Models

The GLMM assumes a linear effect of both the continuous and categorical variables (Nelder & Wedderburn, 1972; Hosmer et al., 1997). The outcome variable Y is assumed to be a member of any exponential families (Nelder & Wedderburn, 1972) given as:

$$f_Y(y; \theta; \varphi) = \exp\left\{a(y, \varphi) + \frac{y\theta - b(\theta)}{c(\varphi)}\right\} \tag{10.1}$$

where a, b, and c are arbitrary functions, φ and θ, respectively, are the scale and natural parameters.

Let observations of the ith of n ($n = 352{,}322$) subjects consist of the response variable $\boldsymbol{y}_i$ and the p independent variables $\boldsymbol{x}_i = (1, x_{i1}, \ldots, x_{ip})^T$ associated with fixed effects, and a $c \times 1$ vector of covariates z_i associated with random effects.

$$g\left\{E\left(\boldsymbol{y}_i|\boldsymbol{X}\right)\right\} = \beta_0 + \boldsymbol{x}_i\boldsymbol{\beta} + z_i\boldsymbol{u} \tag{10.2}$$

where $\boldsymbol{\beta} = (\beta_1, \ \ldots, \ \beta_p)$ is a vector of unknown fixed effect parameters and $g(.)$ is the link function, which gives the log-odds of being dead, and it links the mean of the outcome (Y) to the covariates (**X**), vector $\boldsymbol{u}$ a $c \times 1$ is the country-level random effects representing unmeasured contextual factors.

The GAMM is an extension of the GLMM (Hastie & Tibshirani, 1990; Wood, 2017), which assumes linear effects of the categorical variables and the potential nonlinear effects of the functions for the continuous variables. Let $\boldsymbol{W}$ be n by q matrix with the q-dimensional vector of continuous variables with possible nonlinear effects related to children under the age of five.

$$g\left\{\boldsymbol{y}_i|\boldsymbol{X}, \boldsymbol{W})\right\} = \beta_0 + \boldsymbol{x}_i\boldsymbol{\beta} + \sum_{l=1}^{q} f_l\left(\boldsymbol{W}\right) + \boldsymbol{z}_i\boldsymbol{u} = \eta_i \tag{10.3}$$

where a vector of unknown smooth functions is given by $\boldsymbol{f} = (f_1, f_2, \ldots, f_q)^T$, where $g(.)$ is a monotonic differentiable link function, and $f_i(.)$ is a centered twice-differentiable smooth function. Moreover, the random effects $\boldsymbol{u} \sim N\{0, A(\boldsymbol{\psi})\}$ and $\boldsymbol{\psi}$ are $c \times 1$ vectors of variance components. For a given variance component $\boldsymbol{\psi}$, the integrated log-quasi-likelihood function of $(\beta_0, \psi, f_i, i = 1, \ldots, n)$ is given (Lin & Zhang, 1999) by:

$$\exp\left[l\left\{\beta_0, \psi, f_1(.), \ldots, f_p(.)\right\}\right] \propto |A|^{-1/2} \int \exp\left\{-\frac{1}{2\phi}\sum_{i=1}^{n} a_i\left(y_i, \mu_i\right) - \frac{1}{2}\boldsymbol{u}^T\boldsymbol{A}^{-1}\boldsymbol{u}\right\} d\boldsymbol{u} \tag{10.4}$$

where $\boldsymbol{y} = (y_1, \ldots, y_n)^T$ and $a_i\left(y_i, \mu_i\right) \propto -2\int_{y_i}^{\mu_i} n_i\left(y_i - b\right)/v(b)db$ define the conditional deviance function of $\{\beta_0, f_1(.), \ldots, f_p(.)\}$ given $\boldsymbol{u}$, with $\boldsymbol{A}$ as the full rank matrix. The GAMM inferences on nonparametric function $f_i(.)$ need the estimation of the smoothing parameter and the variance component $\boldsymbol{\psi}$ as well. However, in the previous two models, the nonspatial data was carried out using a binary GLM to describe the relationship between the binary variable of interest (child is dead coded as 1 and 0 otherwise) variables and the covariates. The GGAMM is a generalization of GAMM by adding a bivariate spatial function. Let the under-five children belong to country (second level administrative areas) h and cluster (districts) k in terms of location, and the random spatial effects of the GGAMM are generally given as (Wand, 2003; Wand et al., 2011).

$$\phi_{hk} = f_{\text{spat}}\left(\text{lon}_k, \text{lat}_k\right) + U_h.$$

The nonlinear spatial effect $f_{\text{spat}}(\text{lon}_k, \text{lat}_k)$ is a function of geographical coordinates of the kth cluster where lat_k and lon_k are the latitude and longitude of clusters, respectively, where the spatial heterogeneity unobserved parameter is captured by the $f_{\text{spat}}(\text{lon}_k, \text{lat}_k)$ at location k, for which some are spatially unstructured and the others are structured. This is denoted as:

$$f_{\text{spat}(k)} = f_{\text{unst}(\text{lon}_k,\text{lat}_k)} + f_{\text{str}(\text{lon}_k,\text{lat}_k)} \tag{10.5}$$

the posterior distribution is obtained by combining the observed data and the prior distribution (Fenta et al., 2021b).

10.3.2 Natural Cubic Smoothing Spline Estimation

Equation 10.4 is a continuous linear functional of the $f_i(.)$, and one can show that for the given parameters θ and ψ, the natural cubic smoothing spline estimators of the functions $f_i(.)$ maximize the penalized log-quasi-likelihood is given as (O'sullivan et al., 1986; Hastie & Tibshirani, 2017; Green & Silverman, 2019):

$$\begin{aligned} & l\left\{\beta_0, \psi, f_1(.), \ldots, f_p(.)\right\} - \frac{1}{2}\sum_{i=1}^{p}\theta_i \int_{s_i}^{t_i} f_i''(x)^2 dx \\ & = l\left\{\beta_0, \psi, f_1(.), \ldots, f_p(.) - \frac{1}{2}\sum_{i=1}^{p}\theta_i f_i^T \boldsymbol{H}_i f_i\right\} \end{aligned} \tag{10.6}$$

where (s_i, t_i) is the range of the ith covariate and $\boldsymbol{\theta} = (\theta_1, \ \ldots, \theta_p)^T$ is a vector of the smoothing parameters that regulate the trade-off between the goodness of fit and smoothness of the estimated functions (O'sullivan et al., 1986; Green & Silverman, 2019). Besides, the $f_i(.)$ is an $r_i \times 1$ unknown vector of the values of $f_i(.)$ computed at the r_i-ordered different values of $\boldsymbol{x}_{ij}(j = 1, 2, 3, \ldots, n)$, and $\boldsymbol{H}_i$ is the corresponding positive (nonnegative) definite smoothing matrix (Green & Silverman, 2019). The GAMM given in Eq. 10.3 can be formulated in a matrix form as:

$$g\left(\mu_i\right) = \beta_0 + \boldsymbol{x}_i\boldsymbol{\beta} + N_1 f_1 + \cdots + N_q f_q + z_i^T \boldsymbol{u} \tag{10.7}$$

where $g(\mu_i) = \{g(\mu_1), \ldots, g(\mu_p)\}^T$, $z_i = (z_1, \ldots, z_n)^T$, $\boldsymbol{u} = (u_1, \ldots, u_n)^T$, and $N_i f_i$ is the ith component of $f_i(x_{ij})$. In Eq. 10.7, it is difficult to compute the full natural cubic smoothing spline parameters except for the Gaussian case. Therefore, another approach is proposed (Hastie & Tibshirani, 2017, Green & Silverman, 2019).

10.3.3 Prior Distributions

In Bayesian model, the unknown smooth functions(f_l, l = 1, 2. . . q, f_{str}, and f_{unstr}) and the unknown fixed effect parameters and variance ($\boldsymbol{\beta},\boldsymbol{\sigma}^2$) are taken as random variables, and hence it needs specifying the appropriate prior assumptions.

However, for the categorical fixed effect parameters $\boldsymbol{\beta}$ independent diffuse priors, $\pi(\Phi) \propto$ constant is assumed. The nonlinear smooth parameters were modeled by second-order random walk prior (Fenta et al., 2021b) given by $f_l/f_{l-1}, f_{l-2}, \tau_l^2 \sim N\left(2f_{l-1} - f_{l-2}, \tau_l^2\right)$ for $l = 1, 2, \ldots f$ with non-informative priors for f_1, f_2 (Spiegelhalter et al., 2002; Brezger & Lang, 2006; Gosoniu et al., 2006; Bolstad, 2009; Fahrmeir & Kneib, 2009).

The exchangeable normal priors are assumed $f_{\text{ustr}} \sim N\left(0, \gamma_{\text{unst}}^2\right)$ to capture the unstructured spatial random effects (f_{ustr}), where γ_{unst}^2 is a variance component that allows for over-dispersion and heterogeneity (Spiegelhalter et al., 2002, Brezger & Lang, 2006, Gosoniu et al., 2006, Bolstad, 2009, Fahrmeir & Kneib, 2009). The R-INLA assigns a prior to log (γ_{unst}^2) which by default is a log-gamma distribution (Rue et al., 2009). To model the spatial correlation (structured) components, the neighborhoods must be first defined. Two areas are neighbors if they share common boundaries. The spatial autocorrelation is modeled using a normal distribution with mean zero and a precision matrix that controls associations between two neighbors. As a result, the spatial structured effect of correlations between two areas is achieved by considering the f_{str} using the generalized Markov random field (GMRF) priors, where the MRF is defined by Brezger and Lang (2006) and Bolstad (2009).

$$f_{\text{str}/\gamma_{\text{str}}^2)} \sim N\left(0, \gamma_{\text{str}}^2 S^{-1}\right) \tag{10.8}$$

where γ_{str}^2 denotes the unknown precision parameter that captures the degree of similarities, and S is the spatial precision matrix that designates the spatial structure components. Therefore, the *(i.j)*th component of the spatial precision matrix $\boldsymbol{S}$ is expressed as:

$$\boldsymbol{S} = \begin{cases} n_d & d{=}e \\ 1 & d{\sim}e \\ 0 & \text{elsewhere} \end{cases}$$

where *d~e* denotes the country, *d* is adjacent to *e*, and n_d is the number of adjacent countries to *d*. Thus, area *d* with neighboring area *e* would have conditional distributions given by:

$$f_{\text{str}}^d \mid \left\{f_{\text{str}}^e, d \neq e\right\} \sim N(\pi, \varepsilon) \tag{10.9}$$

where $\pi = \frac{1}{n_d}\sum_{e \in m} f_{\text{str}}^d$, $\varepsilon = \frac{\tau_{\text{str}}^2}{n_d}$ and d and e are adjacent areas in the set of all adjacent areas (m) of area s (Spiegelhalter et al., 2002, Brezger & Lang, 2006, Gosoniu et al., 2006, Bolstad, 2009, Fahrmeir & Kneib, 2009). For all unknown variances, the inverse-gamma prior distribution is proposed $IG\ (a_j, b_j)$ (Fahrmeir & Kneib, 2009) with constant parameters $a_i > 0$ and $b_i > 0$ with hyper-parameters $a_i = b_i = 0.001$ is the standard choice for a weakly informative prior (Spiegelhalter et al., 2002, Brezger & Lang, 2006, Gosoniu et al., 2006, Bolstad,

2009, Fahrmeir & Kneib, 2009). Let Φ be the vector of unknown parameters in the model and $L(.)$ be the likelihood, which is the product of individual likelihoods with $\Phi = \{\beta, \sigma^2, f_l, f_{\text{strc}}\}$. Under the Bayesian context, the posterior distribution L(Φ/y) is a function of the prior distribution L(Φ) and the likelihood function L(y/Φ) (Gosoniu et al., 2006; Bolstad, 2009; Wand et al., 2011). Moreover, the DHS provided a sample weight for each survey respondent that accounted for the unequal likelihood of selection and nonresponse. To confirm that our results are representative of the sSA population, the sample weights were included in the analysis through the options pop-up command of "weight" representing the sample weight by "inla" function (Rue et al., 2009).

10.3.4 Model Diagnostics

The model performance was validated through the deviance information criteria (DIC) (Rue et al., 2009; Shimaponda-Mataa et al., 2017), the conditional predictive ordinate (CPO) (Gelfand et al., 1992; Gelman & Meng, 1996), and Watanabe-Akaike information criteria (WAIC) (Watanabe, 2013). Finally, the model with the lowest DIC and WAIC and the highest values of CPO is the preferred one to fit the data (Wand, 2003; Wand et al., 2011).

10.3.5 Model Validation and Evaluation

The test statistic like receiver operating characteristic-area under the curve (ROC-AUC) is used to compare the overall predictive power of the models. The ROC-AUC is used to specify the ability of the model to predict the presences/absences of events correctly: while the specificity is used to assess the percentage of absences correctly predicted, sensitivity measures the percentage of presences correctly predicted (Fielding & Bell, 1997; Allouche et al., 2006; Pearson, 2007).

10.3.6 Sensitivity Analysis for Priors

The sensitivity analysis was performed to check the impact of the different values of variance component priors on the selected (final) model to see whether the result of the parameters remained unchanged. According to different scholars, the following specifications were used as recommended: IG (0.001, 0.001), IG (0.01, 0.01), IG (0.5, 0.0005), and (1, 0.026) of different degrees of uncertainty (Best et al., 1999; Kelsall & Wakefield, 1999; Lunn et al., 2000; Wakefield, 2007; Fahrmeir & Kneib, 2009; Kazembe & Kandala, 2015). Moreover, for modeling the precision of the spatial effects using MRF models, the first two equal prior specifications ($a = b$)

have often been a gold standard preference on the variances of random effects (Lunn et al., 2000), and the third specifications were suggested by Kelsall and Wakefield (1999) and Kazembe and Kandala (2015), respectively. The other remaining prior choice was proposed by Best et al. (1999), Wakefield (2007), and Kazembe and Kandala (2015) for assessing the residual odds of range (0.5, 2.0). Generally, for well-identified parameters and the big dataset, the choice of any of the priors has only minor different effects on the posterior inferences (Fahrmeir & Kneib, 2009). In this work, the R integrated nested Laplace approximation (R-INLA) package was used for analysis purposes; this is due to the time efficiency as compared to MCMC and other estimation techniques (Lang & Brezger, 2000; Spiegelhalter et al., 2002; Martins et al., 2013).

10.4 Results

10.4.1 Descriptive Results

Table 10.1 presents the prevalence of under-five mortality (U5M) among children from 33 sSA countries. A total of 352,322 under-five children were included in the study. The overall prevalence of U5M for all countries was 6.04. However, there are inequalities in the child's U5M rate among children across sSA countries. The three countries with the highest proportion of U5M were Chad (9.79%), Nigeria (9.68%), and Sierra Leone (8.99%), while Gabon (3.33%), Mozambique (3.25), and Ghana (2.98%) were the lead U5M prevalent countries (Table 10.1).

The study sought to find out the potential significant factors and spatial patterns of U5M among children across sSA countries using the most recent DHS datasets. Results from the generalized geo-additive mixed effects model for the linear fixed effect parameters and the posterior mean/standard deviation with 95% credible intervals are given in Fig. 10.4. The negative/positive coefficients correspond to a decreasing/increasing risk for the U5M among children across sSA countries, respectively. More specifically, the finding showed that the U5M status of children below 5 years is positively associated with the male gender. The log-odds of a male child (0.12) with an odds ratio of (1.13) imply that the male under-five children are 13% more likely to die as compared to the female under-five children. Moreover, under-five children from urban areas are less likely to die (log-odds $= -0.11$ and odds ratio $= 0.89$) compared with children from rural areas. The link between the U5M status of under-five children and the educational attainment of their mothers was negatively associated. The estimated log-odds of U5M for children born from mothers with illiterate, primary, and secondary were 2.19, 1.94, and 1.53 compared with under-five children born from mothers with higher educational counterparts. Children born from households with improved sources of drinking water and cleaned fuels were 11 and 14% less likely to die compared with those from the unimproved sources of drinking water and uncleaned use of fuels, respectively. Additionally, under-five children from lower socioeconomic household

Table 10.1 The number of under-five children across the DHS waves for each country and the prevalence of symptoms of respiratory infections among U5C children in sSA

Survey countries	Survey year	Weighted sample	Percent	Under-five mortality n (%)
Angola	2015	14,322	3.84	703(5.15)
Benin	2017	13,589	3.93	938(7.02)
Burkina Faso	2021	12,343	3.54	490(3.7)
Burundi	2016	13,192	3.92	720(5.86)
Cameroon	2018	9734	2.9	648(6.15)
Chad	2015	18,623	5.36	1722(9.79)
Comoros	2012	3149	0.93	127(4.22)
Congo Democratic	2013	18,718	5.29	1488(7.47)
Ivory Coast	2021	10,645	2.81	697(6.14)
Ethiopia	2016	10,641	3.17	635(5.49)
Gabon	2019	6376	1.75	265(3.33)
Gambia	2019	8362	2.2	435(4.65)
Ghana	2019	3004	0.83	76(2.98)
Guinea	2018	8014	2.27	678(8.65)
Kenya	2022	19,530	5.03	694(3.39)
Lesotho	2014	3140	0.9	223(6.94)
Liberia	2019	5704	1.51	459(7.55)
Madagascar	2021	12,500	3.55	719(5.78)
Malawi	2015	17,286	5.01	824(4.87)
Mali	2018	9940	2.97	665(7.16)
Mauritania	2019	11,638	3.36	452(3.59)
Mozambique	2015	5179	1.58	165(3.25)
Namibia	2013	5059	1.38	228(4.48)
Nigeria	2018	33,924	9.84	3211(9.68)
Rwanda	2019	8092	2.4	296(3.66)
Senegal	2019	6719	1.75	274(4.02)
Sierra Leone	2019	9900	2.81	836(8.99)
South Africa	2016	3623	1.03	135(3.59)
Tanzania	2022	10,783	3.13	389(3.56)
Togo	2023	6979	1.93	444(6.26)
Uganda	2016	15,522	4.4	812(5.09)
Zambia	2019	9959	2.83	475(4.88)
Zimbabwe	2015	6133	1.85	325(5.65)
Total		352,322	100	21,248(6.04)

were positively associated with U5M. Particularly, compared against the benchmark category (the medium wealth quintiles), children from households with the richer and richest wealth quintile odds ratio were decreased by 7% and 13%, respectively. In contrast for those from lower and lowest wealth quintiles, the estimated odds ratio increased by 9% and 11%, respectively, as compared to the baseline category (Fig. 10.4).

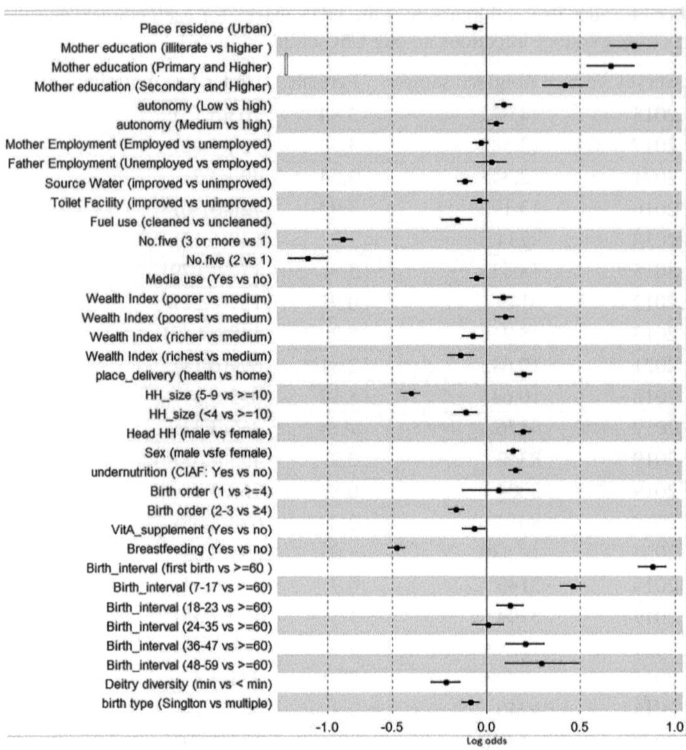

Variable	Odds Ratio	95% Cr. I
Place residene (Urban)	0.94	(0.90,0.99)
Mother education (illiterate vs higher)	2.19	(1.93,2.49)
Mother education (Primary and Higher)	1.94	(1.71,2.20)
Mother education (Secondary and Higher)	1.53	(1.35,1.72)
autonomy (Low vs high)	1.10	(1.05,1.15)
autonomy (Medium vs high)	1.05	(1.01,1.10)
Mother Employment (Employed vs unemployed)	0.97	(0.93,1.02)
Father Employment (Unemployed vs employed)	1.03	(0.95,1.12)
Source Water (improved vs unimproved)	0.89	(0.86,0.93)
Toilet Facility (improved vs unimproved)	0.97	(0.92,1.01)
Fuel use (cleaned vs uncleaned)	0.86	(0.79,0.93)
No.five (3 or more vs 1)	0.40	(0.38,0.42)
No.five (2 vs 1)	0.33	(0.30,0.37)
Media use (Yes vs no)	0.95	(0.91,0.99)
Wealth Index (poorer vs medium)	1.09	(1.04,1.15)
Wealth Index (poorest vs medium)	1.11	(1.05,1.17)
Wealth Index (richer vs medium)	0.93	(0.88,0.98)
Wealth Index (richest vs medium)	0.87	(0.81,0.94)
place_delivery (health vs home)	1.22	(1.17,1.28)
HH_size (5-9 vs >=10)	0.67	(0.64,0.71)
HH_size (<4 vs >=10)	0.90	(0.84,0.95)
Head HH (male vs female)	1.22	(1.17,1.27)
Sex (male vsfe female)	1.16	(1.12,1.20)
undernutrition (CIAF: Yes vs no)	1.17	(1.13,1.21)
Birth order (1 vs >=4)	1.07	(0.88,1.30)
Birth order (2-3 vs ≥4)	0.85	(0.82,0.89)
VitA_supplement (Yes vs no)	0.94	(0.88,1.00)
Breastfeeding (Yes vs no)	0.62	(0.59,0.65)
Birth_interval (first birth vs >=60)	2.42	(2.24,2.60)
Birth_interval (7-17 vs >=60)	1.59	(1.48,1.70)
Birth_interval (18-23 vs >=60)	1.14	(1.06,1.22)
Birth_interval (24-35 vs >=60)	1.01	(0.93,1.10)
Birth_interval (36-47 vs >=60)	1.23	(1.11,1.37)
Birth_interval (48-59 vs >=60)	1.35	(1.10,1.64)
Deitry diversity (min vs < min)	0.81	(0.74,0.87)
birth type (Singlton vs multiple)	0.92	(0.88,0.97)

Fig. 10.4 Posterior estimates of the fixed effect parameters associated with U5M among children across sSA countries

10.4.2 Nonlinear Effects

The nonlinear effects for the given continuous variables estimated log-odds of U5M with a 95% credible interval are presented in Fig. 10.5. Moreover, the estimates log-odds for child's U5M for those variables were different from 0, implying that there are nonlinear effects of the continuous variables on child's mortality among under-five children across the sSA countries (Table 10.2).

Moreover, the estimated log-odds of the under-five children mortality are directly and nonlinearly associated with the age of the child (in months). It reveals that the child's U5M status is negatively correlated with the lower age group (approximately age below 20 months). The estimated log-odds of child's U5M among children are considerably high between the ages of 30 and more months and get static after 55 months. The estimated log-odds of child's U5M seem nonlinearly associated with their weight at birth (in kg). It seems negatively associated with the highest weight and positively correlated with the lowest weight of a child in (kg) (Fig. 10.5).

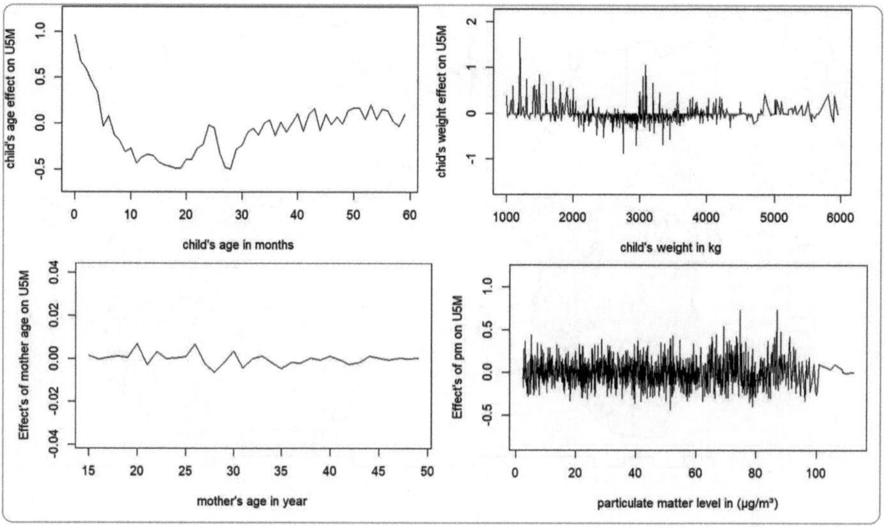

Fig. 10.5 The effects of continuous variables on the under-five child's mortality across sSA countries

Table 10.2 Regression coefficient and variance component estimation of the nonlinear terms

Variables	Estimate	SE	LL	UL
Mother's age	9.07	1.42	5.94	11.47
Child's age	2.11	0.19	1.74	2.50
Child's weight	0.95	0.25	0.46	1.44
Particulate matter ($PM_{2.5}$)	2.67	0.13	2.42	2.92
Nitrogen dioxide (NO_2)	1.07	0.06	0.94	1.20
Country-level random effect	0.67	0.26	1.82	5.95
Country-level spatial effect	4.11	1.06	0.13	1.15

SE standard error of the estimate, *LL* lower level, *UL* upper level

10.4.3 Spatial Effects

The results of the spatial effect from the GGAMM are presented in Figs. 10.6 and 10.7. The estimated log-odd of child's U5M spatially distributed with both positive and negative values across all 33 the sSA countries. Both the estimated clustered (spatial/structured) and unstructured were generated from the GGAMM model for 33 countries in sSA among the under-five children. The variance estimates for the country cluster-level spatial effects (which account for spatial autocorrelation) and random effects were nonzero and statistically significant (Table 10.2). The different color on both structured and unstructured spatial effects reveals the estimated log-odds of a child's U5M across the sSA countries, and the different color shows that each of the country's contribution to the log-odds of U5M is different. The color ranges from red to blue where red denotes the positive effect on the posterior

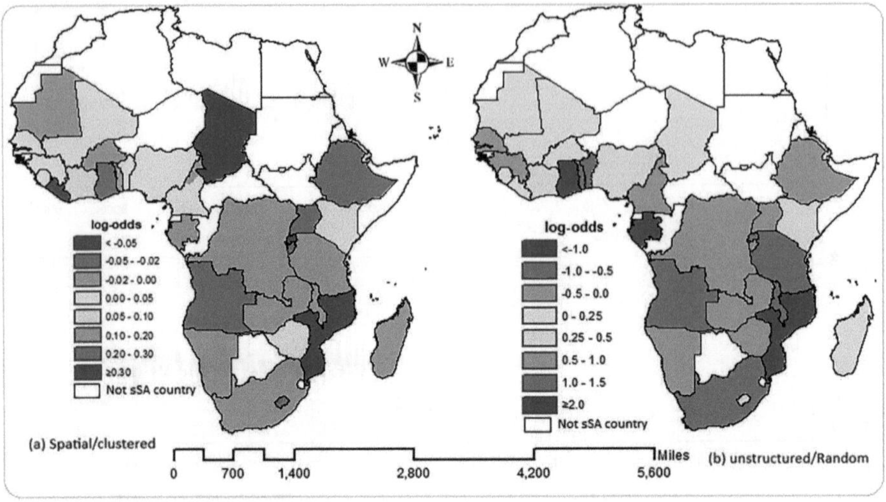

Fig. 10.6 (**a**) Spatial (structured) and (**b**) spatial (unstructured) estimated variation of child's U5M posterior estimates among U5C in sub-Saharan African countries

parameters of the log-odds of the child's U5M across the countries, while yellow and blue colors, respectively, show the decreased negative effect on the child's estimated log-odds of U5M across the sSA countries.

Notably, under-five children from Chad, Liberia, and Gabon in sSA countries were more likely to have the highest estimated odds of child's U5M, but children from Rwanda, Zimbabwe, and Angola have lower estimated log of U5M in the continent (Figs. 10.6 and 10.7).

10.4.4 Model Goodness of Fit and Diagnostics

The model selection was performed based on the computed values of goodness of fit test. The ROC-area under the curve (ROC-AUC) for the proposed three models was given in Fig. 10.8, and all reveal that all the models classify the under-five child's U5M better than chance (diagonal line that is always 0.500). The AUC for the GGAMM is a little bit larger than the other two and implied that it a better model. Moreover, the GGAMM has the lowest WAIC and DIC, and highest CPO revealing that it the best model for classifying child's U5M and identifying the potential risk factors of child's U5M across the sSA countries (Fig. 10.8).

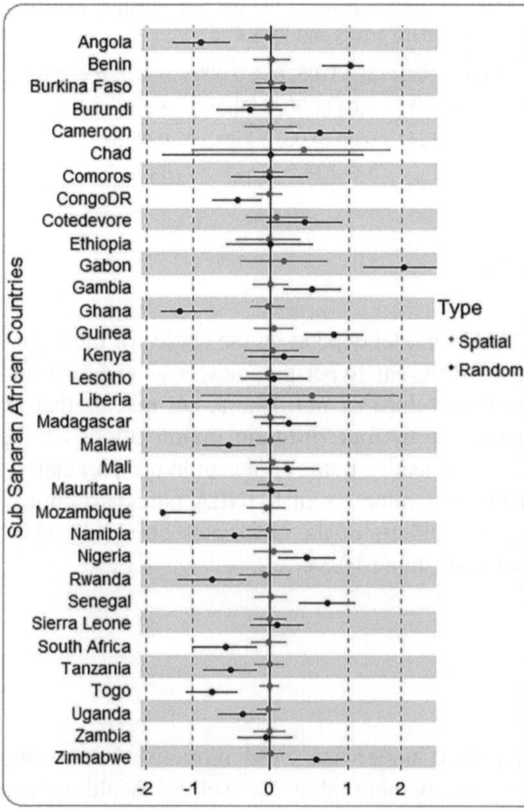

Log-odds (95% Cr.I)	Log-odds (95% Cr.I)
-0.05(-0.39,0.13)	-0.90(-1.24,-0.48)
0.01(-0.22,0.29)	1.02(0.64,1.38)
0.00(-0.22,0.19)	0.15(-0.19,0.50)
-0.02(-0.40,0.30)	-0.27(-0.69,0.18)
0.00(-0.36,0.38)	0.63(0.17,1.08)
0.42(-1.02,1.87)	0.00(-1.41,1.41)
-0.02(-0.26,0.16)	-0.02(-0.51,0.49)
-0.01(-0.22,0.14)	-0.43(-0.75,-0.10)
0.07(-0.26,0.62)	0.43(-0.16,0.87)
-0.03(-0.52,0.40)	-0.01(-0.56,0.57)
0.17(-0.17,0.99)	2.03(1.18,2.55)
0.00(-0.26,0.26)	0.53(0.16,0.91)
-0.03(-0.34,0.15)	-1.17(-1.61,-0.71)
0.04(-0.16,0.39)	0.82(0.39,1.18)
0.02(-0.34,0.46)	0.16(-0.33,0.61)
-0.04(-0.39,0.19)	0.05(-0.37,0.51)
0.54(-0.91,1.98)	0.00(-1.41,1.41)
0.00(-0.23,0.23)	0.23(-0.13,0.60)
-0.01(-0.24,0.19)	-0.54(-0.87,-0.19)
0.02(-0.26,0.36)	0.22(-0.20,0.62)
0.00(-0.20,0.18)	0.02(-0.32,0.35)
-0.05(-0.41,0.13)	-1.39(-1.81,-0.92)
-0.02(-0.35,0.27)	-0.47(-0.91,-0.02)
0.04(-0.17,0.37)	0.47(0.07,0.82)
-0.06(-0.52,0.19)	-0.75(-1.16,-0.23)
0.01(-0.21,0.25)	0.73(0.36,1.10)
0.00(-0.24,0.24)	0.09(-0.27,0.45)
-0.01(-0.30,0.23)	-0.58(-1.00,-0.15)
0.00(-0.22,0.21)	-0.52(-0.87,-0.16)
0.00(-0.16,0.14)	-0.75(-1.07,-0.42)
-0.02(-0.22,0.11)	-0.35(-0.66,-0.03)
-0.01(-0.25,0.23)	-0.06(-0.42,0.31)
0.01(-0.19,0.24)	0.60(0.23,0.96)

Fig. 10.7 The estimated under-five child's log-odds with 95% credible interval (Cr.I) across countries in sSA (**a**) structured (**b**) unstructured

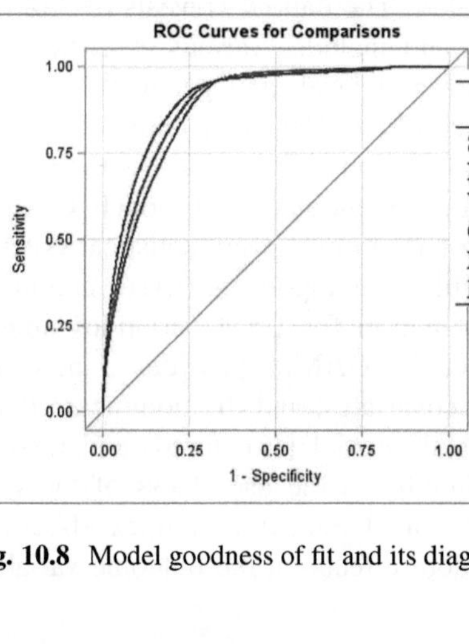

Model Comparisons and Diagnostics

Statistics	GLMM	GAMM	GGAMM
ROC-AUC	0.883	0.892	0.905
WAIC	279,102.4	263,225.3	254,539.9
CPO	0.308	0.3101	0.312
DIC	155,869.1	148,164.9	144,734.9
MLINK	-42,091.5	-43,057.7	-44,914.8

Fig. 10.8 Model goodness of fit and its diagnostics

Table 10.3 The summary of the GGAMM sensitivity analysis for the combination of hyper-parameters with the posterior mean-variance (standard error) and 95% Cr.I

Spatial effects	$a = b = 0.001$	$a = 0.01, b = 0.01$	$a = 0.05, b = 0.0005$	$a = 1, b = 0.026$
γ^2_{str}, 95% Cr.I	3.98 (1.13, 6.16)	4.33 (1.83, 6.98)	4.03 (1.30, 6.78)	3.56 (−0.04, 6.32)
γ^2_{unstr}, 95% Cr.I	0.58 (0.27, 1.11)	0.59 (0.02, 1.12)	0.60 (0.02, 1.11)	0.65 (0.12, 1.14)
DIC	144,818.7	144,838.4	144,838.8	144,846.5

10.4.5 Model Sensitivity Results

The parameters in the selected GGAMM model depend on the choice of the hyper-parameters. For this model, we used different hyper-parameters to examine and check whether the prior specification is robust or not. The result reveals that an almost equivalent result was obtained from four different combinations of the parameter distribution; our model is less sensitive to the choice of hyper-parameters. As a result, the default choice of hyper-parameters in R-INLA (standard choice, a = b = 0.01) was used to explore the effects of the covariates on child's U5M across sSA countries using the GGAMM (Table 10.3).

10.5 Conclusions

In developing countries, especially sSA, under-five child mortality is not only influenced by different socioeconomic, demographic, as well as health-related covariates, but also they vary considerably among administrative areas. This chapter uses a large nationally representative dataset from 33 sSA countries in examining the effect of covariates on the u5M of a child. The most recent demographic and health survey (DHS) dataset from each of 33 countries has been used to investigate the determinant factors of under-five child mortality. The dataset consists of 352,322 under-five children across 33 sSA countries and includes various characteristics such as child level, maternal level, environmental level, and geographical level covariates as determinants of U5M among children. The main objective of this chapter was to find a model that can explain variations in U5M across the region. To achieve this objective, we employed three different statistical models GLMM, GAMM, and GGAMM, and compared them based on a given statistical criteria. According to different criteria, the model with all components (fixed, nonlinear, spatial, and random) provides a better explanation for U5M variations among children across the sSA regions. The selected GGAMM provides a powerful class of modeling the linear/fixed effects of covariates, and the nonlinear effects of continuous variables by accounting for both spatial (structured) and random (unstructured) effects. Hence, this chapter highlights the usefulness of the generalized geo-additive mixed effects model for analyzing the complex effects of covariates: linear, nonlinear, spatial, and random effects on the outcome variable.

The GGAMM model simultaneously measures fixed, nonlinear, spatial, as well random effects. Moreover, the fixed effect components of the categorical variables were modeled using the diffuse priors, the nonlinear effects of continuous variables were modeled via p-spline second-order random walk, and the spatial effects were followed by Markov random field priors with exchangeable normal priors used for random effects of child, parental, and environmental variables. The statistical inference was made using a fully Bayesian technique. The appropriate priors for all the given parameters and functions were assigned and different combinations of parameters for the inverse gamma have been used to check whether these priors are sensitive or not.

The findings of the result show that both the prevalence and model-based estimated under-five child's mortality had substantial geographical variations across the countries in sSA. Variables in the parametric part of the selected GGAM model including sex of children, educational attainment of parents, place of residence, autonomy of mothers, access to water, toilet, and fuel significantly associated with under-five child mortality in the region. Moreover, findings from GGAMM reveal that the mother's age, child's weight, child's age, and particulate matter are significantly nonlinearly associated with the child's U5M across sSA countries.

Compared with the third SDG-3 of ending deaths of under-five children, with countries aiming to reduce U5M to a minimum of 25/100 live births by 2030 (United Nations, 2012; Resolution, 2015), the result revealed most of the sSA countries still have high U5M. The findings of the generalized geo-additive mixed effects model showed that the rates of estimated U5M among children appear to arise largely from households with poor educational attainment, poor sanitation, unimproved uses of toilets and unclean fuel use, lack of autonomy of mothers, and poor wealth indices. This result is highly consistent with the studies (Fenta & Fenta, 2020; MacDonald et al., 2020; Bobo et al., 2022; Fisher et al., 2022). Hence, the findings of this chapter provide important information that can help in planning intervention programs to reduce the U5M of children across the region, which might have significant public health and policy implications. Therefore, from the policy perspective, the study findings call for the need to implement policies aimed at reducing the child's under-five mortality rate in sSA by improving maternal education, improving women's empowerment in decision-making, as well as strengthening access to basic water and sanitation services. Hence, there is a need for both government and nongovernmental organizations in the sub-Saharan African countries to intervene in the community to reduce the U5M of the child by improving the facilities and enhancing the socioeconomic status of households.

This work demonstrated geospatial mixed effect modeling, which includes the potential linear effects of categorical variables, nonlinear effects of continuous covariates, and structured and unstructured spatial effects on estimating the child's under-five mortality rate across sSA countries. However, due to the nature of complex spatial-temporal datasets deal with spatial effects of U5M changing over time. In our context, the Demographic and Health Survey (DHS) data are inherently spatially and temporally autocorrelated among countries across sSA regions. In this regard, there might be a space-time interaction effect. In the coming work, we will focus on the model extensions of the spatial geo-additive model to the spatial-temporal geo-additive model from the Bayesian perspective to analyze this data. In this model, the nonlinear effects of continuous covariates and time trends will be modeled through penalized splines, but the correlated spatial effects will follow the Markov random field priors. Moreover, the spatial-temporal interaction effects on the U5M rate will be investigated.

Though generalized linear models, generalized additive models, and generalized geo-additive mixed effect models provide flexible frameworks for analyzing complex data, they have certain challenges regarding the appropriate distribution and link/smooth function for the response variable(s), validity and accuracy of model assumptions, and computational demands. The other challenges to communicating and explaining the results of those models to nontechnical stakeholders, especially when the models incorporate complex nonlinear effects, interactions, and some data transformation techniques (Hastie & Tibshirani, 1990; Wood, 2017; Wand, 2003; Wand et al., 2011).

Acknowledgments The datasets used in this study were obtained from the DHS program, thanks to the authorization received to download the dataset on the Website. This work is partially based upon research supported by the South Africa Department of Research and Innovation (DSI), National Research Foundation (NRF), and South Africa Medical Research Council (SAMRC) (South Africa DSI-NRF-SAMRC SARChI Research Chair in Biostatistics, Grant number 114613). Opinions expressed and conclusions arrived at are those of the author and are not necessarily to be attributed to the NRF and SAMRC.

Appendix: R and SAS Codes

```
###### Book chapter on Geo-additive mixed effects model:
       Haile Mekonnen Fenta ######
###Required packages#####
#library(rgdal)
library(rgdax)
library(splines)
library(sp)
library(maptools)
library(spdep)
library(INLA)
library(foreign)
library(shapefiles)
library(BayesX)
library(lattice)
library(R2BayesX)
library(sf)
library(ncdf4)
library(raster)
library(rgdal)
library(rasterVis)
library(RColorBrewer)
```

```
###particulate matter data extraction from geotif format and
     merge it with DHS datasets
###Specific country: first load the shapefile from
#https://sedac.ciesin.columbia.edu/data/set/sdei-global-annual-
     gwr-pm2-5-modis-misr-seawifs-aod-v4-gl-03
#specify the year: example for 2019
pm2.5 <- raster("PM2.5/2019/sdei-global-annual-gwr-pm2-5-modis-
     misr-seawifs-aod-v4-gl-03-2019.tif")
###We need to check the crs of each the two files and
     should be same
crs(pm2.5)<- "+proj=longlat +datum=WGS84 +no_defs "# Shapefile
     reprojection
# Create a data.frame with sample site coordinates
#connect it with GPS values from DHS datasets
#gps <- read_csv("C:/Users/hp/Desktop/DSI/gps.csv")###just
     among zones
data2019 <- read_csv("2019.csv")###EAs
data=as.data.frame(data2019)
coordinates(data) <- ~LONGNUM+ LATNUM # change it to
     spatial points
# make sure they have the same crs with the raster
crs(data)<- "+proj=longlat +datum=WGS84 +no_defs "# Shapefile
     reprojection
compareCRS(data, pm2.5)
# Value extraction
data$pm <- extract(pm2.5, data)
data=cbind(data2021,data)
######################Some descriptive statistics for the
     summary statistics################
# install.packages("devtools")
library(rlang)###########
library(devtools)
devtools::install_github("NightingaleHealth/ggforestplot")
####As country
# Load and attach the package
library(ggforestplot)
library(tidyverse)
# dataset
library(readr)
country_CI <- read_csv("E:/Applications/Postdoc/America
     Din/DHS Datasets/country_CI.csv")
country_CI=as.data.frame(country_CI)
### Forest plots for selected result

# Draw a forest plot of cross-sectional, linear associations
ggforestplot::forestplot(
  df =country_CI,
  name =country,
  estimate =prop,
  se =Std.er,
  colour =Type,
  ylab="Sub Saharan African Countries",
```

```
  xlab="Proportion of under-five children with acute
     respiratory symptoms in SSA",
  cex.axis=0.2)
#####################Modeling Sections##############
#inla.version()#To download the most recent stable version
     of the package.
## Importing the shape file
####Download R-INLA package: Activating INLA library and
     its dependence
#install.packages("INLA", repos=c(getOption("repos"),
     INLA="https://inla.r-inla-download.org/R/stable"), dep=TRUE)
# Packages required
###First data source:DHS sub Saharan Africa
###Importing the shapefiles of the study areas
shapef <- st_read("ShapefileH/ssa.shp")
temp <- poly2nb(shapef)
nb2INLA("ssa.graph", temp)
ssa_shape <- paste(getwd(),"/ssa.graph",sep="")
#call the map
H=("ssa.graph")
###Import the individual dataset from the source
library(readr)
dh <- read_csv("dh.csv")
dh=as.data.frame(dh)
table(is.na(dh))### to check the existence of missing values
     from the dataframe
library(data.table)
attach(dh)
table(is.na(dh$b19))
library(tidyr)
library(dplyr)
setDT(dh)
dh[!complete.cases(dh), ]# to see the place of where the
     missing values are located in the data
###Few missing values for the three continuous variables
     were observed.
dh$m19=as.numeric(dh$m19)
dh[, b19 := ifelse(is.na(b19), median(b19, na.rm = TRUE), b19),
    by = country]
dh[, m19 := ifelse(is.na(m19), median(m19, na.rm = TRUE), m19),
    by = country]
dh[, pm := ifelse(is.na(pm), median(pm, na.rm = TRUE), pm),
    by = country]
### Activating INLA library and its dependence
inla.setOption("enable.inla.argument.weights",TRUE)
###Three models used in the analysis
GLMM<-inla(mor_Rate~factor(sex_child)+ factor(Birth_order)
           +factor(birthi)+factor(type_birth)+factor(place_R)
           +factor(Illiteracy_R)
          +factor(occupation_Mother)+factor(occupation_Father)
           +factor(v190)+factor(media)+factor(autonomy)
           +factor(NU5C)+factor(HHS)
```

```
            +factor(head_HH)+factor(breast_feeding)+factor(CIAF)
            +factor(vitA)+factor(DDS)+factor(wateri)
            +factor(toilet)+
            factor(fuel)+factor(plcae_del),family="binomial",
            data=dh,control.compute=list(dic=TRUE,mlik=TRUE,
            cpo=TRUE,waic=TRUE))
GAMM<-inla(mor_Rate~factor(sex_child)+ factor(Birth_order)
            +factor(birthi)+factor(type_birth)+factor(place_R)
            +factor(Illiteracy_R)
            +factor(occupation_Mother)+factor(occupation_Father)
            +factor(v190)+factor(media)+factor(autonomy)
            +factor(NU5C)+factor(HHS)
            +factor(head_HH)+factor(breast_feeding)
            +factor(CIAF)+factor(vitA)+factor(DDS)+factor(wateri)
            +factor(toilet)+
              factor(fuel)+factor(plcae_del)+f(m19)+f(b19)
            +f(age_mother)+f(pm)
            ,family="binomial",data=dh,control.compute=list
            (dic=TRUE,mlik=TRUE,cpo=TRUE,waic=TRUE),verbose=TRUE)
#  including the spatial effect
dh$ssa.unstruct=dh$country2
attach(dh)
GGAMM<-inla(mor_Rate~factor(sex_child)+ factor(Birth_order)
            +factor(birthi)+factor(type_birth)+factor(place_R)+
              factor(Illiteracy_R)+factor(occupation_Mother)
            +factor(occupation_Father)+factor(v190)
            +factor(media)+factor(autonomy)+factor(NU5C)
            +factor(HHS)
            +factor(head_HH)+factor(breast_feeding)+factor(CIAF)
            +factor(vitA)+factor(DDS)+factor(wateri)
            +factor(toilet)+
              factor(fuel)+factor(plcae_del)+f(m19)+f(b19)
            +f(age_mother)+f(pm)+f(country2,model="besag",
            graph.file=H, param=c(1,0.01)) +
              f(ssa.unstruct,model="iid",param=c(1,0.01)),
            family="binomial",data=dh,control.compute=list
                 (dic=TRUE,
                 mlik=TRUE,cpo=TRUE,waic=TRUE),verbose=TRUE,
                 debug = TRUE,safe=FALSE)
###Compare the three models from the summary results
summary(GLMM)
summary(GAMM)
summary(GGAMM)
? inla# will generate the potential results of the model
tt=GGAMM$summary.fixed#Matrix containing the fixed effect
      parameters
write.csv(tt,"tt6.csv")#export the result to csv format and it
      will be saved automatically in the working directory
###Extract the nonlinear effects values of the continuous
      variable in the GGAMM
mean_m19=GGAMM$summary.random$m19 #used to extract the nonlinear
      effects of the parameters
mean_b19=GGAMM$summary.random$b19
mean_agemother=GGAMM$summary.random$age_mother
```

```
mean_pm=GGAMM$summary.random$pm
mean_no2=GGAMM$summary.random$no2
mean_spatial=GGAMM$summary.random$country2 #used to extract
     the structured spatial effect
mean_unstracture=GGAMM$summary.random$ssa.unstruct #used to
     extract unstructured random effect
###plot the nonlinear effects
plot(mean_agemother$mean~mean_agemother$ID,type="l",
    data=mean_agemother,ylim=range(c(mean_agemother$'0.025quant',
    mean_agemother$'0.975quant')))
plot(mean_m19$mean~mean_m19$ID,data=mean_m19,type="l",
    ylim=range(c(mean_m19$'0.025quant',mean_m19$'0.975quant')))
plot(mean_b19$mean~mean_b19$ID, type="l",data=mean_b19,
    ylim=range(c(mean_b19$'0.025quant',mean_b19$'0.975quant')))
plot(mean_pm$mean~mean_pm$ID,type="l",data=mean_pm,
    ylim=range(c(mean_pm$'0.025quant',mean_pm$'0.975quant')))
plot(mean_no2$mean~mean_no2$ID,type="l",data=mean_no2,
    ylim=range(c(mean_no2$'0.025quant',mean_no2$'0.975quant')))

###########Sensitivity Statistical Analysis on the prior section
           of hyper-parameters (
#(for scale and shape) ############
# we used the inverse gamma distributions
####           IG(a,b)         IG(a,b)      IG(a,b)       IG(a,b)
#structured   (0.001, 0.001) (0.01, 0.01) (0.05, 0.0005) (1, 0.026)
#unstructured (0.001, 0.001) (0.01, 0.01) (0.05, 0.0005) (1, 0.026)
##IG (0.001, 0.001)
GGAMM1<-inla(mor_Rate~factor(sex_child)+ factor(Birth_order)
           +factor(birthi)+factor(type_birth)+factor(place_R)
           +factor(Illiteracy_R)
            +factor(occupation_Mother)+factor(occupation_Father)
           +factor(v190)+factor(media)+factor(autonomy)
           +factor(NU5C)+factor(HHS)
            +factor(head_HH)+factor(breast_feeding)
           +factor(CIAF)+factor(vitA)+factor(DDS)
           +factor(wateri)+factor(toilet)+
             factor(fuel)+f(m19)+f(b19)+f(age_mother)+f(pm)
           +f(country2,model="besag",graph.file=H,
            param=c(1,0.01)) +
             f(ssa.unstruct,model="iid",param=c(0.001,0.001)),
           family="binomial",data=dh,control.compute=list
           (dic=TRUE,mlik=TRUE,cpo=TRUE,waic=TRUE),
           verbose=TRUE,weights = weight)
##IG (0.01, 0.01)
GGAMM2<-inla(mor_Rate~factor(sex_child)+ factor(Birth_order)
           +factor(birthi)+factor(type_birth)+factor(place_R)
           +factor(Illiteracy_R)
            +factor(occupation_Mother)+factor(occupation_Father)
           +factor(v190)+factor(media)+factor(autonomy)
           +factor(NU5C)+factor(HHS)
            +factor(head_HH)+factor(breast_feeding)
           +factor(CIAF)+factor(vitA)+factor(DDS)+factor(wateri)
           +factor(toilet)+
```

```
            factor(fuel)+f(m19)+f(b19)+f(age_mother)+f(pm)
            +f(country2,model="besag",graph.file=H,
             param=c(1,0.01)) +
              f(ssa.unstruct,model="iid",param=c(0.01,0.01)),
            family="binomial",data=dh,control.compute=list
            (dic=TRUE,mlik=TRUE,cpo=TRUE,waic=TRUE),
            verbose=TRUE,weights = weight)

###IG (0.5, 0.0005)
GGAMM3<-inla(mor_Rate~factor(sex_child)+ factor(Birth_order)
            +factor(birthi)+factor(type_birth)+factor(place_R)
            +factor(Illiteracy_R)
              +factor(occupation_Mother)+factor(occupation_Father)
            +factor(v190)+factor(media)+factor(autonomy)
            +factor(NU5C)+factor(HHS)
              +factor(head_HH)+factor(breast_feeding)
            +factor(CIAF)+factor(vitA)+factor(DDS)
            +factor(wateri)+factor(toilet)+
               factor(fuel)+f(m19)+f(b19)+f(age_mother)
            +f(pm)+f(country2,model="besag",graph.file=H,
             param=c(1,0.01)) +
               f(ssa.unstruct,model="iid",param=c(0.05,0.0005)),
            family="binomial",data=dh,control.compute=list
            (dic=TRUE,mlik=TRUE,cpo=TRUE,waic=TRUE),
            verbose=TRUE,weights = weight)
###(1, 0.026)
GGAMM4<-inla(mor_Rate~factor(sex_child)+ factor(Birth_order)
            +factor(birthi)+factor(type_birth)
            +factor(place_R)+factor(Illiteracy_R)
              +factor(occupation_Mother)+factor(occupation_Father)
            +factor(v190)+factor(media)+factor(autonomy)
            +factor(NU5C)+factor(HHS)
              +factor(head_HH)+factor(breast_feeding)
            +factor(CIAF)+factor(vitA)+factor(DDS)
            +factor(wateri)+factor(toilet)+
               factor(fuel)+f(m19)+f(b19)+f(age_mother)+f(pm)
            +f(country2,model="besag",graph.file=H,
             param=c(1,0.01))
 +f(ssa.unstruct,model="iid",param=c(1,0.026)),
            family="binomial",data=dh,control.compute=list
            (dic=TRUE,mlik=TRUE,cpo=TRUE,waic=TRUE),
            verbose=TRUE,weight=weight)
###3compare the results
summary(GGAMM); summary(GGAMM1); summary(GGAMM2);summary(GGAMM3);
   summary(GGAMM4)
####For the ROC_AUC plot, we used SAS for predicted values from
      the three models###
##############
proc logistic data=dh_predicted;
model dh_mor_Rate(event="1")=pred_glmm pred_gamm
      pred_ggamm/nofit ;
roc "GLMM" pred_glmm;
roc "GAMM" pred_gamm;
```

```
roc "GGAMM" pred_ggamm;
roccontrast " Comparing the given models" /estimate=allpairs;
run;
```

References

Adebowale, A. S., Fagbamigbe, A. F., Morakinyo, O., Obembe, T., Afolabi, R. F., & Palamuleni, M. E. (2020). Parental educational homogamy and under-five mortality in sub-Saharan Africa: Clarifying the association's intricacy. *Scientific African, 7*, e00255.

Agresti, A. (2012). *Categorical data analysis*. Wiley.

Aliaga, A., & Ren, R. (2006). *The optimal sample sizes for two-stage cluster sampling in demographic and health surveys*. ORC Macro.

Allouche, O., Tsoar, A., & Kadmon, R. (2006). Assessing the accuracy of species distribution models: Prevalence, kappa and the true skill statistic (TSS). *Journal of Applied Ecology, 43*(6), 1223–1232.

Assunçao, R. M. (2003). Space varying coefficient models for small area data. *Environmetrics: The Official Journal of the International Environmetrics Society, 14*(5), 453–473.

Best, N. G., Arnold, R. A., Thomas, A., Waller, L. A., & Conlon, E. M. (1999). Bayesian models for spatially correlated disease and exposure data. *Bayesian Statistics, 6*, 131–156.

Bobo, F. T., Asante, A., Woldie, M., Dawson, A., & Hayen, A. (2022). Child vaccination in sub-Saharan Africa: Increasing coverage addresses inequalities. *Vaccine, 40*(1), 141–150.

Bolstad, W. M. (2009). *Understanding computational Bayesian statistics*. Wiley.

Brezger, A., & Lang, S. (2006). Generalized structured additive regression based on Bayesian P-splines. *Computational Statistics & Data Analysis, 50*(4), 967–991.

Brockerhoff, M., & Hewett, P. (2000). Inequality of child mortality among ethnic groups in sub-Saharan Africa. *Bulletin of the World Health Organization, 78*, 30–41.

Brunsdon, C., Fotheringham, A., & Charlton, M. (2002). Geographically weighted summary statistics—A framework for localised exploratory data analysis. *Computers, Environment and Urban Systems, 26*(6), 501–524.

Bryce, J., Victora, C. G., & Black, R. E. (2013). The unfinished agenda in child survival. *The Lancet, 382*(9897), 1049–1059.

Child, Y. (2011). Infant and young child feeding. In *Nutrition* (pp. 11–13).

Cressie, N., Calder, C. A., Clark, J. S., Hoef, J. M. V., & Wikle, C. K. (2009). Accounting for uncertainty in ecological analysis: The strengths and limitations of hierarchical statistical modeling. *Ecological Applications, 19*(3), 553–570.

Fahrmeir, L., & Kneib, T. (2009). Propriety of posteriors in structured additive regression models: Theory and empirical evidence. *Journal of Statistical Planning and Inference, 139*(3), 843–859.

Fenta, S. M., & Fenta, H. M. (2020). Risk factors of child mortality in Ethiopia: Application of multilevel two-part model. *PLoS One, 15*(8), e0237640.

Fenta, S. M., Fenta, H. M., & Ayenew, G. M. (2020). The best statistical model to estimate predictors of under-five mortality in Ethiopia. *Journal of Big Data, 7*(1), 1–14.

Fenta, H. M., Zewotir, T., & Muluneh, E. K. (2021a). Disparities in childhood composite index of anthropometric failure prevalence and determinants across Ethiopian administrative zones. *PLoS One, 16*(9), e0256726.

Fenta, H. M., Zewotir, T., & Muluneh, E. K. (2021b). Spatial data analysis of malnutrition among children under-five years in Ethiopia. *BMC Medical Research Methodology, 21*(1), 1–13.

Fenta, S. M., Ayenew, G. M., Fenta, H. M., Biresaw, H. B., & Fentaw, K. D. (2022). Community and individual level determinants of infant mortality in rural Ethiopia using data from 2016 Ethiopian demographic and health survey. *Scientific Reports, 12*(1), 16879.

Fielding, A. H., & Bell, J. F. (1997). A review of methods for the assessment of prediction errors in conservation presence/absence models. *Environmental Conservation, 24*, 38–49.

Finley, A. O. (2011). Comparing spatially-varying coefficients models for analysis of ecological data with non-stationary and anisotropic residual dependence. *Methods in Ecology and Evolution, 2*(2), 143–154.

Fisher, C. B., Bragard, E., Jaber, R., & Gray, A. (2022). COVID-19 vaccine hesitancy among parents of children under five years in the United States. *Vaccine, 10*(8), 1313.

Gelfand, A. E., Dey, D. K., & Chang, H. (1992). *Model determination using predictive distributions with implementation via sampling-based methods.* Stanford University Department of Statistics.

Gelman, A., & Meng, X.-L. (1996). Model checking and model improvement. In *Markov chain Monte Carlo in practice* (pp. 189–201). Springer.

Gosoniu, L., Vounatsou, P., Sogoba, N., & Smith, T. (2006). Bayesian modelling of geostatistical malaria risk data. *Geospatial Health,1*, 127–139.

Green, P. J., & Silverman, B. W. (2019). *Nonparametric regression and generalized linear models: a roughness penalty approach.* Chapman and Hall/CRC.

Hammer, M. S., van Donkelaar, A., Li, C., Lyapustin, A., Sayer, A. M., Hsu, N. C., Levy, R. C., Garay, M. J., Kalashnikova, O. V., & Kahn, R. A. (2020). Global estimates and long-term trends of fine particulate matter concentrations (1998–2018). *Environmental Science & Technology, 54*(13), 7879–7890.

Hastie, T. J., & Tibshirani, R. J. (1990). *Generalized additive models.* CRC Press.

Hastie, T. J., & Tibshirani, R. J. (2017). *Generalized additive models.* Routledge.

Hosmer, D. W., Hosmer, T., Le Cessie, S., & Lemeshow, S. (1997). A comparison of goodness-of-fit tests for the logistic regression model. *Statistics in Medicine, 16*(9), 965–980.

Hu, Y., Wang, J., Zhu, J., & Ren, D. (2011). Mapping under-five mortality in the Wenchuan earthquake using hierarchical Bayesian modeling. *International Journal of Environmental Health Research, 21*(5), 364–371.

Hug, L., Mishra, A., Lee, S., You, D., Moran, A., Strong, K. L., & Cao, B. (2020). *A neglected tragedy The global burden of stillbirths: report of the UN inter-agency group for child mortality estimation, 2020.* United Nations Children's Fund.

Kazembe, L. N., & Kandala, N.-B. (2015). Estimating areas of common risk in low birth weight and infant mortality in Namibia: A joint spatial analysis at sub-regional level. *Spatial and Spatio-temporal Epidemiology, 12*, 27–37.

Kelsall, J., & Wakefield, J. (1999). Discussion of 'Bayesian models for spatially correlated disease and exposure data', by Best et al. *Bayesian Statistics, 6*, 151.

Khatab, K., & Fahrmeir, L. (2008). *Analysis of childhood morbidity with geoadditive probit and latent variable model: A case study for Egypt.* (Technical Report Number 021, 2008). Department of Statistics, University of Munich.

Krainski, E., Gómez-Rubio, V., Bakka, H., Lenzi, A., Castro-Camilo, D., Simpson, D., Lindgren, F., & Rue, H. (2018). *Advanced spatial modeling with stochastic partial differential equations using R and INLA.* Chapman and Hall/CRC.

Lang, S., & Brezger, A. (2000). *Bayesx-software for Bayesian inference based on Markov chain Monte Carlo simulation techniques.*

Lin, X., & Zhang, D. (1999). Inference in generalized additive mixed models by using smoothing splines. *Journal of the royal statistical society: Series B (Statistical Methodology), 61*(2), 381–400.

Lindgren, F., & Rue, H. (2015). Bayesian spatial modelling with R-INLA. *Journal of Statistical Software, 63*(19).

Lunn, D. J., Thomas, A., Best, N., & Spiegelhalter, D. (2000). WinBUGS-a Bayesian modelling framework: concepts, structure, and extensibility. *Statistics and Computing, 10*(4), 325–337.

MacDonald, N., Mohsni, E., Al-Mazrou, Y., Andrus, J. K., Arora, N., Elden, S., Madrid, M.-Y., Martin, R., Mustafa, A. M., & Rees, H. (2020). Global vaccine action plan lessons learned I: Recommendations for the next decade. *Vaccine, 38*(33), 5364–5371.

Martins, T. G., Simpson, D., Lindgren, F., & Rue, H. (2013). Bayesian computing with INLA: New features. *Computational Statistics & Data Analysis, 67*, 68–83.

Miaou, S.-P., Song, J. J., & Mallick, B. K. (2003). Roadway traffic crash mapping: A space-time modeling approach. *Journal of Transportation and Statistics, 6*, 33–58.
Nelder, J. A., & Wedderburn, R. W. (1972). Generalized linear models. *Journal of the Royal Statistical Society: Series A (General), 135*(3), 370–384.
O'sullivan, F., Yandell, B. S., & Raynor, W. J., Jr. (1986). Automatic smoothing of regression functions in generalized linear models. *Journal of the American Statistical Association, 81*(393), 96–103.
Pearson, R. G. (2007). Species' distribution modeling for conservation educators and practitioners. *Synthesis American Museum of Natural History, 50*, 54–89.
Resolution, G. A. (2015). Transforming our world: The 2030 agenda for sustainable development. UN Doc. A/RES/70/1 (September 25, 2015).
Rue, H., Martino, S., & Chopin, N. (2009). Approximate Bayesian inference for latent Gaussian models by using integrated nested Laplace approximations. *Journal of the Royal Statistical Society: Series B (Statistical Methodology), 71*(2), 319–392.
Rutherford, M. E., Mulholland, K., & Hill, P. C. (2010). How access to health care relates to under-five mortality in sub-Saharan Africa: Systematic review. *Tropical Medicine & International Health, 15*(5), 508–519.
Shimaponda-Mataa, N. M., Tembo-Mwase, E., Gebreslasie, M., Achia, T. N., & Mukaratirwa, S. (2017). Modelling the influence of temperature and rainfall on malaria incidence in four endemic provinces of Zambia using semiparametric Poisson regression. *Acta Tropica, 166*, 81–91.
Spiegelhalter, D. J., Best, N. G., Carlin, B. P., & Van Der Linde, A. (2002). Bayesian measures of model complexity and fit. *Journal of the Royal Statistical Society: Series B (Statistical Methodology), 64*(4), 583–639.
United Nations. (2012). *The millennium development goals report 2012*. (Millennium Development Goals Report).
Van Malderen, C., Amouzou, A., Barros, A. J., Masquelier, B., Van Oyen, H., & Speybroeck, N. (2019). Socioeconomic factors contributing to under-five mortality in sub-Saharan Africa: A decomposition analysis. *BMC Public Health, 19*, 1–19.
Van Niekerk, J., Bakka, H., Rue, H., & Schenk, O. (2019). New frontiers in Bayesian modeling using the INLA package in R. arXiv preprint arXiv:1907.10426.
Wakefield, J. (2007). Disease mapping and spatial regression with count data. *Biostatistics, 8*(2), 158–183.
Wand, M. P. (2003). Smoothing and mixed models. *Computational Statistics, 18*(2), 223–249.
Wand, H., Whitaker, C., & Ramjee, G. (2011). Geoadditive models to assess spatial variation of HIV infections among women in Local communities of Durban, South Africa. *International Journal of Health Geographics, 10*(1), 28.
Watanabe, S. (2013). A widely applicable Bayesian information criterion. *Journal of Machine Learning Research, 14*(Mar), 867–897.
Wheeler, D. C., & Waller, L. A. (2009). Comparing spatially varying coefficient models: a case study examining violent crime rates and their relationships to alcohol outlets and illegal drug arrests. *Journal of Geographical Systems, 11*, 1–22.
Wood, S. N. (2017). *Generalized additive models: An introduction with R*. CRC Press.
Zike, D. T., Fenta, H. M., Workie, D. L., & Swain, P. K. (2018). Determinants of under-five mortality in Ethiopia: An application of cox proportional hazard and frailty models. *Turkiye Klinikleri Journal of Biostatistics, 10*(2), 123.

Chapter 11
Survey Design Effect in the Prediction of Events for Categorical Health Outcomes Through Regression Methods: Evidence from Malawi Under-Five Mortality Survey Data: 2000–2016

Tsirizani M. Kaombe and Gracious A. Hamuza

11.1 Introduction

Health systems worldwide use the under-five death rate as one of the metrics for deciding about the general health of a population (Ahmad et al., 2000; Joos et al., 2016). The sub-Saharan African region, however, faces challenges with weak vital registration systems, including inaccurate child birth and death registers, as well as a high prevalence of underreporting of deaths at hospitals (Morris et al., 2003; Groenewald et al., 2016; Maïga et al., 2019; Yaya et al., 2019). Nonetheless, considerable effort is being made by researchers to estimate the under-five mortality rate in the region using national surveys, such as the Demographic and Health Survey (DHS) (Lehtonen & Pahkinen, 2004; Silva et al., 2012; Li et al., 2019; Rerimoi et al., 2019; Kaombe & Manda, 2022, 2023b,a). Yet, most of the applications are design-insensitive, which might bias the estimations (Rutkowski et al., 2010; Kazembe & Mpeketula, 2010; Rajaratnam et al., 2010; Renschler et al., 2015; Wakefield et al., 2019).

The accurate estimation of health outcomes from large and complex surveys can be realised if a study involves survey weights (Koch et al., 1980; Kneipp & Yarandi, 2002; Brenning et al., 2005). The sample weight is the reciprocal of the selection probability for a unit in a sample (Seaman & White, 2013). It measures the number of individuals each sampled unit represents in the population (Winship & Radbill, 1994). For regression-based methods, the sample weight is incorporated

---

T. M. Kaombe (✉)
Department of Mathematical Sciences, School of Natural and Applied Sciences, University of Malawi, Zomba, Malawi
e-mail: tkaombe@unima.ac.mw

G. A. Hamuza
National Statistics Office, Zomba, Malawi

D.-G. Chen, C. A. Coelho (eds.), *Biostatistics Modeling and Public Health Applications*, Emerging Topics in Statistics and Biostatistics,
https://doi.org/10.1007/978-3-031-69690-9_11

as a functional of covariates. The weights compensate for the use of unequal sample inclusions in complex surveys, nonresponse, and under-coverage of the sampling frame in the estimation (Zieschang, 1990; Pfeffermann, 1993; Faiella, 2010; Chen et al., 2014; Vandendijck et al., 2016; Kaombe & Hamuza, 2023).

The disregard of survey design effects in the analysis of binary health response data has not only impacted under-five mortality estimation but also affects studies on diabetes, diarrhoea, schistosomiasis, and malaria (Nsowah-Nuamah et al., 2001; Guimarães et al., 2006; Nyambe et al., 2020; Mwanga et al., 2019; Talukder et al., 2020). When the goal of the study is to describe the relationship between certain factors and a binary health outcome, the factors can still be accurately identified using an unweighted regression model. However, the sizes of the effects may not be accurately measured (Kayode et al., 2012; Fagbamigbe & Nnanatu, 2022; Yaya et al., 2018; Kaombe & Hamuza, 2023). The infrequent application of the survey design effect in studies that estimate or predict under-five mortality may become standard practice, but it could reflect a scarcity of literature demonstrating the technical use of sampling weights in this area.

When using a binary logistic regression model for prediction, the logarithm of the odds of an event in each individual is a linear combination of the covariates, which may be affected by the survey weights (Kaombe & Hamuza, 2023). However, it is currently unclear how much bias a study incurs if the weights are ignored when predicting the under-five mortality rate or other binary outcomes using survey data. This chapter aims to estimate the bias in predicting the under-five mortality rate in Malawi using unweighted and weighted logistic regression models. The prediction bias for under-five mortality rate is the difference between the predicted rate from the model and the actual rate from administrative data. A more accurate prediction occurs when the bias approaches zero (Quenouille, 1956). This present study used the three recent Malawi Demographic and Health Survey (MDHS) datasets for the years 2004, 2010, and 2015–16, and the United Nations Children's Fund (UNICEF) (Unicef-Malawi, 2022) annual routine under-five mortality monitoring data for the same years to compute the biases. The three surveys were engaged in order to yield consistent conclusions from this study. The predictions were made using 100%, 75%, 50%, and 25% sample sizes of the MDHS data in order to account for sample size effects in the estimations.

The need for a health researcher to know the value of the design effect of a survey in the binary regression model cannot be overemphasised, as it can guide the researcher in deciding whether or not to include the survey weights in the analysis (Faiella, 2010). When predicting under-five mortality, knowledge of the prediction bias from this study will provide health researchers with information about the level of accuracy gained in using unweighted and weighted statistical methods for the prediction. The next section of this chapter presents the statistical methods and data used. Then, in Sect. 11.3, we present the results. In Sect. 11.4, there is discussion of findings, whereas Sect. 11.5 gives conclusions.

11.2 Methods

11.2.1 Data Description

This chapter generated evidence about the value (or lack of it) of the sampling design effect when predicting the under-five mortality rate. It used secondary data from the "kids" records file of the Malawi Demographic and Health Survey (MDHS). Three sets of data were used, in order to concretise the evidence: the 2004, 2010, and 2015–16 MDHSs data. The 2004 MDHS was conducted between October 2004 and January 2005, and it estimated the child health status of the country for the period 2000 up to 2005, whereas the 2010 MDHS took place between June and November 2010, and it covered the health situation of the country from 2005 up to 2010. Then, the 2015–16 MDHS was conducted between October 2015 and February 2016, and it estimated the health status of the country spanning the years 2010–2016. Each MDHS used two-stage cluster stratified sampling, in which 522, 849, and 850 clusters were, respectively, selected from the country at first stage in 2004, 2010, and 2015–16. Then 15,091, 27,345, and 27,516 households were sampled at second stage from the sampled clusters in the respective years, while taking into account the rural and urban stratifications (National Statistical Office (NSO) [Malawi] and ORC Macro, 2005; National Statistical Office (NSO) and ICF Macro, 2011; National Statistical Office (NSO) [Malawi] and ICF, 2017). Children aged below 5 years in the sampled households formed the sample in this study. These were, respectively, 10,914, 19,967, and 17,286 children in 2004, 2010, and 2015–16 MDHSs. The birth histories of the children, such as details about under-five mortality, were provided by the mothers or adult caregivers aged between 15 and 49 years. As indicated in Sect. 11.1, we accounted for effects of sample sizes in the predictions of under-five mortality in this study through using resampled 75%, 50% and 25% of the sampled clusters, in addition to the original sample size (Jaki et al., 2019; Kaombe & Hamuza, 2023). This was done with the help of the STATA function "bsample", that was applied on the cluster number variable (Vergouwe et al., 2005).

The study used the variable "whether or not an under-five child died in a household within the 5 years preceding the survey" as an outcome variable in the regression model. While the following explanatory variables, which were chosen based on findings from previous studies, were used: child sex, birth order, whether the birth was singleton or multiple, type of delivery (regular or caesarean), maternal age, maternal education, maternal occupation, place of residence, place of delivery, preceding birth interval, contraceptive use, and region (Manda, 1999; Kazembe & Mpeketula, 2010; Kayode et al., 2012; Getachew & Bekele, 2016; Argawu & Mekebo, 2022; Dadi, 2015; Tuoyire & Amo-Adjei, 2022). We cleaned the data and fitted the models using STATA version 12.0 and computed the predicted national under-five mortality rate using R version 3.6.3 software. The UNICEF annual data showed that the under-five mortality rates in Malawi were, respectively, 119.7, 84.2, and 49.5 per 1000 live births in 2004, 2010, and 2015 (Unicef-Malawi,

2022). Therefore, we used these values and those predicted from the fitted logistic regression models on the MDHS data to calculate the bias (Kaombe & Hamuza, 2023). The MDHS data that were used in this study are publicly and freely available for users at www.DHSprogram.com.

11.2.2 Logistic Regression Model and Predicted Mortality Rate Without Weights

Suppose Y denotes a binomial random variable capturing the total number of children aged below 5 years who died in some cluster in the country during some period of time within the 5 years prior to the MDHS. Let y_{ic} be the specific outcome for the i-th child in c-th cluster, $i = 1, 2, ..., n_c$; $c = 1, 2, ..., k$, which was $y_{ic} = 1$ if the observed outcome was death, and $y_{ic} = 0$ otherwise. If the probability that i-th child died in a household that was in c-th cluster was $\pi_{ic} = P(Y = 1)$, then $Y \sim Binomial(n, \pi)$, whose probability mass function is given by

$$f(y_{ic}|n, \pi_{ic}) = \exp\left[y_{ic} \log\left(\frac{\pi_{ic}}{1-\pi_{ic}}\right) + n\log(1-\pi_{ic}) + \log\binom{n}{y_{ic}} \right]. \quad (11.1)$$

If $x_{ick}^T = (x_{ic0}, x_{ic1}, x_{ic2}, ..., x_{icp})$ is a vector of observed values of each explanatory variable on the i-th child in cluster c, with $x_{ic0} = 1$, then the probability of a child dying, i.e., π_{ic}, can be determined upon considering the covariates $\mathbf{x}$, i.e., $\pi_{ic} = P(Y = 1|\mathbf{x})$. For all the children, the function of this conditional probability of the child dying given the covariates, i.e., $\pi_{ic} = P(Y = 1|\mathbf{x})$, will mimic the logistic curve when plotted against the covariates $\mathbf{x}$, whose unweighted form is given by

$$\pi_{ic}(\mathbf{x}) = P(Y = 1|\mathbf{x}) = \frac{\exp(\beta^T \mathbf{x})}{1+\exp(\beta^T \mathbf{x})}, \quad (11.2)$$

where $\beta^T = (\beta_0, \beta_1, ..., \beta_p)$ is a vector of regression coefficients and $\mathbf{x} = (1, x_{ic1}, x_{ic2}, ..., x_{icp})^T$ is a vector of covariates. The log-odds (or logit) form of the unweighted logistic regression model follows from Eq. (11.2), and it is given by

$$\log\left(\frac{\pi_{ic}(\mathbf{x})}{1-\pi_{ic}(\mathbf{x})}\right) = \beta^T \mathbf{x} = \beta_0 + \beta_1 x_{ic1} + ... + \beta_p x_{icp}. \quad (11.3)$$

The likelihood function of β for the model in Eqs. (11.2–11.3) is obtained by multiplying the values of probabilities in Eq. (11.1) for all the children in all the clusters. The estimation of β is found by first taking the logarithm of the likelihood function and then finding the partial derivatives of the log-likelihood function with respect to β. Then, upon equating to zero the partial derivatives so obtained, the maximum likelihood (ML) estimates $\hat{\beta}$ are solved through numerical methods due to the fact that the equations are usually not in closed forms (Carroll & Pederson, 1993). The ML estimate $\hat{\beta}$ was interpreted as the change in logarithm of odds of death of a child corresponding to the change in the level of a covariate X, while the exponentiated ML estimate $exp\left(\hat{\beta}\right)$ was interpreted as the odds ratio of death of a child when comparing two levels of X.

Now, the obtained ML estimates $\hat{\beta}$ can be inputted back into Eq. (11.2) to determine the predicted probability of death for each child, i.e., $\hat{\pi}_{ic}\left(\mathbf{x}\right)$. In turn, the overall unweighted predicted probability of death for all under-five children in the country was estimated by taking average of all fitted probabilities from the model (Kaombe & Hamuza, 2023) as

$$\hat{\pi}\left(\mathbf{x}\right) = \frac{\Sigma_{i=1}^{n_c}\Sigma_{c=1}^{k}\hat{\pi}_{ic}\left(\mathbf{x}\right)}{\Sigma_{c=1}^{k}n_c}, \quad (11.4)$$

where $\hat{\pi}_{ic}\left(\mathbf{x}\right) = \frac{exp\left(\hat{\beta}^T\mathbf{x}\right)}{1+exp\left(\hat{\beta}^T\mathbf{x}\right)}$ is the fitted probability of death of the i-th child in c-th cluster given the covariates values $\mathbf{x}$, and given the fitted model. The estimate of under-five mortality in Eq. (11.4) is the usual point estimate of the proportion of under-five deaths across all clusters in the country. Based on sampling distribution theory for sample proportions, the unweighted variance of $\hat{\pi}\left(\mathbf{x}\right)$ had to be estimated by

$$var\left(\hat{\pi}\left(\mathbf{x}\right)\right) = \frac{\hat{\pi}\left(\mathbf{x}\right)\left(1-\hat{\pi}\left(\mathbf{x}\right)\right)}{\Sigma_{c=1}^{k}n_c}. \quad (11.5)$$

Since the predicted mortality rate in Eq. (11.4) is calculated separately once the fitted probabilities $\hat{\pi}_{ic}\left(\mathbf{x}\right)$ from the fitted model are obtained, the model's ML estimates $\hat{\beta}$ that are used to compute $\hat{\pi}\left(\mathbf{x}\right)$ can be from a unweighted or weighted model (Kaombe & Hamuza, 2023). In the case of the quantity in Eq. (11.4), $\hat{\beta}$ was unweighted, and so was the mortality estimate $\hat{\pi}\left(\mathbf{x}\right)$. But we also considered a scenario of weighting $\hat{\pi}\left(\mathbf{x}\right)$, based on methods given in the next section, using ML estimates from the unweighted model. Taking the square root of the variance in Eq. (11.5) provided the standard error of the estimated under-five mortality rate.

From the estimate of under-five mortality rate in Eq. (11.4), we computed the bias of the estimate as follows (Kaombe & Hamuza, 2023):

$$bias\left(\hat{\pi}\left(\mathbf{x}\right)\right) = \hat{\pi}\left(\mathbf{x}\right) - \pi, \quad (11.6)$$

where $\hat{\pi}\left(\mathbf{x}\right)$ is the predicted under-five mortality rate in Eq. (11.4) and π is the raw annual under-five mortality rate from UNICEF report (Unicef-Malawi, 2022). The model fitting and all other calculations as given above were done on all three MDHS datasets in order to confirm the findings and were repeated at 75%, 50%, and 25%

of each MDHS data in order to account for sample size effect in the estimated bias (Vergouwe et al., 2005; Jaki et al., 2019).

11.2.3 Logistic Regression Model and Predicted Mortality Rate with Survey Weights

Defining the binomial random variable as in Sect. 11.2.2, let $w_{ic} = \frac{N_c}{n_c}$ be the sample weight for i-th child in c-th cluster, where N_c is the total number of children aged below 5 years in a cluster c and n_c the sample size of selected children in the cluster c. From the 2018 Malawi population and housing census, there were 2,552,406 children who were aged below 5 years in the country, and these were studied in 18,772 equally sized clusters (or enumeration areas) ((2019), NSO). Using this information, we estimated the population of under-five children in each cluster during the 2015–16 MDHS as $N_c = \frac{2{,}555{,}406}{18{,}772} = 135.969$ children. Therefore, each sampled child in the 2015–16 MDHS represented information for $w_{ic} = \frac{135.969}{n_c}$ children in their location, depending on the size of the sampled cluster. With the 2008 Malawi population and housing census, the population of children aged below 5 years in the country was 2,370,011 then, and these were located in 12,631 equally sized clusters ((2009), NSO). Hence, the cluster-specific population of children during the 2004 or 2010 MDHS was estimated at $N_c = \frac{2{,}370{,}011}{12{,}631} = 187.634$. Then, the sampling weight when using the 2004 or 2010 MDHS data was $w_{ic} = \frac{187.634}{n_c}$ (Kaombe & Hamuza, 2023).

Using the information in the foregoing paragraph, the weighted conditional probability of death of i-th child given the covariates $\mathbf{x}$ was defined by

$$\pi_{ic}^{*}(\mathbf{x}) = P(Y = 1|\mathbf{x}) = \frac{\exp\left(\beta^T \mathbf{x} w_{ic}\right)}{1+\exp\left(\beta^T \mathbf{x} w_{ic}\right)}, \tag{11.7}$$

where $w_{ic} = \frac{135.969}{n_c}$ if the model was applied on 2015–16 MDHS data, and $w_{ic} = \frac{187.634}{n_c}$ when the analysis was done on 2004 or 2010 MDHS data, and the other involved quantities were as defined in the unweighted conditional probability of event in Eq. (11.2). Therefore, the weighted logit model (Zeng, 2017) is given by

$$\log\left(\frac{\pi_{ic}^{*}(\mathbf{x})}{1-\pi_{ic}^{*}(\mathbf{x})}\right) = \beta^T \mathbf{x} w_{ic} = \left[\beta_0+\beta_1 x_{ic1}+\cdots+\beta_p x_{icp}\right] w_{ic}, \tag{11.8}$$

where $\pi_{ic}^{*}(\mathbf{x})$ was the weighted probability of event given in Eq. (11.7), $w_{ic} = \frac{135.969}{n_c}$ when dealing with the 2015–16 MDHS dataset, and $w_{ic} = \frac{187.634}{n_c}$ when analysing the 2004 or 2010 MDHS data, with $w_{00} = 1$ as baseline weight. During model fitting, these sampling weights ensured that each child's likelihood contribution accounts for the survey design effect when computing ML estimates, with the aim of balancing off the unequal sample selection, nonresponse, or under-coverage of the sampling frame from cluster to cluster in the computation of ML estimates (Pfeffermann, 1993; Faiella, 2010; Chen et al., 2014; Vandendijck et al., 2016).

We used the STATA survey function *svy* to define the sampling weights during the model fitting. The ML estimates $\hat{\beta}\,(w_{ic})$ were solved in a similar manner as in Sect. 11.2.2. However, the standard errors of the ML estimates were calculated using the jackknife technique (Markatou et al., 1997). Since each sampled child in a cluster was not replaced in the population before selecting the next child, then the population became finite as sampling continued. Therefore, a hypergeometric probability distribution was supposed to be assumed for the observed number of under-five deaths at any period of survey time rather than the binomial probability distribution. The standard deviation of the hypergeometric random variable is larger than that of a binomial random variable by a factor, fpc $= \sqrt{\frac{N-n}{N-1}}$. Therefore, multiplying this quantity with the standard errors of ML estimates from a binomial regression model is termed finite population correction (fpc) factor that approximates the standard errors to the hypergeometric model. When the finite population correction (fpc) factor is approximately 1, the fpc does not change anything to the standard errors of a binomial regression model and can be ignored. This was checked in our case, and the fpc was close to 1 for each dataset, so we ignored it. For the 2015–16 MDHS and using 2018 national census, $\text{fpc}_{(2015)} = \sqrt{\frac{2{,}552{,}406-17{,}286}{2{,}552{,}406-1}} = 0.9966$, whereas for 2004 MDHS and considering 2008 census, $\text{fpc}_{(2004)} = \sqrt{\frac{2{,}370{,}011-10{,}914}{2{,}370{,}011-1}} = 0.9976$. Then, for the 2010 MDHS and using 2008 census, $\text{fpc}_{(2010)} = \sqrt{\frac{2{,}370{,}011-19{,}967}{2{,}370{,}011-1}} = 0.9958$ (Kaombe & Hamuza, 2023).

Upon obtaining the weighted ML estimates $\hat{\beta}\,(w_{ic})$ from the weighted model in Eq. (11.8) or unweighted ML estimates $\hat{\beta}$ from the unweighted model in Eq. (11.3), we considered a second set of cluster-strata weights that were applied during the computation of the overall predicted national under-five death rate. Either way, this required estimating the cluster-specific mortality rates $\hat{\pi}_c\,(\mathbf{x})$ from either model. Then, the weighted predicted under-five mortality rate is found as follows (Kaombe & Hamuza, 2023):

$$\hat{\pi}\,(\mathbf{x}) = \frac{\Sigma_{c=1}^{k}\hat{\pi}_c\,(\mathbf{x})\left(\frac{n_c}{\bar{m}}\right)}{k}, \tag{11.9}$$

where $\bar{m} = \frac{\Sigma_{c=1}^{k} n_c}{k}$ is the average number of children per cluster, $\hat{\pi}_c\,(\mathbf{x}) = \frac{\Sigma_{i=1}^{n_c}\hat{\pi}_{ic}(\mathbf{x})}{n_c}$ is the cluster-specific estimated probability of death of a child if the model was unweighted, and $\hat{\pi}_c\,(\mathbf{x}) = \frac{\Sigma_{i=1}^{n_c}\hat{\pi}^*_{ic}(\mathbf{x}w_{ic})}{n_c}$ for weighted model, with $\hat{\pi}_{ic}$ as fitted probabilities of death obtained from the model, and $\frac{n_c}{\bar{m}}$ is the weighting term per cluster. The weighted variance of the overall mortality rate was computed as follows (Kaombe & Hamuza, 2023):

$$var\left(\hat{\pi}\left(\mathbf{x}\right)\right) = \frac{1}{k}\Sigma_{c=1}^{k}\frac{\left(\hat{\pi}_c\left(\mathbf{x}\right) - \hat{\pi}\left(\mathbf{x}\right)\right)^2}{k-1}\left(\frac{n_c}{\bar{m}}\right)^2, \tag{11.10}$$

where $\hat{\pi}_c(\mathbf{x})$ is as defined in Eq. (11.9), and $\hat{\pi}(\mathbf{x})$ is weighted predicted under-five mortality rate in Eq. (11.9). After obtaining the weighted predicted mortality rate estimates in Eq. (11.9), the computations of bias in the mortality estimate were done as in Eq. (11.6) in Sect. 11.2.2, and we used R version 3.6.3 for the calculations.

We computed the predicted probabilities of death, $\hat{\pi}_{ic}(\mathbf{x})$, using the best model as determined by the Akaike Information Criterion (AIC), i.e., $AIC = 2p - 2l(.)$, with p as total regression model coefficients and $l(.)$ the estimated log likelihood. The AIC was only applicable to the unweighted model, as the STATA *svy* function does not produce AIC values for survey weighted models. The initial model used all available covariates as in Sect. 11.2.1. The second model dropped the variables that were worst fit in the first model based on the p-values.

11.3 Results

We present the results of the survey weighting techniques and bias computation methods for the predicted under-five mortality presented in Sect. 11.2, as demonstrated in Kaombe and Hamuza (2023). We first present the unweighted and weighted models' estimation results. Thereafter, we present results of the predicted under-five mortality rate from the fitted model and the estimated bias upon applying the methods given in Sect. 11.2.

11.3.1 Data Summary

The summary of the data is given in Table 11.1. It is shown that the percentages of deaths in under-five children have been below 10% for the past 15 years in Malawi, with a decreasing trend during this period, such that the proportion was almost halved between 2010 and 2015–16. In addition, there was a higher proportion of under-five deaths in male babies compared to females, in birth order of 1 or 6 and above compared to 2–5, caesarean compared to regular births, twin or multiple births compared to singleton births, and in home-based deliveries. Further, the majority of under-five deaths were observed in babies who were born to mothers aged below 20 years or 35 years and above, mothers whose preceding birth interval was less than 24 months, mothers who were not using modern contraceptive methods, mothers who had no formal education qualification, and mothers who were working. Furthermore, the proportions of under-five deaths were larger in children from rural areas, and children from central and southern regions of the study country. The Chi-square test of independence showed that all the studied explanatory variables had

Table 11.1 Distribution of under-five deaths by socio-demographic characteristics of a child across the three surveys.

	2004 MDHS			2010 MDHS			2015 MDHS		
Characteristics	*n* (%)	Died (%)	χ^2 *p*-val	*n* (%)	Died (%)	χ^2 *p*-val	*n* (%)	Died (%)	χ^2 *p*-val
Overall sample	10,914 (100)	1,056 (9.68)		19,967 (100)	1,607 (8.05)		17,286 (100)	824 (4.77)	
Child's sex			< 0.0001			0.001			0.003
Male	5,523 (50.60)	593 (10.74)		9,979 (49.98)	865 (8.67)		8,687 (50.25)	455 (5.24)	
Female	5,391 (49.40)	463 (8.59)		9,988 (50.02)	742 (7.43)		8,599 (49.75)	369 (4.29)	
Birth order			< 0.0001			< 0.0001			< 0.0001
1	2,469 (22.62)	290 (11.75)		3,925 (19.66)	363 (9.25)		4,400 (25.45)	267 (6.07)	
2–5	6,403 (58.67)	566 (8.84)		12,049 (60.34)	876 (7.27)		10,370 (59.99)	414 (3.99)	
6+	2,042 (18.71)	200 (9.79)		3,993 (20.00)	368 (9.22)		2,516 (14.56)	143 (5.68)	
Caesarean birth			0.641			0.012			0.006
No	10,575 (97.01)	1,021 (9.65)		19,002 (95.44)	1,507 (7.93)		16,122 (93.53)	749 (4.65)	
Yes	326 (2.99)	34 (10.43)		907 (4.56)	93 (10.25)		1,116 (6.47)	72 (6.45)	
Delivery type			< 0.0001			< 0.0001			< 0.0001
Singleton	10,547 (96.64)	938 (8.89)		19,104 (95.68)	1,396 (7.31)		16,618 (96.14)	707 (4.25)	
Multiple	367 (3.36)	118 (32.15)		863 (4.32)	211 (24.45)		668 (3.86)	117 (17.51)	
Birth place			0.013			0.482			0.007
Home or other	3,205 (29.73)	343 (10.70)		4,934 (25.46)	400 (8.11)		1,354 (7.83)	85 (6.28)	
Health facility	7,576 (70.27)	694 (9.16)		14,446 (74.54)	1,126 (7.79)		15,932 (92.17)	739 (4.64)	
Maternal age			0.161			< 0.0001			< 0.0001
<20	713 (6.53)	80 (11.22)		1,179 (5.90)	102 (8.65)		1,246 (7.21)	85 (6.82)	
20-34	8,254 (75.63)	775 (9.39)		14,792 (74.08)	1,109 (7.50)		12,647 (73.16)	558 (4.41)	
35-49	1,947 (17.84)	201 (10.32)		3,996 (20.01)	396 (9.91)		3,393 (19.63)	181 (5.33)	
Preceding birth interval			< 0.0001			< 0.0001			< 0.0001
<24 months	1,538 (18.26)	218 (14.17)		2,281 (14.25)	306 (13.42)		1,446 (11.26)	113 (7.81)	
24–36 months	2,994 (35.55)	252 (8.42)		6,327 (39.52)	429 (6.78)		3,705 (28.85)	169 (4.56)	
>36 months	3,890 (46.19)	291 (7.48)		7,400 (46.23)	503 (6.80)		7,690 (59.89)	264 (3.43)	

(continued)

Table 11.1 (continued)

	2004 MDHS			2010 MDHS			2015 MDHS		
Characteristics	*n* (%)	Died (%)	χ^2 *p*-val	*n* (%)	Died (%)	χ^2 *p*-val	*n* (%)	Died (%)	χ^2 *p*-val
Contraceptive use			< 0.0001			< 0.0001			< 0.0001
Not using	7,957 (72.91)	863 (10.85)		11,484 (57.51)	1,037 (9.03)		7,021 (40.62)	436 (6.21)	
Using	2,957 (27.09)	193 (6.53)		8,483 (42.49)	570 (6.72)		10,265 (59.38)	388 (3.78)	
Maternal educ			< 0.0001			0.002			0.076
No education	2,870 (26.30)	308 (10.73)		3,372 (16.89)	289 (8.57)		2,161 (12.50)	101 (4.67)	
Primary	6,967 (63.84)	678 (9.73)		13,865 (69.44)	1,145 (8.26)		11,456 (66.27)	573 (5.00)	
Secondary or above	1,077 (9.87)	70 (6.50)		2,730 (13.67)	173 (6.34)		3,669 (21.23)	150 (4.09)	
Maternal job status			0.767			0.026			0.013
Not working	4,449 (40.77)	435 (9.78)		8,194 (41.12)	617 (7.53)		5,938 (34.35)	250 (4.21)	
Working	6,464 (59.23)	621 (9.61)		11,733 (58.88)	986 (8.40)		11,348 (65.65)	574 (5.06)	
Residence			< 0.0001			0.696			0.033
Urban	1,137 (10.42)	76 (6.68)		1,896 (9.50)	157 (8.28)		2,766 (16.00)	110 (3.98)	
Rural	9,777 (89.58)	980 (10.02)		18,071 (90.50)	1,450 (8.02)		14,520 (84.00)	714 (4.92)	
Region			0.049			< 0.0001			0.018
Northern	1,349 (12.46)	106 (7.86)		3,560 (17.83)	232 (6.52)		3,208 (18.56)	126 (3.93)	
Central	4,141 (37.94)	418 (10.09)		6,866 (34.39)	544 (7.92)		6,023 (34.84)	316 (5.25)	
Southern	5,424 (49.70)	532 (9.81)		9,541 (47.78)	831 (8.71)		8,055 (46.60)	382 (4.74)	

individual significant association with under-five child death variable, evidenced in at least two of the DHS datasets.

11.3.2 Unweighted and Weighted Maximum Likelihood Estimates

The results in Table 11.2 provided the model estimates upon using all the available covariates from Table 11.1 for describing under-five child death. It is shown, in both unweighted and weighted models across all the years, that the odds of death of the child were lower in female children, preceding birth interval of 24 months and above, and in children born to mothers that used modern contraceptives. The odds of death were higher in caesarean births, twin or multiple delivered births, children born to working class mothers, children born to mothers aged 35–49 years, children from rural areas, and in children born in central and southern regions. The effects of birth order, place of delivery, and place of residence were not significant in determining death of the child in a model that had the other factors mentioned above. Hence, these were dropped in the final model that was used for prediction of the under-five mortality rate. The AIC values in Table 11.2 were reserved for comparisons with those of the models fitted to data in the respective years upon dropping the three worst-fitted variables.

Upon fitting the reduced logit models to the datasets, with the three worst-fitted covariates dropped jointly, it was shown that the AIC values came close to the values of those in original models in Table 11.2 in respective years, see Table 11.3. Trying to drop any one of the three covariates alone worsened the fit of the model, with very large AIC values observed, hence the model estimates in Table 11.3 were used for computation of predicted mortality rate and biases in this study. The model's ML estimates in Table 11.3 showed that the *p*-values for the reduced models got lower compared to those in original models in Table 11.2. But the sizes and directions of the estimates did not change. Thus, the odds of death of the child were significantly lower in female compared to male children, children born to mothers who had preceding birth interval of 24 months and above, children born to mothers who used modern contraceptive methods, and mothers whose highest level of education was secondary and above. Whereas the odds of child death were higher in caesarean births, twin or multiple births, children born to mothers aged 35–49 years, children born to mothers who were working, and children from central and southern regions. In addition, both the ML estimates and their *p*-values slightly adjusted upwards or downwards in the weighted models when compared with those from unweighted models for the respective years. This implied that the fixed-effect sizes from the unweighted logistic regression models were somehow biased if the aim of the model was to estimate risk factors of under-five mortality and the sizes of the risk.

Table 11.2 Effects of child characteristics on death outcome upon fitting full logit model to DHS data

	Unweighted full logit model			Weighted full logit model		
Variable	2004 DHS OR (*p*-value)	2010 DHS OR (*p*-value)	2015 DHS OR (*p*-value)	2004 DHS OR (*p*-value)	2010 DHS OR (p-value)	2015 DHS OR (*p*-value)
Child's sex						
Male*						
Female	0.7544 (<0.0001)	0.8462 (0.007)	0.8104 (0.019)	0.8166 (0.025)	0.8605 (0.030)	0.8005 (0.016)
Birth order						
1*						
2–5	1.2420 (0.076)	1.1372 (0.189)	0.9252 (0.582)	1.2458 (0.067)	1.0922 (0.325)	0.9145 (0.492)
6+	0.8027 (0.067)	0.9156 (0.325)	1.0935 (0.492)	0.8051 (0.076)	0.8793 (0.189)	1.0808 (0.582)
Caesarean birth						
No*						
Yes	1.3248 (0.249)	1.4604 (0.010)	1.6474 (0.003)	1.1775 (0.633)	1.3497 (0.077)	1.6441 (0.011)
Delivery type						
Singleton *						
Multiple	5.6246 (< 0.0001)	4.6150 (< 0.0001)	4.7779 (< 0.0001)	5.9002 (< 0.0001)	4.4839 (< 0.0001)	4.6865 (< 0.0001)
Birth place						
Home or other *						
Health facility	0.9947 (0.951)	1.0514 (0.482)	0.8084 (0.129)	1.0675 (0.507)	1.0193 (0.809)	0.8215 (0.205)
Maternal age						
<20 *						
20–34	1.0443 (0.903)	1.4958 (0.277)	1.1806 (0.751)	0.9885 (0.975)	1.3500 (0.418)	1.2088 (0.729)
35–49	1.4239 (0.345)	2.2416 (0.033)	1.5579 (0.406)	1.3860 (0.406)	1.9696 (0.070)	1.5396 (0.453)
Preceding birth interval						
<24 months *						
24–36 months	0.5357 (<0.0001)	0.4603 (<0.0001)	0.5472 (<0.0001)	0.5541 (<0.0001)	0.4667 (<0.0001)	0.5426 (<0.0001)
>36 months	0.4378 (<0.0001)	0.4273 (<0.0001)	0.3988 (<0.0001)	0.4316 (<0.0001)	0.4707 (<0.0001)	0.3890 (<0.0001)

Contraceptive use						
Not using ∗						
Using	0.6477 (< 0.0001)	0.7147 (< 0.0001)	0.6115 (< 0.0001)	0.6302 (0.0001)	0.7076 (< 0.0001)	0.5816 (< 0.0001)
Maternal educ						
No education ∗						
Primary	0.9342 (0.435)	1.0630 (0.452)	1.1556 (0.258)	0.9096 (0.323)	1.0198 (0.835)	1.1768 (0.249)
Secondary or above	0.6042 (0.815)	0.9052 (0.447)	1.0800 (0.663)	0.7141 (0.189)	0.7962 (0.145)	1.0972 (0.621)
Maternal job status						
Not working ∗						
Working	1.0192 (0.815)	1.1004 (0.139)	1.4117 (0.001)	1.0176 (0.857)	1.0990 (0.203)	1.3871 (0.004)
Residence						
Urban ∗						
Rural	1.2405 (0.171)	0.8741 (0.226)	1.2794 (0.101)	1.3155 (0.165)	0.9070 (0.448)	1.2590 (0.173)
Region						
Northern ∗						
Central	1.1205 (0.419)	1.2287 (0.039)	1.1974 (0.177)	1.1490 (0.374)	1.3335 (0.008)	1.1663 (0.265)
Southern	1.1563 (0.290)	1.4375 (< 0.0001)	1.0839 (0.535)	1.2889 (0.101)	1.5457 (< 0.0001)	1.1100 (0.430)
AIC	4786.213	7904.787	4285.794	–	–	–

OR odd ratio, (∗) reference level

Table 11.3 Effects of child characteristics on death outcome upon fitting reduced logit model to DHS data

	Unweighted reduced logit model			Weighted reduced logit model		
Variable	2004 DHS OR (*p*-value)	2010 DHS OR (*p*-value)	2015 DHS OR (*p*-value)	2004 DHS OR (*p*-value)	2010 DHS OR (*p*-value)	2015 DHS OR (*p*-value)
Child's sex						
Male*						
Female	0.7354 (< 0.0001)	0.8406 (0.004)	0.8137 (0.021)	0.8023 (0.014)	0.8567 (0.022)	0.8033 (0.017)
Caesarean birth						
No*						
Yes	1.2981 (0.282)	1.4652 (0.009)	1.5624 (0.008)	1.1766 (0.631)	1.3473 (0.076)	1.5601 (0.022)
Delivery type						
Singleton *						
Multiple	5.5135 (< 0.0001)	4.5837 (<0.0001)	4.8281 (<0.0001)	5.8221 (<0.0001)	4.4277 (<0.0001)	4.7329 (<0.0001)
Maternal age						
<20 *						
20-34	1.0311 (0.932)	1.5191 (0.258)	1.2021 (0.725)	0.9781 (0.953)	1.3752 (0.390)	1.2309 (0.704)
35-49	1.2147 (0.593)	2.2192 (0.033)	1.6638 (0.334)	1.1830 (0.667)	1.9254 (0.076)	1.6304 (0.380)
Preceding birth interval						
<24 months *						
24–36 months	0.5415 (<0.0001)	0.4561 (<0.0001)	0.5479 (<0.0001)	0.5661 (<0.0001)	0.4650 (<0.0001)	0.5434 (<0.0001)
>36 months	0.4502 (<0.0001)	0.4247 (<0.0001)	0.3889 (<0.0001)	0.4473 (<0.0001)	0.4640 (<0.0001)	0.3797 (<0.0001)
Contraceptive use						
Not using *						
Using	0.6442 (<0.0001)	0.7249 (<0.0001)	0.6047 (<0.0001)	0.6259 (<0.0001)	0.7203 (<0.0001)	0.5754 (<0.0001)
Maternal educ						
No education *						
Primary	0.9365 (0.441)	1.1119 (0.177)	1.1204 (0.369)	0.9208 (0.391)	1.0751 (0.419)	1.1430 (0.337)
Secondary or above	0.5847 (0.007)	0.9481 (0.671)	1.4339 (<0.0001)	0.6926 (0.139)	0.8464 (0.250)	0.9824 (0.922)

Maternal job status						
Not working *						
Working	1.0234 (0.773)	1.0841 (0.199)	1.4339 (<0.0001)	1.0307 (0.754)	1.0808 (0.279)	1.4118 (0.003)
Region						
Northern *						
Central	1.1179 (0.420)	1.2480 (0.023)	1.1909 (0.190)	1.1371 (0.419)	1.3669 (0.003)	1.1636 (0.271)
Southern	1.1327 (0.356)	1.4714 (<0.0001)	1.0804 (0.552)	1.2403 (0.172)	1.5933 (<0.0001)	1.1079 (0.438)
AIC	4870.063	8268.383	4285.641	–	–	–

OR odd ratio, (*) reference level

11.3.3 Predicted National Under-Five Mortality Rate and Bias of the Predicted Value

The results for predicted value as well as bias of under-five mortality estimate are given in Table 11.4. It is shown that the bias was considerably lower in the weighted overall predicted under-five mortality rate than in the unweighted case, regardless of whether or not the fitted model was weighted. Further, the results showed that the standard errors for the weighted overall predicted mortality rate were also smaller compared to those for unweighted counterpart, irrespective of weighting status of the fitted model. In addition, it was shown that the bias for the 2004 mortality estimates was largest compared to the 2010 and 2015 results, holding constant the weighting status of the fitted model and of the overall predicted mortality. Furthermore, the results showed that the standard errors for the predicted mortality rates increased with decreasing sample size of the survey.

11.4 Discussion

In this chapter, the usefulness of survey probability weights in the prediction of under-five mortality through regression methods was investigated. The results showed that weighting the model causes some positive and negative changes in the maximum likelihood (ML) estimates that were originally obtained from the unweighted model, which confirmed the presence of some bias in ML estimates from the unweighted model (Pfeffermann, 1993; Faiella, 2010). However, the study has found that ignoring the model weighting has little impact on the accuracy of estimation of the overall predicted under-five mortality rate. It is the survey design weighting that is applied on the overall predicted mortality estimates from each cluster that has significant effect on the bias of the overall national under-five mortality estimate. This implies that the up and down shifts in the fixed-effect estimates for various explanatory variables cancel the weighting effect in the model's fitted probabilities, leaving the predicted mortality rate the same as the one obtained from the unweighted model. Hence, the need for applying second-stage survey weights on the cluster-specific predicted probabilities of event in order to achieve a less-biased overall under-five mortality estimate (Kaombe & Hamuza, 2023).

The biases in mortality estimates from the 2004 MDHS data were much higher compared to those from 2010 and 2015 MDHS datasets. This reflects the fact that the 2004 MDHS data had more missing values in a number of explanatory variables than they were in the 2010 and 2015 datasets, which might have disturbed the randomness and representativeness of the sample for 2004 data, when calculating the overall mortality estimate. The study has also observed that reducing sample size of the MDHS only led to increase in standard errors of the predicted mortality rates and not in the sizes of the overall predicted mortality rates themselves, as they

Table 11.4 Bias in under-5 mortality rate using unweighted and weighted logit model or predicted rate.

n	$\hat{\pi}(\mathbf{x})\ (S.E.)$	π	$bias\left(\hat{\pi}(\mathbf{x})\right)$	$\hat{\pi}(\mathbf{x})\ (S.E.)$	π	$bias\left(\hat{\pi}(\mathbf{x})\right)$
	2004 unweighted model, unweighted $\hat{\pi}(\mathbf{x})$			2004 weighted model, weighted $\hat{\pi}(\mathbf{x})$		
10,914	0.00424 (0.00062)	0.1197	**−0.11546**	0.08601 (0.00002)	0.1197	**−0.03369**
8,292	0.00427 (0.00085)	0.1197	**−0.11543**	0.09061 (0.00002)	0.1197	**−0.02909**
5,624	0.00402 (0.00095)	0.1197	**−0.11568**	0.08711 (0.00000)	0.1197	**−0.03259**
2,878	0.00397 (0.00127)	0.1197	**−0.11573**	0.08950 (0.00003)	0.1197	**−0.03020**
	2004 unweighted model, weighted $\hat{\pi}(\mathbf{x})$			2004 weighted model, unweighted $\hat{\pi}(\mathbf{x})$		
10,914	0.08982 (0.00002)	0.1197	**−0.02988**	0.00407 (0.00061)	0.1197	**−0.11563**
8,292	0.09101 (0.00003)	0.1197	**−0.02869**	0.00427 (0.00085)	0.1197	**−0.11543**
5,624	0.08876 (0.00002)	0.1197	**−0.03094**	0.00398 (0.00094)	0.1197	**−0.11572**
2,878	0.09023 (0.00005)	0.1197	**−0.02947**	0.00397 (0.00127)	0.1197	**−0.11573**
	2010 unweighted model, unweighted $\hat{\pi}(\mathbf{x})$			2010 Weighted Model, Weighted $\hat{\pi}(\mathbf{x})$		
19,967	0.00321 (0.00040)	0.0842	**−0.08099**	0.07680 (0.00001)	0.0842	**−0.00740**
15,064	0.00321 (0.00055)	0.0842	**−0.08099**	0.07587 (0.00002)	0.0842	**−0.00833**
10,153	0.00311 (0.00062)	0.0842	**−0.08109**	0.07351 (0.00003)	0.0842	**−0.01069**
5,030	0.00304 (0.00083)	0.0842	**−0.08116**	0.07012 (0.00000)	0.0842	**−0.01408**
	2010 unweighted model, weighted $\hat{\pi}(\mathbf{x})$			2010 weighted model, unweighted $\hat{\pi}(\mathbf{x})$		
19,967	0.07687 (0.00001)	0.0842	**−0.00733**	0.00321 (0.00040)	0.0842	**−0.08099**
15,064	0.07734 (0.00002)	0.0842	**−0.00687**	0.00315 (0.00054)	0.0842	**−0.08105**
10,153	0.07517 (0.00002)	0.0842	**−0.00903**	0.00304 (0.00062)	0.0842	**−0.08116**
5,030	0.07192 (0.00001)	0.0842	**−0.01228**	0.00296 (0.00082)	0.0842	**−0.08124**

(continued)

Table 11.4 (continued)

n	$\hat{\pi}(\mathbf{x})\ (S.E.)$	π	$bias\left(\hat{\pi}(\mathbf{x})\right)$	$\hat{\pi}(\mathbf{x})\ (S.E.)$	π	$bias\left(\hat{\pi}(\mathbf{x})\right)$
	2015 unweighted model, unweighted $\hat{\pi}(\mathbf{x})$			2015 weighted model, weighted $\hat{\pi}(\mathbf{x})$		
17,286	0.00201 (0.00034)	0.0495	**−0.04749**	0.04010 (0.00000)	0.0495	**−0.00850**
13,099	0.00186 (0.00044)	0.0495	**−0.04764**	0.03807 (0.00001)	0.0495	**−0.01143**
8,644	0.00190 (0.00052)	0.0495	**−0.04760**	0.03834 (0.00002)	0.0495	**−0.01116**
4,314	0.00219 (0.00075)	0.0495	**−0.04731**	0.04456 (0.00004)	0.0495	**−0.00494**
	2015 unweighted model, weighted $\hat{\pi}(\mathbf{x})$			2015 weighted model, unweighted $\hat{\pi}(\mathbf{x})$		
17,286	0.04211 (0.00000)	0.0495	**−0.00739**	0.00196 (0.00034)	0.0495	**−0.04754**
13,099	0.03940 (0.00001)	0.0495	**−0.01010**	0.00180 (0.00043)	0.0495	**−0.04770**
8,644	0.03996 (0.00002)	0.0495	**−0.00954**	0.00183 (0.00051)	0.0495	**−0.04767**
4,314	0.04553 (0.00004)	0.0495	**−0.00397**	0.00214 (0.00075)	0.0495	**−0.04736**

$\hat{\pi}(\mathbf{x})$ predicted mortality, $S.E.$ std. error, π raw mortality, $bias\left(\hat{\pi}(\mathbf{x})\right)$ $\hat{\pi}(\mathbf{x}) - \pi$

stayed constant despite lowering the sample size. Further, it has been observed that the sample size of as low as 2% of the population of all children in the country could still yield less-biased mortality estimates, provided that the sample was random and representative of the population, and provided that the computation of the overall mortality estimate was weighted. This was expected as the variance statistic for a sample proportion, such as mortality rate has sample size in the denominator, which makes the variance to become larger in lower sample sizes, but this may not affect the value of mortality estimate due to weighting effect and representativeness of the sample.

The model's ML estimates showed that the risk of under-five mortality was lower in female babies compared to male children, in children whose mothers had preceding birth interval of 24 months and above, children whose mothers used modern contraceptive methods, and children whose mothers attended up to secondary education and above. The risk was higher in caesarean births, twin or multiple births, in children whose mothers were aged 35–49 years, children born to working class mothers, and children residing in central and southern regions of Malawi. These results are consistent with previous findings, and there are also clear biological and social explanations in literature for these observations (Manda, 1999; Kazembe & Mpeketula, 2010; Pongou, 2013; Smith et al., 2007; Shearer, 1993; Kaombe & Manda, 2022, 2023b). For example, the well-educated mothers have an upper hand in terms of knowledge and skills about child healthcare, which benefits the baby's health compared to the less-educated mothers (Manda, 1999). The high risk of death in twin births largely reflects an increased risk of intrapartum anoxia in second twins born at term that reduce their survival (Smith et al., 2007). With the caesarean births, the high risk of death stems from increased chances of iatrogenic prematurity or respiratory disease (Shearer, 1993). While the lower death rates in female babies are attributed to their genetic and biological make-up together with preconception environments that lowers their risk against most diseases compared to male babies (Pongou, 2013). Furthermore, the high risk of under-five deaths in children from working class mothers is attributed to inadequate breastfeeding that working mothers subject the babies to Amir-ud Din et al. (2022).

11.5 Conclusion

This chapter studied impact of survey sampling design on predicted under-five mortality rate using demographic and health survey data from three consecutive surveys in Malawi. The findings showed that the risk factors for under-five mortality have not changed from those observed in previous studies in the sub-Saharan African region and other developing countries. The study has found that the model's probability weights have very little effect on the bias of the predicted mortality rate, such that ignoring the weighting in the fitted model will not change the predicted mortality value. However, it has been observed that weighting the cluster-specific overall predicted mortality rates has significant effect in minimising the bias of the overall predicted national under-five mortality rate. The study has also found that a random and representative sample of size at least 2% of the population is enough to obtain low-biased national under-five mortality estimate, provided the computation of the overall predicted mortality estimate considers cluster weights. Low sample size only affects standard errors of the estimated mortality, which become large and hence widen confidence intervals for the estimates.

This chapter therefore recommends applying cluster sampling weights to cluster-specific predicted probabilities of event, when computing overall predicted probability of the event in a model that analyses the binary health outcome, without regard of weighting during the model fitting process. Although this study focused on models for binary response variable, the findings apply to other models for categorical data with more than two levels. Future research could incorporate methods for addressing missing data in explanatory variables such as birth weight and antenatal care visits, so that the models use as many covariates as possible while observing the effect of sampling design in predicting under-five mortality rate.

Acknowledgments We are sincerely thankful to the National Statistical Office of Malawi and Measure DHS program for the data we used in this study.

References

Ahmad, O. B., Lopez, A. D., & Inoue, M. (2000). The decline in child mortality: A reappraisal. *Bulletin of the World Health Organization, 78*, 1175–1191.

Amir-ud Din, R., Zafar, S., Muzammil, M., Shabbir, R., Malik, S., & Usman, M. (2022). Exploring the relationship between maternal occupation and under-five mortality: Empirical evidence from 26 developing countries. *The European Journal of Development Research, 34*(5), 2373–2399.

Argawu, A. S., & Mekebo, G. G. (2022). Risk factors of under-five mortality in Ethiopia using count data regression models, 2021. *Annals of Medicine and Surgery, 82*, 104764.

Brenning, A., Gruber, S., & Hoelzle, M. (2005). Sampling and statistical analyses of BTS measurements. *Permafrost and Periglacial Processes, 16*(4), 383–393.

Carroll, R. J., & Pederson, S. (1993). On robustness in the logistic regression model. *Journal of the Royal Statistical Society: Series B (Methodological), 55*(3), 693–706.

Chen, C., Wakefield, J., & Lumely, T. (2014). The use of sampling weights in Bayesian hierarchical models for small area estimation. *Spatial and Spatio-Temporal Epidemiology, 11*, 33–43.

Dadi, A. F. (2015). A systematic review and meta-analysis of the effect of short birth interval on infant mortality in Ethiopia. *PloS One, 10*(5), e0126759.

Fagbamigbe, A. F., & Nnanatu, C. C. (2022). Modelling the spatial distribution and the factors associated with under-five mortality in Nigeria. *Spatial Demography, 10*(2), 255–282.

Faiella, I. (2010). The use of survey weights in regression analysis, *Bank of Italy Temi di Discussione (Working Paper) No 739*.

Getachew, Y., & Bekele, S. (2016). Survival analysis of under-five mortality of children and its associated risk factors in Ethiopia. *J Biosens Bioelectron, 7*(213), 2.

Groenewald, P., Bradshaw, D., Neethling, I., Martin, L. J., Dempers, J., Morden, E., Zinyakatira, N., & Coetzee, D. (2016). Linking mortuary data improves vital statistics on cause of death of children under five years in the western cape province of South Africa. *Tropical Medicine & International Health, 21*(1), 114–121.

Guimarães, R. J., Freitas, C. C., Dutra, L. V., Moura, A., Amaral, R. S., Drummond, S. C., Guerra, M., Scholte, R. G., Freitas, C. R., & Carvalho, O. S. (2006). Analysis and estimative of schistosomiasis prevalence for the state of Minas Gerais, Brazil, using multiple regression with social and environmental spatial data. *Memórias do Instituto Oswaldo Cruz, 101*, 91–96.

Jaki, T., Kim, M., Lamont, A., George, M., Chang, C., Feaster, D., & Van Horn, M. L. (2019). The effects of sample size on the estimation of regression mixture models. *Educational and Psychological Measurement, 79*(2), 358–384.

Joos, O., Amouzou, A., Silva, R., Banda, B., Park, L., Bryce, J., Kanyuka, M., & Group, R. M. W. (2016). Strengthening community-based vital events reporting for real-time monitoring of under-five mortality: lessons learned from the Balaka and Salima districts in Malawi. *PloS One, 11*(1), e0138406.

Kaombe, T. M., & Hamuza, G. A. (2023). Impact of ignoring sampling design in the prediction of binary health outcomes through logistic regression: Evidence from Malawi demographic and health survey under-five mortality data; 2000–2016. *BMC Public Health, 23*(1), 1–12.

Kaombe, T. M., & Manda, S. O. (2022) , Identifying outlying and influential clusters in multivariate survival data models. In *Modern biostatistical methods for evidence-based global health research* (pp. 377–410). Springer.

Kaombe, T. M., & Manda, S. O. (2023a). Detecting influential data in multivariate survival models. *Communications in Statistics-Theory and Methods, 52*(11), 3910–3926.

Kaombe, T. M., & Manda, S. O. (2023b). A novel outlier statistic in multivariate survival models and its application to identify unusual under-five mortality sub-districts in Malawi. *Journal of Applied Statistics, 50*(8), 1836–1852.

Kayode, G. A., Adekanmbi, V. T., & Uthman, O. A. (2012). Risk factors and a predictive model for under-five mortality in Nigeria: evidence from Nigeria demographic and health survey. *BMC Pregnancy and Childbirth, 12*(1), 1–11.

Kazembe, L. N., & Mpeketula, P. M. (2010). Quantifying spatial disparities in neonatal mortality using a structured additive regression model. *PloS One, 5*(6), e11180.

Kneipp, S. M., & Yarandi, H. N. (2002). Complex sampling designs and statistical issues in secondary analysis. *Western Journal of Nursing Research, 24*(5), 552–566.

Koch, G. G., Gillings, D. B., & Stokes, M. E. (1980). Biostatistical implications of design, sampling, and measurement to health science data analysis. *Annual Review of Public Health, 1*(1), 163–225.

Lehtonen, R., & Pahkinen, E. (2004). *Practical methods for design and analysis of complex surveys*. Wiley.

Li, Z., Hsiao, Y., Godwin, J., Martin, B. D., Wakefield, J., Clark, S. J., With Support from the United Nations Inter-agency Group for Child Mortality Estimation and Its Technical Advisory Group. (2019). Changes in the spatial distribution of the under-five mortality rate: Small-area analysis of 122 DHS surveys in 262 subregions of 35 countries in Africa. *PloS One, 14*(1), e0210645.

Maïga, A., Jiwani, S. S., Mutua, M. K., Porth, T. A., Taylor, C. M., Asiki, G., Melesse, D. Y., Day, C., Strong, K. L., Faye, C. M., et al. (2019). Generating statistics from health facility data: The state of routine health information systems in eastern and Southern Africa. *BMJ Global Health, 4*(5), e001849.

Malawi National Statistical Office (NSO). (2009). *2008 Malawi Population and Housing Census: Main Report*. Zomba.

Malawi National Statistical Office (NSO). (2019). *2018 Malawi Population and Housing Census: Main Report*. Zomba.

Manda, S. (1999). Birth intervals, breastfeeding and determinants of childhood mortality in Malawi. *Social Science & Medicine, 48*(3), 301–312.

Markatou, M., Basu, A., & Lindsay, B. (1997). Weighted likelihood estimating equations: The discrete case with applications to logistic regression. *Journal of Statistical Planning and Inference, 57*(2), 215–232.

Morris, S. S., Black, R. E., & Tomaskovic, L. (2003). Predicting the distribution of under-five deaths by cause in countries without adequate vital registration systems. *International Journal of Epidemiology, 32*(6), 1041–1051.

Mwanga, E. P., Minja, E. G., Mrimi, E., Jiménez, M. G., Swai, J. K., Abbasi, S., Ngowo, H. S., Siria, D. J., Mapua, S., Stica, C., et al. (2019). Detection of malaria parasites in dried human blood spots using mid-infrared spectroscopy and logistic regression analysis. *Malaria Journal, 18*(1), 1–13.

National Statistical Office (NSO) and ICF Macro. (2011). *Malawi demographic and health survey 2010', Zomba, Malawi, and Calverton, Maryland.* NSO and ICF Macro.

National Statistical Office (NSO) [Malawi] and ICF. (2017). *2015-16 Malawi demographic and health survey: Key findings', Zomba, Malawi, and Rockville, Maryland.* NSO and ICF.

National Statistical Office (NSO) [Malawi] and ORC Macro. (2005). *Malawi demographic and health survey 2004', Zomba, Malawi, and Calverton, Maryland.* NSO and ORC Macro.

Nsowah-Nuamah, N., Mensah, G., Aryeetey, M. E., Wagatsuma, Y., & Bentil, G. (2001). Urinary schistosomiasis in southern Ghana: A logistic regression approach to data from a community-based integrated control program. *The American Journal of Tropical Medicine and Hygiene, 65*(5), 484–490.

Nyambe, S., Agestika, L., & Yamauchi, T. (2020). The improved and the unimproved: factors influencing sanitation and diarrhoea in a peri-urban settlement of Lusaka, Zambia. *PloS One, 15*(5), e0232763.

Pfeffermann, D. (1993). The role of sampling weights when modeling survey data. *International Statistical Review/Revue Internationale de Statistique, 61*, 317–337.

Pongou, R. (2013). Why is infant mortality higher in boys than in girls? A new hypothesis based on preconception environment and evidence from a large sample of twins. *Demography, 50*(2), 421–444.

Quenouille, M. H. (1956). Notes on bias in estimation. *Biometrika, 43*(3/4), 353–360.

Rajaratnam, J. K., Tran, L. N., Lopez, A. D., & Murray, C. J. (2010). Measuring under-five mortality: validation of new low-cost methods. *PLoS Medicine, 7*(4), e1000253.

Renschler, J. P., Walters, K. M., Newton, P. N., & Laxminarayan, R. (2015). Estimated under-five deaths associated with poor-quality antimalarials in Sub-Saharan Africa. *The American Journal of Tropical Medicine and Hygiene, 92*(Suppl 6), 119.

Rerimoi, A. J., Jasseh, M., Agbla, S. C., Reniers, G., Roca, A., & Timæus, I. M. (2019). Under-five mortality in the Gambia: Comparison of the results of the first demographic and health survey with those from existing inquiries. *Plos One, 14*(7), e0219919.

Rutkowski, L., Gonzalez, E., Joncas, M., & Von Davier, M. (2010). International large-scale assessment data: Issues in secondary analysis and reporting. *Educational Researcher, 39*(2), 142–151.

Seaman, S. R., & White, I. R. (2013). Review of inverse probability weighting for dealing with missing data. *Statistical Methods in Medical Research, 22*(3), 278–295.

Shearer, E. L. (1993). Cesarean section: Medical benefits and costs. *Social Science & Medicine, 37*(10), 1223–1231.

Silva, R., et al. (2012). Child mortality estimation: Consistency of under-five mortality rate estimates using full birth histories and summary birth histories. *PLOS Medicine, 9*(8), 1–14.

Smith, G. C., Fleming, K. M., & White, I. R. (2007). Birth order of twins and risk of perinatal death related to delivery in England, Northern Ireland, and Wales, 1994–2003: Retrospective cohort study. *BMJ, 334*(7593), 576.

Talukder, A., Hossain, M., et al. (2020). Prevalence of diabetes mellitus and its associated factors in Bangladesh: Application of two-level logistic regression model. *Scientific Reports, 10*(1), 1–7.

Tuoyire, D. A., & Amo-Adjei, J. (2022). Preceding birth interval, timing and number of antenatal contacts in Africa, 2010–2020. *International Health, 15*, 445–452.

Unicef-Malawi (2022). *Monitoring the situation of children and women: Key demographic indicators*. https://data.unicef.org/country/mwi/

Vandendijck, Y., Faes, C., Kirby, R., Lawson, A., & Hens, N. (2016). Model-based inference for small area estimation with sampling weights. *Spatial Statistics, 18*, 455–473.

Vergouwe, Y., Steyerberg, E. W., Eijkemans, M. J., & Habbema, J. D. F. (2005). Substantial effective sample sizes were required for external validation studies of predictive logistic regression models. *Journal of Clinical Epidemiology, 58*(5), 475–483.

Wakefield, J., Fuglstad, G.-A., Riebler, A., Godwin, J., Wilson, K., & Clark, S. J. (2019). Estimating under-five mortality in space and time in a developing world context. *Statistical Methods in Medical Research, 28*(9), 2614–2634.

Winship, C., & Radbill, L. (1994). Sampling weights and regression analysis. *Sociological Methods & Research, 23*(2), 230–257.

Yaya, S., Bishwajit, G., Okonofua, F., & Uthman, O. A. (2018). Under five mortality patterns and associated maternal risk factors in Sub-Saharan Africa: A multi-country analysis. *PloS One, 13*(10), e0205977.

Yaya, S., Uthman, O. A., Okonofua, F., & Bishwajit, G. (2019). Decomposing the rural-urban gap in the factors of under-five mortality in Sub-Saharan Africa? evidence from 35 countries. *BMC Public Health, 19*(1), 1–10.

Zeng, G. (2017). On the existence of maximum likelihood estimates for weighted logistic regression. *Communications in Statistics-Theory and Methods, 46*(22), 11194–11203.

Zieschang, K. D. (1990). Sample weighting methods and estimation of totals in the consumer expenditure survey. *Journal of the American Statistical Association, 85*(412), 986–1001.

Chapter 12
Issues in Multivariate Spatial Analysis of Multiple Diseases Using Complex Health Survey Data

Sheyla Rodrigues Cassy and Samuel Manda

12.1 Introduction

Nowadays, collecting multiple disease measures in an area is becoming more common when health surveys are conducted. Most spatial statistics analyses of such data use univariate disease mapping approaches. However, the collected multiple diseases could be interrelated and share similar risk factors (Wong et al., 2014; Chang et al., 2011), and thus incorporating data from related diseases could be useful from both an epidemiological and a statistical perspectives (Held et al., 2005). A major limitation of univariate disease mapping models is their inability to account for the possible correlation among related diseases in the same area and to consider neighborhood dependency in disease risks. Recent developments in spatial methods for disease mapping have included models that consider the correlation between diseases to improve the estimates of disease risks. Several multivariate disease mapping models have been proposed in the literature, including the shared spatial component models (Dabney & Wakefield, 2005; Knorr-Held & Best, 2001) and multivariate conditionally autoregressive (MCAR) models (Feltbower et al., 2005; Manda et al., 2009). For example, the shared component model jointly analyses all related diseases and separates the specific risks of each disease into a shared component, which captures the underlying general spatial disease risk pattern common to all diseases and one disease-specific spatial component, which deviates from the shared spatial pattern. Identifying similar patterns in geographical variation of related conditions in a multivariate model potentially provides more convincing

S. R. Cassy
DMI, Faculdade de Ciências, Universidade Eduardo Mondlane, Maputo, Mozambique

S. Manda (✉)
Department of Statistics, University of Pretoria, Pretoria, South Africa
e-mail: samuel.manda@up.ac.za

D.-G. Chen, C. A. Coelho (eds.), *Biostatistics Modeling and Public Health Applications*, Emerging Topics in Statistics and Biostatistics,
https://doi.org/10.1007/978-3-031-69690-9_12

evidence of any spatial pattern of underlying risks than would otherwise have been possible using the analysis of any single disease separately. These joint disease mapping models have been used to model and estimate risks of related cancers (Gómez-Rubio et al., 2019; Carroll et al., 2017; Downing et al., 2008; Held et al., 2005) childhood illnesses (Kazembe et al., 2007), and childhood cancer and diabetes (Manda et al., 2009; Feltbower et al., 2005).

Recent methodological research in spatial analyses of complex health survey data has shown limitations of not accounting for the survey designs. However, while correctly employing joint disease mapping models, most analyses have not accounted for the survey designs (Orunmoluyi et al., 2022; Manda et al., 2020; Kinyoki et al., 2018, 2017; Adebayo et al., 2016; Kinyoki et al., 2016; Kandala et al., 2014; Kazembe et al., 2009b; Kandala et al., 2008). Limited research has shown how survey designs such as sampling weights could be accounted for in disease mapping analyses of health survey data (Watjou et al., 2017; Chen et al., 2014; Mercer et al., 2014). These studies have shown that ignoring sampling weight in a disease mapping analysis could lead to biased estimates of the spatial distributions of disease risk, which could negatively affect policy decisions based on them. This chapter deals with two issues, namely multivariate disease mapping models and adjustments for survey design in the estimation of spatial patterns when several interrelated diseases are analysed using health survey data. These issues are exemplified by a bivariate disease mapping analysis of childhood fever and diarrhea data from the 2015 Mozambique Immunization Indicators, Malaria, and HIV/AIDS Survey (IMASIDA 2015) (MISAU, 2016).

12.2 Spatial Models for Health Survey Data

12.2.1 Model Specification

Suppose there are J health outcomes in area $i : i = 1, 2, ..., N$ and the sample size for outcome $j : j = 1, 2, ..., J$ is m_{ij}. We denote y_{ijk} as the binary response value for subject k to health outcome j in area i ($k = 1, ..., m_{ij}$), with n_{ij} being the total number of subjects that are positive to health outcome j in area i. The unknown prevalence of health outcome j in area i is given by P_{ij}.

A well-known model for estimating the area prevalence rates is based on the area-level approaches that assume a model conditional on the sampled observations. A common area-level model is a binomial distribution given as

$$n_{ij} \sim \text{Binomial}(m_{ij}, P_{ij}). \tag{12.1}$$

For this model, accounting for both spatial dependence and heterogeneity is done with the random effects specifications. This specification produces indirect estimates and area-specific estimates based on borrowing information from other areas as well. Thus, in separate models, random effects are introduced as follows:

$$\text{logit}(P_{i1}) = \beta_{01} + u_{i1} + v_{i1}, \tag{12.2}$$

$$\text{logit}(P_{i2}) = \beta_{02} + u_{i2} + v_{i2}, \tag{12.3}$$

where β_{01} and β_{02} are the intercepts for disease 1 and disease 2, respectively; $\mathbf{u}_{i1}$ and $\mathbf{u}_{i2}$ are the spatially structured random effects variables, while $\mathbf{v}_{i1}$ and $\mathbf{v}_{i2}$ are heterogeneity random effects.

However, as discussed in the Introduction section, diseases with similar etiologies may present similar risk profiles, i.e., similar spatial variation, and a multivariate spatial analysis has proven to be a more appropriate alternative to obtain better estimates of the spatial patterns. In this chapter, we use the shared spatial component model (Held et al., 2005; Knorr-Held & Best, 2001) and set it up for the case of two disease measures in an area. To capture the similar spatial patterns in the two outcomes, spatial structured spatial random components are decomposed into specific and shared effects. Thus, the resulting model is given by

$$\text{logit}(P_{i1}) = \beta_{01} + s_i\delta + s_{i1} + v_{i1}, \tag{12.4}$$

$$\text{logit}(P_{i2}) = \beta_{02} + \frac{s_i}{\delta} + v_{i2}, \tag{12.5}$$

where β_{01} and β_{02} are the intercepts for disease 1 and disease 2, respectively; s_1 is the shared component, while s_{i1} is the component specific to the first disease only.

The extra parameter δ ($\delta > 0$) is included to allow differential gradient from the shared component for the two diseases. The reason for the parameters of scales δ to $\frac{1}{\delta}$ compares the weight of disease 1 relative to disease 2 associated with the shared component. In this model, common spatial trends are investigated using the shared component, and divergent trends are investigated through the disease specific component. The scaling parameters allow each disease to have a unique association with the overall pattern of the disease. For interpretation of the shared component, a value of δ close to 1 indicates that disease 1 and disease 2 have a similar magnitude of association with the general pattern of the disease, while a large and positive δ indicates that disease 1 has a stronger association with the general disease pattern than disease 2.

Several studies that have used the shared spatial component model using health survey data failed to account for disproportionate sample design of the surveys (Orunmoluyi et al., 2022; Adebayo et al., 2016; Kinyoki et al., 2016; Kazembe et al., 2009a; Kandala et al., 2008). It is well established that when the survey design is informative, ignoring the complex survey design in the spatial analyses of the data may result in biases (Pfeffermann & Sverchkov, 2007). Recently, Models (2) and (3) have been adjusted to account for the survey weights (Cassy et al., 2022; Vandendijck et al., 2016; Chen et al., 2014; Mercer et al., 2014). The approach has been to model the spatial dependence by allowing spatial smoothing of the Horvitz-Thompson estimator $\hat{P}_{ij}^{HW}$ with a hierarchical spatial smoothing model after an appropriate transformation such as a logarithm or logit transformation (Vandendijck et al., 2016; Chen et al., 2014; Mercer et al., 2014). The transformed estimate is assumed normal, and spatial smoothing is done on the mean of this normal distribution.

However, in this chapter we consider pseudo-likelihood (PL), which uses a weighted likelihood (Chen et al., 2014; Mercer et al., 2014). In pseudo-likelihood models, the total number of individuals with disease j in area i (n_{ij}) is weighted using the normalized design weights $(\tilde{w}^d_{ijk})$. Thus, rather than using binomial outcomes used in Eq. (12.1), here, we consider

$$n_{ij} = \sum_{k \in s_i} \tilde{w}^d_{ijk} y_{ijk}, \tag{12.6}$$

and the resulting model can be described as

$$\begin{aligned} n^{PL}_{ij} | P^*_{ij} &\sim \text{Binomial}\left(m_{ij}, P^*_{ij}\right) \\ \text{logit}(P^*_{i1}) &= \beta_{01} + s_i\delta + s_{i1} + v_{i1}, & (12.7) \\ \text{logit}(P^*_{i2}) &= \beta_{02} + \frac{s_i}{\delta} + v_{i2}, & (12.8) \end{aligned}$$

where β_{01} and β_{02} are the intercept for disease 1 and disease 2, respectively.

12.2.2 Parameters Estimation

We now outline Bayesian methods of parameter estimation for the model. Accordingly, all the unknown parameters in the model are assumed to be random variables, and the prior distributions of the parameters have to be specified.

The parameter estimation involved evaluation of the posterior distribution, which is the conditional distribution of the model parameters given the observed data is obtained by taking the product of likelihood function together with the prior and hyperprior distribution.

Likelihood Function

For the binomial distribution, we have defined the likelihood function as

$$L(n^{PL}_{ij} | \mathbf{s}, \mathbf{v}) \propto \prod_{i=1}^{N} \prod_{j=1}^{J} \binom{m_{ij}}{n^{PL}_{ij}} \left(P^*_{ij}\right)^{y_i} \left(P^*_{ij}\right)^{m_{ij}-n_{ij}}. \tag{12.9}$$

Prior Specification

In this analysis, improper uniform priors were assigned to the two disease-specific intercept parameters β_{0k}.

The prior distribution for the spatially unstructured **v** is assumed to follow a normal distribution with zero mean and variance σ_v^2, that is,

$$v_{ij} \sim N(0, \sigma_v^2), \tag{12.10}$$

whereas we considered an intrinsic conditional autoregressive (ICAR) distribution (Rue et al., 2009; Besag et al., 1991) for the spatially structured s_i and s_i' as follows:

$$s_i|s_{i',i\neq i'} \sim N\left(\frac{1}{a_i}\sum_{i'\in ne(i)} s_{i'}, \frac{\sigma_s^2}{a_i}\right), \tag{12.11}$$

$$s_i1|s_{i1',i\neq i'} \sim N\left(\frac{1}{a_i}\sum_{i1'\in ne(i1)} s_{i1'}, \frac{\sigma_{s_i}^2}{a_i}\right), \tag{12.12}$$

where $ne(i)$ indicates the set of neighbors and a_i the number of neighbors for a given area i. Here, two areas are considered neighbors if they share a common boundary, according to common convention.

In addition, the logarithm of the scaling parameters assumes normal distribution with mean 0 and a small fixed variance of σ^2, i.e.,

$$\log \delta \sim N(0, 0.17). \tag{12.13}$$

This prior assumes that both δ and $\frac{1}{\delta}$ are positive, which is supported by the positive correlations between the two diseases according to Knorr-Held and Best (2001). As a motivation to the choice of the prior, we refer to Knorr-Held and Best (2001).

Typically, gamma priors are assigned to the precision of the both structured and unstructured effects Gamma(0.5,0.008) as

$$\frac{\beta^\alpha}{(\alpha-1)!}\sigma^{(\alpha-1)}\exp(-\beta\sigma), \tag{12.14}$$

for $\sigma > 0$, where $\alpha > 0$ is the shape scale parameter and $\beta > 0$ is the inverse scale parameter.

Posterior Distribution

Under assumptions of conditional independence and considering all priors above, the posterior distribution is given by

$$p(\theta|n_{ij}) \propto \prod_{i=1}^{N}\prod_{j=1}^{J}\binom{m_{ij}}{n_{ij}^{PL}}\left(P_{ij}^{*}\right)^{y_i}\left(P_{ij}^{*}\right)^{m_{ij}-n_{ij}} \times p(s_i|\sigma_s^2) \times p(s_{i1}|\sigma_{s_1}^2)$$
$$\times p(v_{i1}|\sigma_{v_1}^2) \times p(\sigma_{v_{i2}}^2|\sigma_{v_2}^2) \times p(\log\delta) \times p(\beta_{0j}), \quad (12.15)$$

where θ is the vector of all parameters.

Typically, the marginal posterior distributions cannot be carried out in closed form and, therefore, to avoid the analytic intractable integral problem involved in the marginalized functions.

Several approaches are available, including Markov chain Monte Carlo (MCMC) methods. In this method, a sample from the joint posterior distribution is obtained, and inference is made based on a posterior sample. However, MCMC methods are computationally intensive, and, in general, it takes a long time to achieve convergence. An attractive alternative for MCMC methods is accomplished via Integrated Nested Laplace Approximation (INLA) (Rue et al., 2009). The INLA criterion is a relatively new technique developed to circumvent these shortfalls.

Integrated Nested Laplace Approximation

Instead of considering the full posterior distributions, INLA proceeds on the basis of approximations to the marginal posterior distributions. The posterior distribution for the latent Gaussian model is

$$\pi(\mathbf{x},\theta|\mathbf{y}) \propto \pi(\theta)\pi(x|\theta)\prod \pi(y_i|x_i,\theta)$$
$$\propto \pi(\theta)|\mathbf{Q}(\theta)|^{\frac{n}{2}} \exp\left(-\frac{1}{2}x^T Q(\theta)x + \sum_{i\in I}\log\pi(y_i|x_i,\theta)\right), \quad (12.16)$$

where $\mathbf{x}$ is the class of latent fields, θ is the set of hyperparameters, and $\mathbf{y}$ is the data. In the INLA approach, the posterior marginals of interest are

$$\pi(x_i|\mathbf{y}) = \int \pi(x_i|\theta,\mathbf{y})\pi(\theta|\mathbf{y})d\theta \quad (12.17)$$

and

$$\pi(\theta_j|\mathbf{y}) = \int \pi(\theta|y)d\theta_{-j}, \quad (12.18)$$

and these are used to construct the nested approximations:

$$\tilde{\pi}(x_i|\mathbf{y}) = \int \tilde{\pi}(x_i|\boldsymbol{\theta},\mathbf{y})\tilde{\pi}(\boldsymbol{\theta}|\mathbf{y})d\boldsymbol{\theta} \quad (12.19)$$

and

$$\tilde{\pi}(\theta_j|\mathbf{y}) = \int \tilde{\pi}(\boldsymbol{\theta}|\mathbf{y})d\boldsymbol{\theta}_{-j}, \tag{12.20}$$

where $\boldsymbol{\theta}_{-j}$ is all of θs, except θ_j.

For more details on this method, see Blangiardo and Cameletti (2015); Rue et al. (2009).

12.2.3 *Model Assessment*

The models were compared using the deviance information criterion (DIC). For each model, we calculated DIC and their effective number of parameters (pD) in order to select the best model. DIC was proposed by Spiegelhalter et al. (2002) to account for the complexity of the model. The DIC value is obtained as

$$\text{DIC} = \overline{D} + pD, \tag{12.21}$$

where $\overline{D}$ is the posterior mean of the deviance that measures the goodness of fit, while pD gives the effective number of parameters in the model, which penalizes for the complexity of the model. Model with lower DIC value is preferred (Spiegelhalter et al., 2002).

12.3 Application to Joint Mapping Childhood Malaria and Diarrhea in Mozambique

Although Mozambique has experienced substantial improvements in child health, preventable child deaths continue to be unacceptably high to achieve the Sustainable Development Goals (Sachs et al., 2022; Unicef et al., 2021; Faso, 2019). Understanding the local epidemiology of diseases in these two countries is critical for defining and prioritizing interventions that can contribute to accelerating the reduction of morbidity and mortality in children under 5 years of age in the country. We used shared component model (Model 1) and shared component model adjusted for survey weights (Model 2), presented above, to estimate the geographical distribution of childhood fever and diarrhea at the province level in Mozambique.

12.3.1 Study Area

In this chapter, we used publicly available dataset from Mozambique IMASIDA 2015. Mozambique is located in the southeastern part of the African continent, between the parallels 10°27′ and 26°52′ south latitude and between the meridians 30°12′ and 40°51′ longitude. It has a surface area of 801,590 km^2, and to the North it borders with Tanzania, to the West with Malawi, Zambia, Zimbabwe, and Eswatini, and to the South with South Africa. It has three main regions, namely northern, central, and southern regions. The country is divided into ten provinces and the City of Maputo: to the North, Niassa, Cape Delgado, and Nampula, to the Center, Zambézia, Tete, Manica, and Sofala, and to the South, Inhambane, Gaza, Maputo, and Maputo City (Fig. 12.1).

12.3.2 Sampling Design and Data Collection

The IMASIDA 2015 is a cross-country survey that is conducted to assess the general health of the population with emphasis on maternal health, child health, and population health indicators of global health importance, such as HIV prevalence. Data collection was done by the National Statistical Office of Mozambique in partnership with the Ministry of Health and the Community Health Services Unit of

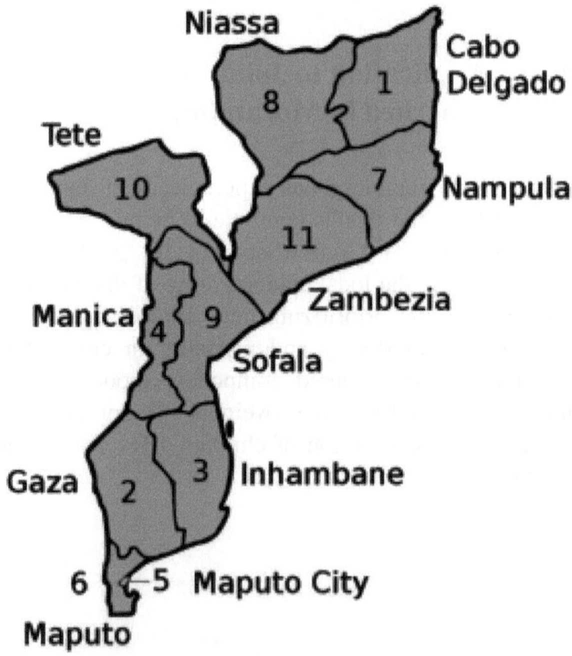

Fig. 12.1 Mozambique map showing the provinces

Mozambique. The census frame included in the 2015–2016 MDHS is the total list of standard enumeration areas (clusters) demarcated for the 2008 Malawi Population and Housing Census. The 2016 MDHS data is collected using a multistage sampling involving the selection of clusters in the first stage and subsequent selection of households in the second stage. Cluster selection was also stratified by province and place of residence (i.e., rural/urban).

A total of 307 EAs were randomly sampled, in which 134 were urban and 173 were rural. In the second sampling stage, all households within the EA were listed followed by random selection of households. A total of 24 households were systematically selected per EA. In total, 7,368 households were selected. Women aged 15–49 years and children aged 6–59 months, who were habitually resident or had spent the night before the survey in the household, were eligible for interview. The response rate was 98%.

Our study focuses on prevalence of diarrhea and fever at province level in Mozambique. For the aim of this study, we used the children under 5 years (KR) dataset.

12.3.3 Outcomes

Two outcome variables were considered (diarrhea and fever statuses). Children under 5 years old who had their mother answer whether they had diarrhea or fever within the past 2 weeks were included in the analysis. The remaining children with missing values for the outcomes were excluded from our analysis.

12.3.4 Computation

The disease-specific intercepts β_k are assigned improper uniform priors. Furthermore, we assign a zero-mean normal distribution with a high variance for the baseline parameter and $Gamma$ (0.5, 0.008) priors for both the spatial and nonspatial precision parameters, σ_u^{-2} and σ_v^{-2}, following the ideas in previous studies as in Chen et al. (2014). The logarithm of the scaling parameter (i.e., $\log \delta$) has been assigned a normal distribution with zero mean and precision 1/5.9.

All models were performed in `R` software (R Core Team, 2020) and the available package such as `survey` (Lumley, 2020) and `INLA` (Blangiardo & Cameletti, 2015; Schrödle & Held, 2011). We fitted the shared component model using the observed number of subjects with the respective diseases (Model 1) and shared component bivariate model using pseudo-likelihood (Model 2). The parameters of the models were then estimated using the INLA approach (Blangiardo & Cameletti, 2015; Bivand et al., 2015; Rue et al., 2009) and the INLAMSM package (https://CRAN.R-project.org/package=INLAMSM) that was recently developed by Palmí-Perales et al. (2019) to implement multivariate spatial models for area data using `R-INLA`.

According to Rue et al. (2009), INLA provides a faster alternative to Markov Chain Monte Carlo (MCMC) methods for approximating the marginal posterior distributions of Markov random field (MRF) models.

12.3.5 Results

Of the total 4,969 children included in the study, 26.34% had fever, 11.11% had diarrhea, while 5.74% had fever and diarrhea simultaneously (Table 12.1). The results mapped in Fig. 12.2 clearly show some hotspots concerning the distribution of fever and diarrhea in the different provinces. Furthermore, fever was more prevalent than diarrhea.

Shared component models were adjusted without survey weights and accounted for survey weights to produce provincial-level estimates of fever and diarrhea prevalence. When comparing the models with DIC for fit and complexity, it is

Table 12.1 Cross-table of childhood fever and diarrhea prevalence in Mozambique, using IMASIDA data

	Diarrhea		
Fever	No	Yes	Total
No	3,393 (68.28)	267 (5.37)	3,660 (5,73)
Yes	1,024 (20.61)	285 (5.74)	1,309 (26,34)
Total	4,417 (88,89)	552 (11,11)	4,969 (100.0)

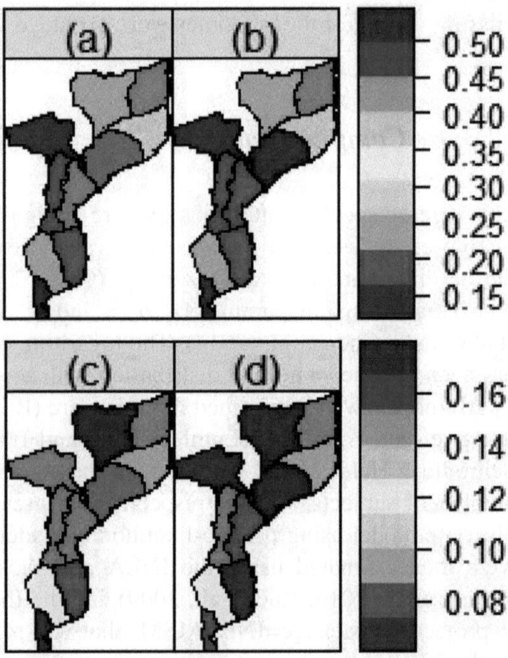

Fig. 12.2 Maps of observed (unweighted and weighted) prevalence of fever ((**a**) and (**b**)) and diarrhea ((**c**) and (**d**)) by province in Mozambique using IMASIDA

verified that Model 2 adjusted to the weights has a better performance in relation to Model 1 that does not take into account the survey weights (Table 12.2). The relative effect of shared variations due to fever prevalence compared to diarrhea prevalence is measured by δ. This is estimated as $\delta = 1.12$ and suggests that unobserved risk factors have a relatively greater effect on fever than diarrhea (Model 2). In fact, $\delta^2 = 1.25$ demonstrates that the gradient of fever prevalence in each area was higher than diarrhea.

Figure 12.3 presents the area-specific estimates for diarrhea and fever in Mozambique. The left column gives the unweighted estimates, while the right column gives the weighted estimates. The disease-specific spatial effects show areas where fever and diarrhea differed (Fig. 12.3). There appear to be fever *hotspots* in the northern part of Mozambique (Nampula and Zambézia) and low prevalence in Maputo City, Maputo Province, and Tete (Fig. 12.3). Additionally, it is observed that the provinces of Zambézia and Niassa are the most affected by diarrhea, and the least affected area of the country is the province of Inhambane (Fig. 12.3). The shared spatially structured random effects are shown in Fig. 12.4. The shared effects were high mainly in the provinces of Zambézia and Nampula. In addition, when comparing weighted and unweighted estimates, some difference is observed in the maps, which may have an impact on policy intervention.

Table 12.2 Comparison measures of models

	Model 1	Model 2
DIC	168.08	167.23
pd	19.92	19.91
−2LL	−135.98	−136.31

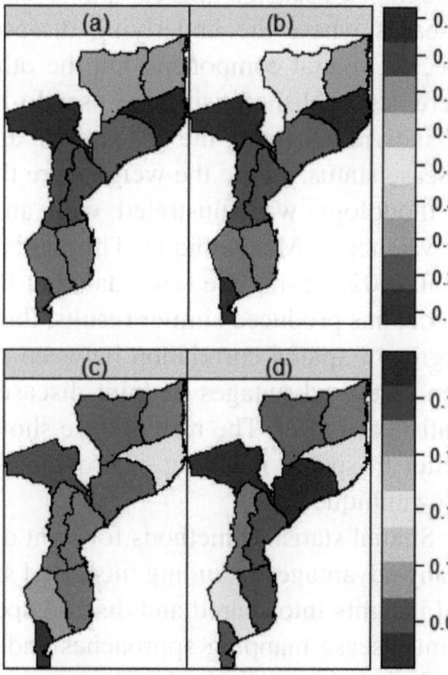

Fig. 12.3 Maps of estimated prevalence of fever (unweighted (**a**) and weighted (**b**)) and diarrhea (unweighted (**c**) and weighted (**d**)) by provinces in Mozambique using IMASIDA 2015

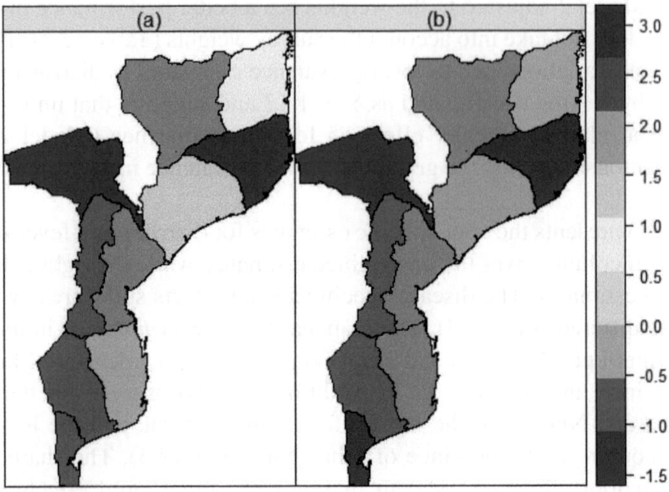

Fig. 12.4 Maps of a posteriori estimates of shared spatial effects of fever (**a**) and diarrhea (**b**) by provinces in Mozambique using IMASIDA 2015

12.4 Discussion and Conclusion

This chapter has explored how joint disease mapping approaches for binomial data could be combined with adjustments for survey designs when analyzing several interrelated diseases simultaneously using health survey data. For the joint spatial model, we used the shared spatial component model simultaneously interrelated diseases where the underlying disease spatial risk is split into a common and specific spatial component. On the other hand, adjustments for the survey design were accomplished using the pseudo-likelihood (PL) approach where the number of individuals with the disease in an area was a weighted sum of individual disease status, where the weights are the normalized survey weights. The explored methodology was illustrated with an analysis of childhood fever and diarrhea prevalence in Mozambique. This study was based on a previous analysis by Cassy et al. (2022) using the same data but fitted separately. Although the joint mapping model has produced similar results, the joint analysis has additionally measured the degree of spatial correlation between the prevalence of fever and diarrhea. That is one of the advantages of joint disease mapping models, in addition to increased statistical power. The results have shown that weight-adjusted methods provided a better fit spatial mapping of provincial-level comorbidity of fever and diarrhea in Mozambique.

Spatial statistics methods for joint disease mapping of interrelated diseases have many advantages including increased statistical power and providing epidemiological insights into shared and disease-specific disease spatial risks. There are several joint disease mapping approaches and several survey design adjustments aimed at exploring the spatial risk of two or more health outcomes simultaneously when survey data is analyzed. The maps of shared effects could be used to plan integrated disease management of the related diseases. This map can also be useful for testing hypotheses related to the epidemiological profiles of the studied diseases. In this way, joint spatial modeling could be used effectively in supporting decision-making for prevention and control strategies.

Acknowledgments We thank the Editor and the referee for their comments. We also extend thanks to DHS Measure, for allowing us to use 2015 IMASIDA dataset for this study.

References

Adebayo, S. B., Gayawan, E., Heumann, C., & Seiler, C. (2016). Joint modeling of anaemia and malaria in children under five in Nigeria. *Spatial and Spatio-Temporal Epidemiology, 17*, 105–115.

Besag, J., York, J., & Mollié, A. (1991). Bayesian image restoration with two applications in spatial statistics. *Annals of the Institute of Statistics and Mathematics, 43*, 1–59. https://doi.org/10.1007/bf00116466

Bivand, R. S., Gomez-Rubio, V., & Rue, H. (2015). Spatial data analysis with R-INLA with some extensions. *Journal of Statistical Software, 63*(20), 1–31.

Blangiardo, M., & Cameletti, M. (2015). *Spatial and spatio-temporal Bayesian models with R-INLA*. Wiley.

Carroll, R., Lawson, A. B., Faes, C., Kirby, R. S., Aregay, M., & Watjou, K. (2017). Extensions to multivariate space time mixture modeling of small area cancer data. *International Journal of Environmental Research and Public Health, 14*(5), 503.

Cassy, S. R., Manda, S., Marques, F., & Martins, M. D. R. O. (2022). Accounting for sampling weights in the analysis of spatial distributions of disease using health survey data, with an application to mapping child health in Malawi and Mozambique. *International Journal of Environmental Research and Public Health, 19*(10), 6319.

Chang, C.-D., Wang, C.-C., & Jiang, B. C. (2011). Using data mining techniques for multi-diseases prediction modeling of hypertension and hyperlipidemia by common risk factors. *Expert Systems with Applications, 38*(5), 5507–5513.

Chen, C., Wakefield, J., & Lumley, T. (2014). The use of sampling weights in Bayesian hierarchical models for small area estimation. *Spatial and Spatio-Temporal Epidemiology, 11*, 33–43. https://doi.org/10.1016/j.sste.2014.07.002

Dabney, A. R., & Wakefield, J. C. (2005). Issues in the mapping of two diseases. *Statistical Methods in Medical Research, 14*(1), 83–112.

Downing, A., Forman, D., Gilthorpe, M. S., Edwards, K. L., & Manda, S. O. M. (2008). Joint disease mapping using six cancers in the Yorkshire region of England. *International Journal of Health Geographics, 7*, 1–14.

Faso, B. (2019). Institute for health metrics and evaluation. *Institute for Health Metrics and Evaluation*.

Feltbower, R. G., Manda, S. O. M., Gilthorpe, M. S., Greaves, M. F., Parslow, R. C., Kinsey, S. E., Jonathan Bodansky, H., & McKinney, P. A. (2005). Detecting small-area similarities in the epidemiology of childhood acute lymphoblastic leukemia and diabetes mellitus, type 1: A Bayesian approach. *American Journal of Epidemiology, 161*(12), 1168–1180.

Gómez-Rubio, V., Palmí-Perales, F., López-Abente, G., Ramis-Prieto, R., & Fernández-Navarro, P. (2019). Bayesian joint spatio-temporal analysis of multiple diseases. *SORT-Statistics and Operations Research Transactions, 43*(1), 51–74.

Held, L., Natário, I., Fenton, S. E., Rue, H., & Becker, N. (2005). Towards joint disease mapping. *Statistical Methods in Medical Research, 14*(1), 61–82.

Kandala, N. B., Ji, C., Stallard, N., Stranges, S., & Cappuccio, F. (2008). Morbidity from diarrhoea, cough and fever among young children in Nigeria. *Annals of Tropical Medicine & Parasitology, 102*(5), 427–445.

Kandala, N. B., Manda, S. O., Tigbe, W. W., Mwambi, H., & Stranges, S. (2014). Geographic distribution of cardiovascular comorbidities in south Africa: a national cross-sectional analysis. *Journal of Applied Statistics, 41*(6), 1203–1216.

Kazembe, L. N., Appleton, C. C., & Kleinschmidt, I. (2007). Spatial analysis of the relationship between early childhood mortality and malaria endemicity in Malawi. *Geospatial Health, 2*(1), 41–50.

Kazembe, L. N., Muula, A. S., & Simoonga, C. (2009a). Joint spatial modelling of common morbidities of childhood fever and diarrhoea in Malawi. *Health & Place, 15*(1), 165–172.

Kazembe, L. N., Muula, A. S., & Simoonga, C. (2009b). Joint spatial modelling of common morbidities of childhood fever and diarrhoea in Malawi. *Health & Place, 15*(1), 165–172.

Kinyoki, D. K., Kandala, N. B., Manda, S. O., Krainski, E. T., Fuglstad, G. A., Moloney, G. M., & Noor, A. M. (2016). Assessing comorbidity and correlates of wasting and stunting among children in Somalia using cross-sectional household surveys: 2007 to 2010. *BMJ Open, 6*(3), e009854.

Kinyoki, D. K., Manda, S. O., Moloney, G. M., Odundo, E. O., Berkley, J. A., Noor, A. M., & Kandala, N. B. (2017). Modelling the ecological comorbidity of acute respiratory infection, diarrhoea and stunting among children under the age of 5 years in Somalia. *International Statistical Review, 85*(1), 164–176.

Kinyoki, D. K., Moloney, G. M., Uthman, O. A., Odundo, E. O., Kandala, N. B., Noor, A. M., & Berkley, J. A. (2018). Co-morbidity of malnutrition with falciparum malaria parasitaemia among children under the aged 6–59 months in Somalia: a geostatistical analysis. *Infectious Diseases of Poverty, 7*, 1–9.

Knorr-Held, L., & Best, N. G. (2001). A shared component model for detecting joint and selective clustering of two diseases. *Journal of the Royal Statistical Society: Series A (Statistics in Society), 164*(1), 73–85. https://doi.org/10.1186/s12936-018-2509-9

Lumley, T. (2020). *Package 'survey'*. https://cran.r-project.org

Manda, S., Haushona, N., & Bergquist, R. (2020). A scoping review of spatial analysis approaches using health survey data in sub-Saharan Africa. *International Journal of Environmental Research and Public Health, 17*(9), 3070. ISSN 16604601. https://doi.org/10.3390/ijerph17093070

Manda, S. O., Feltbower, R. G., & Gilthorpe, M. S. (2009). Investigating spatio-temporal similarities in the epidemiology of childhood leukaemia and diabetes. *European Journal of Epidemiology, 24*(12), 743–752.

Mercer, L., Wakefield, J., Chen, C., & Lumley, T. (2014). A comparison of spatial smoothing methods for small area estimation with sampling weights. *Spatial Statistics, 8*, 69–85.

I. MISAU (2016). Inquérito de indicadores de imunização, malária e hiv/sida em moçambique (IMASIDA) 2015: Relatório de indicadores básicos.

Orunmoluyi, O. S., Gayawan, E., & Manda, S. (1838). Spatial co-morbidity of childhood acute respiratory infection, diarrhoea and stunting in Nigeria. *International Journal of Environmental Research and Public Health, 19*(3), 2022.

Palmí-Perales, F., Gómez-Rubio, V., & Martinez-Beneito, M. A. (2019). Bayesian multivariate spatial models for lattice data with INLA. *arXiv preprint arXiv:1909.10804*.

Pfeffermann, D., & Sverchkov, M. (2007). Small-area estimation under informative probability sampling of areas and within the selected areas. *Journal of the American Statistical Association, 102*(480), 1427–1439.

R Core Team. (2020). R: A language and environment for statistical computing. *Published online, 1*, 371–78.

Rue, H., Martino, S., & Chopin, N. (2009). Approximate Bayesian inference for latent Gaussian models by using integrated nested Laplace approximations. *Journal of the Royal Statistical Society: Series B (Statistical Methodology), 71*(2), 319–392.

Sachs, J., Kroll, C., Lafortune, G., Fuller, G., & Woelm, F. (2022). *Sustainable development report 2022*. Cambridge University Press.

Schrödle, B., & Held, L. (2011). Spatio-temporal disease mapping using INLA. *Environmetrics, 22*(6), 725–734.

Spiegelhalter, D. J., Best, N. G., Carlin, B. P., & Van Der Linde, A. (2002). Bayesian measures of model complexity and fit. *Journal of the Royal Statistical Society: Series B (Statistical Methodology), 64*(4), 583–639. https://doi.org/10.1111/1467-9868.00353

Unicef, et al. (2021). *Levels and trends in child malnutrition: Joint child malnutrition estimates*. UNIVED.

Vandendijck, Y., Faes, C., Kirby, R. S., Lawson, A., & Hens, N. (2016). Model-based inference for small area estimation with sampling weights. *Spatial Statistics, 18*, 455–473.

Watjou, K., Faes, C., Lawson, A., Kirby, R. S., Aregay, M., Carroll, R., & Vandendijck, Y. (2017). Spatial small area smoothing models for handling survey data with nonresponse. *Statistics in Medicine, 36*(23), 3708–3745.

Wong, C. W., Wong, T. Y., Cheng, C.-Y., & Sabanayagam, C. (2014). Kidney and eye diseases: Common risk factors, etiological mechanisms, and pathways. *Kidney International, 85*(6), 1290–1302.

Index

D.-G. Chen, C. A. Coelho (eds.), *Biostatistics Modeling and Public Health Applications*, Emerging Topics in Statistics and Biostatistics,
https://doi.org/10.1007/978-3-031-69690-9

MIX
Papier aus verantwortungsvollen Quellen
Paper from responsible sources
FSC® C105338

If you have any concerns about our products,
you can contact us on
ProductSafety@springernature.com

In case Publisher is established outside the EU,
the EU authorized representative is:
Springer Nature Customer Service Center GmbH
Europaplatz 3, 69115 Heidelberg, Germany

Printed by Libri Plureos GmbH
in Hamburg, Germany